Mental Health Care and National Health Insurance

A Philosophy of and an Approach to
Mental Health Care for the Future

Mental Health Care and National Health Insurance

A Philosophy of and an Approach to
Mental Health Care for the Future

David Upton

With commentaries by
Richard H. Beinecke and Bertram S. Brown, Robert L. DuPont,
Henry A. Foley, Robert W. Gibson, Milton Greenblatt,
Zigmond M. Lebensohn, Judd Marmor, Philip R. A. May,
Mildred Mitchell-Bateman, Morris B. Parloff, and
Jack Weinberg[†] and Theodora Fine

PLENUM PRESS • NEW YORK AND LONDON

Library of Congress Cataloging in Publication Data

Upton, David, 1943 –
  Mental health care and national health insurance.

  Bibliography: p.
  Includes index.
  1. Mental health. 2. Insurance, Mental health. I. Title. [DNLM: 1. Mental health ser-
vices—Trends—United States. 2. National health insurance, United States—Trends.
WM 30 U806m]
RA790.U67 1983   368.4'2   83-8049
ISBN-13: 978-1-4684-4453-7   e-ISBN-13: 978-1-4684-4451-3
DOI: 10.1007/978-1-4684-4451-3

©1983 Plenum Press, New York
Softcover reprint of the hardcover 1st edition 1983

A Division of Plenum Publishing Corporation
233 Spring Street, New York, N.Y. 10013

For Ellen, with love

Contributors

David Upton, M.D.

David Upton, M.D., formerly served as Consultant to the United States Senate Veterans' Affairs Committee, Chief of Psychiatry, the United States Army Mental Health Clinic, Fort Belvoir, Virginia, and Visiting Physician, Los Angeles County Community Mental Health Center Systems. Dr. Upton is currently engaged in writing a textbook on psychotherapy and a book on the psychological aspects of hospital care.

Richard H. Beinecke, ACSW

Program Development Officer, Horizon Health Group, Inc., Washington, D.C.

Vice President, Research and Development, Institute for New Challenges, Washington, D.C.

Former Director, Adult and Emergency Services, United Counseling Service, Bennington, Vermont.

Bertram S. Brown, M.D.

President and Chief Executive Officer, Hahnemann University, Philadelphia, Pennsylvania.

Robert L. Sutherland Professor of Mental Health and Social Policy, University of Texas at Austin, Austin, Texas.

Former Director, National Institute of Mental Health, U.S. Department of Health and Human Services, Washington, D.C.

Robert L. DuPont, M.D.

President, American Council on Marijuana and Other Psychoactive Drugs, Inc., Washington, D.C.

Clinical Professor of Psychiatry, Georgetown Medical School, Washington, D.C.

Former Director, National Institute on Drug Abuse, U.S. Department of Health and Human Services, Washington, D.C.

Theodora Fine, M.A.

Assistant Director of Government Relations, American Psychiatric Association, Washington, D.C.

Program Analyst, Administration on Aging, U.S. Department of Health and Human Services, Washington, D.C.

Legislative Assistant, United States Senator John Tunney, Washington, D.C.

Henry A. Foley, Ph.D.

Adjunct Professor and Senior Scholar, Institute for Health Policy Studies, University of California, San Francisco, California.

Former Administrator, Health Resources Administration, U.S. Department of Health and Human Services, Washington, D.C.

Former Executive Director, Colorado State Department of Social Services, Denver, Colorado.

Robert W. Gibson, M.D.

President and Chief Executive Officer, the Sheppard and Enoch Pratt Hospital, Baltimore, Maryland.

Past President, National Association of Private Psychiatric Hospitals.

Past President, American Psychiatric Association.

Milton Greenblatt, M.D.

Director, Neuropsychiatric Institute Hospital and Clinics Professor and Executive Vice Chairman, Department of Psychiatry and Behavioral Sciences, University of California, Los Angeles, California.

Distinguished Service Award, American Psychiatric Association, 1981.

Former Commissioner of Mental Health, Commonwealth of Massachusetts.

Zigmond M. Lebensohn, M.D.

Clinical Professor of Psychiatry, Georgetown University School of Medicine, Washington, D.C.

Chief Emeritus, Department of Psychiatry, Sibley Memorial Hospital, Washington, D.C.
Past Member, Board of Trustees, American Psychiatric Association.

Judd Marmor, M.D.

Adjunct Professor of Psychiatry, University of California at Los Angeles School of Medicine, Los Angeles, California.
Franz Alexander Professor of Psychiatry, Emeritus, University of Southern California School of Medicine, Los Angeles, California.
Past President, American Psychiatric Association.

Philip R. A. May, M.D.

Professor of Psychiatry, Neuropsychiatric Institute, Center for Health Sciences, University of California, Los Angeles, California.

Mildred Mitchell-Bateman, M.D.

Professor and Chairman, Department of Psychiatry, Marshall University School of Medicine, Huntington, West Virginia.
Consultant, Huntington Veterans Administration Medical Center, Psychiatry Service, Huntington, West Virginia.
Life Fellow, American Psychiatric Association.

Morris B. Parloff, Ph.D.

Chief, Psychosocial Treatments Research Branch, Division of Extramural Research Programs, National Institute of Mental Health, U.S. Department of Health and Human Services, Rockville, Maryland.
Chief, Psychotherapy and Behavioral Intervention Section, Clinical Research Branch, Division of Extramural Research Programs, National Institute of Mental Health, U.S. Department of Health and Human Services, Washington, D.C.
Chief, Section on Personality, Laboratory on Psychology, National Institute of Mental Health, U.S. Department of Health and Human Services, Washington, D.C.

Paul F. Slawson, M.D.

Professor of Psychiatry, University of California at Los Angeles Neuropsychiatric Institute, Los Angeles, California.
Member, Board of Trustees, American Psychiatric Association.

Jack Weinberg, M.D.†

Director, Illinois Mental Health Institutes, Chicago, Illinois.
Chair, Council on Aging, American Psychiatric Association.
Past President, American Psychiatric Association.

Louis Jolyon West, M.D.

Professor and Chairman, Department of Psychiatry and Biobehavioral Sciences, University of California at Los Angeles School of Medicine.
Director, the Neuropsychiatric Institute, University of California at Los Angeles Center for the Health Sciences, Los Angeles, California.
Professor and Head, Department of Psychiatry, Neurology and Biobehavioral Sciences, University of Oklahoma School of Medicine (1954–1959).
The H. B. Williams Memorial Travelling Professor of the Royal Australian and New Zealand College of Psychiatrists (1979).

Foreword

The burial societies of the Romans were, essentially, private group insurance programs. So were the protection funds of medieval guilds. Largely through the efforts of labor unions, by 1968 more than two-thirds of the labor force in U.S. industry was covered by group life and health insurance plans mostly provided (as fringe benefits) by employers. Today the proportion is even higher, and the establishment of national health insurance, to be sponsored by government, is being debated in the halls of Congress.

Complete medical care for the citizenry, with health professionals partly or wholly salaried by a government agency, is now standard in many countries, including those of eastern Europe, most of the British commonwealth (including Australia, Canada, and New Zealand), several Latin American countries, Greece, Turkey, Sweden, and of course China, the USSR, and eastern Europe. The major alternative scheme, in which the government provides reimbursement for private care, is employed by several other Western nations, including Norway, Denmark, Austria, West Germany, and Spain.

Both of these methods of government coverage exist for certain groups in the United States: the former for military personnel, service-connected or impecunious veterans, and the indigent mentally ill; the latter for those covered under the 1965 amendment to the Social Security Act. However, most health insurance in the United States is private, much of it operating on a group basis.

Like other insurance, health insurance is a type of risk sharing. In its pure form, it is a scheme to protect against large expenses or losses by having a number of people periodically pay small amounts of money into a fund, the resources of which may later be used to offset losses, if and when they occur. This procedure is called underwriting. From the insurers' point of view, however, certain requirements must be met if the plan is to be economically feasible.

1. *Size* is a critical requirement. The more people whose risks are underwritten, the more securely the risk can be shared, and the more money can be pooled. In other words, the objects or persons insured must be numerous enough, and homogenous enough, so that the probable frequency and severity of losses can be projected.

2. The *type* of risk is also important. Insurance works best when the risk for which protection is sought is a relatively infrequent occurrence and lies outside the control of the person insured. If the event is indeed infrequent, even an occasional large loss will still allow for a low premium. The idea is to offer protection and derivative peace of mind referable to unexpected events.

3. The *time* covered must be taken into account. Only a small proportion of the insured objects or persons should be at risk at any given time. If the entire group claimed full recovery for maximum loss at the same time, the insurance plan would be wiped out. In other words, the risk should be spread as widely as possible, not only by the size of the group but through time as well.

4. An objective and relatively standardized *method* must obtain to determine whether a claim is appropriate, both qualitatively and quantitatively. Insurance policies (contracts) usually go into considerable detail in describing what events must take place, what shall be deemed a loss, and how it is to be measured, before a claim will be settled and paid.

This is basically the system that was devised in the 18th century to insure sailing ships and their cargos bound to and from ports in England. In fact, the primary insuring clause in most modern marine insurance policies still closely resembles the original form written more than 200 years ago by Lloyd's of London in 1779:

> Touching the adventures and perils which we the assurers are contented to bear and do take upon us in this voyage: they are of the seas, men-of-war, fire, enemies, pirates, rovers, thieves, jettisons, letters of mart and countermart, surprisals, takings at sea, arrests, restraints, and detainments of all kings, princes, and people, of what nation, condition, or quality soever, barratry of the master and mariners, and of all other perils, losses, and misfortunes, that have or shall come to the hurt, detriment, or damage of the said goods and merchandises, and ship, etc., or any part thereof.

Health insurance differs in certain respects from the picture described above. As sold today, most health insurance is a rather complicated product of which only one element, the so-called catastrophic coverage, fits the traditional insurance model. Catastrophic health insurance pays most of the costs of medical treatment after a predetermined (deductible) amount has been paid by the patient. In this way, it restricts payment to severe illness, which represents large but infrequent losses.

However, the bulk of the personal or family health care plan, as such offerings are usually called, deviates from the traditional insurance format. It covers what can, in all fairness, be seen as *anticipated medical expense* rather than the more traditional *random loss*. Minor ailments and injuries occur with such frequency and regularity as to be a relatively predictable expense, even within a small group over a short period of time. As medical expense payments become more uniform and regular, the plan shifts away from the casualty model of insurance and becomes instead a form of social indemnity. (Depending upon the goals of the program, this may or may not be a desirable feature.) Whether intended or not, such a shift has inevitable fiscal consequences, because large premiums are required to support regular payments for medical care in behalf of a large number of the insured persons. The attendant cash flow carries proportional administrative expense (and also profit) with consequent diversion of health care dollars. If the premiums are paid by the employer, as is the case in many group health insurance plans, the employee-consumer may be well insulated from the actual cost of the provided benefits. This insulation, coupled with an understandable sense of entitlement often encouraged by the employer or by fellow consumers, can lead to a very high demand for and consumption of health services. When, as a result, premiums are increased, the pattern becomes cyclical and feeds on its own demand. This aggravates the inflationary uptrending to which the plan is already subject.

As noted above, most health insurance in the United States is sold in the form of group plans, generally associated with employment. This arrangement has many advantages: It provides the requisite large number of participants; it guarantees prompt payment of premium from payroll sources; and it militates against adverse selection, because plan enrollment is restricted to active workers who, as a group, are less likely to require benefits than the general public with its reservoir of chronic disability. However, while a particular plan may have enough participants to approach normative experience through prevention of adverse selection, its fiscal stability nevertheless depends on the prevention of excessive utilization.

Copayment was an initial effort to minimize overutilization of health insurance. This was based on the idea that sharing the cost would give pause to the claimant's assertion of need, thereby restricting his utilization to the most legitimate and pressing instances of illness or injury. Unfortunately, with the trend toward more inclusive and liberal plans as part of "employee benefit packages," the deterent effect of copayment has often been sharply compromised.

Primary control of health care benefit utilization has always been based on the idea that no one will get sick just to collect a benefit, and that doctors will restrict treatment to those who are truly ill. This idea, if valid, should mean that utilization is largely based on involuntary or randomized experiences, and thus is consistent with a casualty insurance model. However, it does place the benefit structure at the disposal of the health care provider, and it permits deliberate or unwitting collusion between providers (e.g., physicians and hospitals) and consumers (patients). At first, this was not thought to be much of a problem. Surely doctors were not going to invent illness, and treat it, just to collect a professional fee from an insurance company! Most doctors have too many patients anyway, it was said, so there would be scant motive for such dubious practice. But a few venal exceptions to an honor-bound rule can run up costs very fast. Experience has proved that providers must be monitored to prevent abuses. Thus, peer review has now become a central factor in utilization control.

For many years, most health plans excluded coverage of the so-called nervous and mental disorders. Various reasons were given for this arbitrary exclusion. Perhaps the most important reason was a putative lack of demand. Unlike medical and surgical treatment, which could be accepted as inevitable, the need for psychiatric treatment was not always readily perceived, and could be easily dismissed in many cases. Most people were inclined to see mental illness as a remote possibility in which government, in the form of the state hospital, would ultimately provide care if necessary. Certainly the insurance companies, well aware that serious mental illness tends to be chronic, and that its treatment is costly, could hardly have been expected to promote the inclusion of psychiatric benefits, especially in the absence of a strong expression of demand.

However, as time and progress brought steadily better diagnosis and treatment, it became apparent that some mental and emotional disorders did respond to specific therapies, that chronicity was not inevitable, and that prophylactic intervention was feasible in many cases. As a result, insurance benefits were expanded to include psychiatric illness. Naturally, utilization went up. Interestingly enough, although long-term inpatient care still presented a potential problem, it was outpatient treatment that emerged as the focus of major concern. In the 1950s, prior to the liberalization of coverage, psychoanalysis achieved unprecedented popularity, both as a scientific psychology and as a mode of clinical practice. From this followed a broad general interest in intensive psychotherapy as a means of treating a wide variety of mental complaints. The result was a selective utilization of outpatient benefits far beyond what had been anticipated.

To make matters worse, there were almost no guidelines. There was no clear indication of which individuals should receive psychotherapy (not to mention psychoanalysis), or when it should stop. Added to this was the powerful taboo against any breach of confidentiality in the doctor–patient relationship where psychiatry was concerned. Psychoanalytic therapists were disinclined to share *any* clinical information about patients whose treatment was based on such a personal and sensitive relationship. The attitude of many therapists was one of entitled indifference. Translated into economic terms, this meant "Pay until we stop therapy, and don't ask questions."

Such a demand was obviously incompatible with responsible underwriting. It was inevitable that benefits would be cut back. Well-meaning psychotherapists had blurred the distinction between wish and need and had rendered uncertain the critical distinction between treatment, which is medically indicated, psychotherapy, which is discretionary or elective, and counseling, which is essentially for self-improvement or even basically educational in character. The insurance model does not work if the beneficiary has free and uncontrolled access to the benefit.

The insurance industry viewed this whole picture as one of overutilization; excessive and inappropriate use of benefits could not be tolerated. The unavoidable consequence would be underwriting losses followed by larger premiums. The major portions of most health premiums are paid by employers, who, of necessity, must be cost-sensitive. Their immediate complaints about higher premiums were met by the insurance industry's automatic suggestion that benefits be cut. Psychiatric benefits, being considered difficult to control, or appearing to be too discretionary, were the first to go. Ironically, medical and surgical care was seen as inviolate, even though the cost for such care had increased disproportionately compared with psychiatric treatment with respect to inflation and had, in fact, contributed substantially to the experienced and projected losses.

Inevitably, the restriction of benefits threw many insured persons into the public sector when psychiatric treatment was needed. Unfortunately, at about the same time (during the late 1960s and early 1970s) many state governments were already set upon a course of dismantling or drastically reducing their state hospital systems in favor of community-based programs. These were supposed to substitute regional and local treatment centers, with emphasis on more intensive (and thus briefer) forms of care, for the prolonged and expensive mental hospital treatment model. However, equivalent funding was not shifted from state hospital systems to community programs. As a result, the amount and quality of service available to many patients was sharply reduced.

At first, complaints about this shift were relatively infrequent and isolated. This was probably because the quest for service in the mental health field presents serious tactical problems for employed prospective patients. Moreover, as inflation continued to increase the cost of medical care, even further compromise was needed. Because employers were not receptive to an increase in premium contributions, a trade-off of benefits was inevitable. Employees subject to the same inflationary pressure started to seek sponsored assistance with other types of health expense such as dentistry, eyeglasses, and foot care. These alternatives appeared attractive both to the insured individuals (who were relieved of unwelcome personal expenses) and to the insurance companies (which could easily write policies controlling utilization and ultimate cost of such services through carefully chosen deductibles and limits). Such plans carry little of the traditional underwriting risk. Because utilization rates are high in these plans, the program cost can be quite accurately predicted and a profit insured. For the insurance company, this is far more attractive business than dealing with patients who may require prolonged treatment for a severe but poorly defined mental illness.

In the first section of this book, Dr. David Upton argues that while National Health Insurance may be delayed, it will come in its own time as a partnership between government and the private sector. Whatever form it takes, it will be based on an insurance model. No reasonable person would seriously question the level of mental health care advocated by Dr. Upton and the others who have contributed to this volume. But health care, never cheap, now looms enormous in the national economy. It appears that the portion of delegated resources that will go for mental health in any forthcoming national scheme must, to a significant degree, depend on the willingness of providers more effectively to adapt to the reality of the marketplace. This reality, together with the considerations of fairness, equity, and humanity so warmly expressed by Dr. Upton and his colleagues, will determine the shape of things to come in mental health coverage for the American people.

Paul F. Slawson, M.D.
Louis Jolyon West, M.D.

Contents

Points of View

Introduction

The aim, intent, and purpose of my white paper are amply expressed in Chapter 1. I would only expand here on my underlying philosophy of mental illness/emotional problems and mental health care, a philosophy that prompted me to write this paper and edit this book.

I hope and believe that our attitudes toward what constitutes illness, health, and health care are changing. We must come to view mental illness/emotional problems as real and "legitimate," as just like any other form of illness. We must come to view the symptoms of emotional distress as being as painful and potentially as debilitating as the symptoms of any so-called physical illness. [Mental illness/emotional problems are "physical." They involve pathological alterations or derangements of brain physiology, even if this does not require specific medical (psychiatric), as opposed to nonmedical, i.e., purely psychological, treatment.] We should realize that the symptoms of emotional distress, ignored or not properly treated, can lead to as many serious medical complications for a person as can physical symptoms, ignored or improperly treated. We attempt to treat the pains and aches of major and minor physical illness to the full limits of our medical knowledge and capabilities. We should be prepared to do the same as regards mental illness/emotional problems.

At the same time, it is clear that we cannot and should not treat *all* emotional pain any more than we should treat *all* physical pain. There are limits to what we can and cannot treat and how much we can improve any patient's health by psychological or medical means. In this connection, a significant part of any treatment must be directed toward enabling the patient to function to the maximum extent possible even with the pain and limitations his illness causes him. In fact, much medical care, as well as mental health care, is of a supportive nature. We must be careful not to deprive the patient of this aspect of care. As I point out in my paper, it is often as meaningful and helpful to the patient as any specific medical test or procedure we can perform on him or any medicine we can prescribe for him. It is a vital part of treatment.

Obviously, as a psychiatrist, I hold a strong belief in the validity and importance of mental health care. Nevertheless, I would be the first to caution that we should not extend unnecessary mental health care to a person, any more than we should extend him unnecessary medical-surgical care. (We do provide much unnecessary medical care of all kinds. Not only is it expensive, it is often harmful to the patient.) Mental health care *per se* must be reserved solely for the person who suffers mental illness/emotional problems. Nevertheless, a person does not have to suffer emotional distress to make use of the process of mental health care. It is in every person's interest to know and understand himself (or herself), to constantly seek to grow, and to work toward leading a fulfilling, meaningful life in every sense. I believe strongly in psychological self-investigation—call it psychotherapy if you will—as a method to achieve these ends. (Of course, there are a multitude of ways and experiences that can promote self-growth.) It is, in my opinion, of great value, no matter how emotionally healthy a person is. Still, persons who enter into psychotherapy or psychoanalysis for "self-investigation" as opposed to treatment should be expected to finance it themselves.

In fact, although many persons might undertake a short course of psychotherapy solely for the purpose of self-investigation, very few would endure a long course. Psychotherapy, properly carried out, is a demanding and rigorous process. One must be motivated by a considerable degree of suffering to enter it and carry it through. We must be very careful not to deny complete mental health care to any person because he *appears* emotionally healthy to the nonprofessional observer. Mental illness/emotional problems is often not as apparent as certain types of medical-surgical illness. On the other hand, certain types of medical-surgical illnesses are not that apparent, either. Thus, a person may suffer severe back pain for which he requires extensive treatment, including surgery. Yet, if he is of a particular constitution, he can appear to be in only slight distress, or he may seem "normal" to the casual observer. In fact, only the person who is suffering—from *any* illness or problem—truly knows how much he is suffering. Pain from any cause or condition is often not perceptible or is only minimally perceptible to the observer, often even when that observer is professionally trained. In view of this, the role of the physician or other health professional is not so much to ascertain absolutely the *specific level* of a patient's pain as it is to diagnose the patient's illness or problem and determine if there is any medical and/or psychological treatment he can employ to alleviate the patient's distress, as he relates it. The whole point of my discussion here is to emphasize that it is too easy to classify a person as emotionally healthy when he indeed suffers from significant, painful symptoms of mental illness/emotional problems that deserve a full course of treatment, treatment that is carefully planned and judiciously applied, treatment that makes appropriate use of the full spectrum of mental health care. Thus, the patient can often benefit from a medical as well as a psychological approach to his mental illness/emotional problem—e.g., the prescription of psychotropic medication, either separate from or as an adjunct to psychotherapy.

Mental health care, and especially psychotherapy, has its critics, just as medical care of every type has its critics. Undoubtedly, some of the criticism of psychotherapy is valid and deserved. Psychotherapy, it is safe to say, is not yet refined as a treatment method. We need to improve our psychotherapeutic technique. (Let us not look at psychotherapy in a vacuum. All medical care can be refined and improved.) In the process, I think we must clarify exactly what psychotherapy can and cannot achieve. Expectations, perhaps, are too high, much as expectations of what different modalities of medical care can achieve are often too high. Too many psychotherapists, I believe, hold expectations of psychotherapy that are unrealistic. Further, many psychotherapists, especially those who are less well trained, often do not practice psychotherapy *per se* so much as they offer their patients (or clients) emotional support and advice. Certainly, these are crucial components of the psychotherapeutic process, but psychotherapy itself extends beyond this for most, but certainly not all, patients. As I suggest in the text of my paper, I think we can reduce the cost of mental health care by properly defining psychotherapy and by offering emotional support and advice, if this is all a person needs, through less costly mechanisms (such as "counseling").

The field of mental health care is young, indeed. Thus, we are constantly learning when and how to apply psychotherapy. It is a healing method that, properly used, can offer symptom relief for many persons who suffer major and minor mental illness/emotional problems. If psychotherapy does not work all the time or if it "only" maintains the status quo for a patient (client), if the results of psychotherapy (or of any variety of mental health care) are not dramatic, then psychotherapy is no different from any type of medical care.

One final point: It is certainly possible to play roulette with illness, health, and medical care—and I include mental health care in the latter category. By this I mean that it is possible to decide that a person will or will not receive a modality of medical care based on the whim (or, more politely, philosophy) of those who decide what type and level of health care it is "permissible" or "necessary" or "advisable" or "affordable" to deliver. In my view, however, it is not logical to indict, prosecute, and lock away from those who need it mental health care, or any modality of health care, purely on the basis that it can be lengthy or expensive or both. It seems to me that the validity and value of any modality of health care must be judged not so much on how much it costs or whether it is cost-effective, but rather on whether it "works." (By "works," I mean such care has the realistic potential to enhance the total health of those persons who receive it; not only can it cure or ameliorate or stabilize symptoms of the specific illness or injury for which it is employed, but it can also prevent the onset of other illness.) Health care *is* expensive, and as the state of the art of health care technology becomes ever more complex, health care will inevitably become even more expensive. Yet, simply, this is the price we must pay—even as we strive to make health care more efficient and control its expense. So long as we view health as a supreme premium, so long as we wish to promote and maintain the highest level of health possible for any individual person, we must expect health care *of all kinds* to grow in scope, method, and, ultimately, cost. This is not "bad or wrong"; rather, it reflects our priorities, both as individual persons and as a society, priorities that I believe are fundamentally sound and correct.

ACKNOWLEDGMENTS.   I especially wish to thank Ms. Carolyn Thompson for her expert deciphering and skillful typing of my manuscript, and Ms. Teddi Fine for helping me bring this book to its full fruition.

D.U.

The White Paper

Overview

1

The enactment of National Health Insurance (NHI) may be delayed for a lengthy period of time due to the state of the national economy. In addition, legislation to fully effect NHI may lie temporarily dormant as a consequence of the recent conservative philosophical trend in national politics. The best guess, though, is that comprehensive NHI is coming sooner or later—organized in terms of a greater or lesser partnership between the private sector and government and instituted in a single package or in graduated phases—e.g., the institution first of health insurance for catastrophic illness or injury. Indeed, the first phase of NHI has already arrived in the form of Medicare, Medicaid, and the Veterans Administration health benefits program. In addition, substantial government subsidies to health insurance plans for federal workers can also be considered to be a form of NHI. The federal government, then, is currently sponsoring, on a full or partial basis, health care for a significant percentage of Americans through both the private and public sectors.

Despite the fact that further legislation regarding NHI may face significant delays, health planners and legislators today are busy defining what amounts of mental health care the American public shall receive under NHI. They are deciding as well who shall deliver such health care and where it shall be delivered. Now, therefore, is the time for psychiatrists, other mental health professionals (MHPs),* and the health care community† at large to consider and to become involved in the review and planning process for the delivery of mental health care under National Health Insurance. The general public also has a large stake—a vested interest in the health care to which it shall be entitled—in understanding and attempting to influence the status of mental health care vis-à-vis NHI.

---

*The term *mental health professional* used herein refers mainly to psychiatrists, licensed clinical psychologists (Ph.D.s), social workers with a master's degree (M.S.W.s) or above, and psychiatric nurses with a master's degree or above. In addition, some highly qualified "clinical psychotherapists" would qualify as mental health professionals.

†*Health care community* as used herein refers to all those persons directly involved in providing health care services of any kind, as well as all persons concerning with planning, legislating, administering, and/or evaluating such health care services.

I should also note that my aim in this paper is to provide a balanced, comprehensive view of mental illness/emotional problems and mental health care to the health care community and to the public independent of a discussion of the requirements for such care under NHI. In other words, I seek to present herein a full and proper hearing on the present state and the future of mental health care in our nation. Such a hearing is mandatory now. Even if, as is highly unlikely, NHI does not ultimately eventuate, health planners and legislators will still be faced with the requirement of revising and updating existing health programs, policies, and insurance for mental health care. The discussion and arguments in this paper are applicable to and can serve as a basis for such a total reappraisal and restructuring.

Whatever the current status of National Health Insurance, the entire health care community—and the American public too—must be alerted to the already existing crisis concerning the availability and delivery of mental health care. The crisis only threatens to get worse under NHI, which, as currently conceived, is likely to further compromise and sacrifice mental health care. For many Americans, access to adequate mental health care will be denied rather than promoted by NHI. (Indeed, this has already occurred under "Phase I" of NHI.)

In essence, the current deliberations over mental health care coverage under NHI feature a nonmedical, political body deciding what mental health care is important and how the psychiatrist and other mental health professionals should practice. Unfortunately, the mental health community has not been well integrated into the decision-making process. As a result, the psychiatrist (and other MHPs) finds himself in a position where he must "lobby" for his patients' rights to mental health care. These rights are in serious jeopardy as all NHI plans currently under consideration by the Congress would sharply curtail mental health care, severely penalizing the many persons who require such care. Indeed, the most liberal plan would authorize a maximum of only 20 outpatient full-session visits per year per patient to a "private" psychiatrist and a maximum of 45 days' coverage for hospitalization for mental illness.* Although formal limits for outpatient care will probably not be strictly mandated by law for all provider agencies (i.e., Community Mental Health Centers and Health Maintenance Organizations), NHI legislation will effect *de facto* limits for care delivered by these agencies, as I shall demonstrate later in this paper.

I should point out here that severe limits on mental health care services are already in effect under Medicare and Medicaid. All NHI legislation introduced to date provides only token and inadequate liberalization of such limits. Current Health Maintenance Organization (HMO) enabling legislation is

---

*Kennedy–Waxman bill (1720), "Health Care for All Americans," 1979. I should also note that the Kennedy–Waxman bill allows the 20 full sessions to be applied as 40 half-sessions, 80 quarter-sessions, etc.

similarly negligent in mandating coverage for mental health care. For outpatient care, such legislation requires only that the HMO provide a patient a minimum number of visits ("not to exceed twenty") to a mental health professional.* Even then, this requirement is only applicable if the HMO seeks federal certification in order to be eligible to receive federal assistance. Lastly, benefits for mental health care under most private health insurance plans are hardly on a par with benefits for treatment of "physical illness." Coverage for outpatient mental health care ranges from minimal under many plans to totally absent in others. Although the American Medical Association now supports the concept of equivalent health insurance benefits for psychiatric care,[1] the fact is that there has been a recent trend toward a reduction as opposed to an increase in mental health care (or psychiatric) benefits available under many private health insurance plans. For example, the Blue Cross/Blue Shield Federal Employees Health Benefits (BCBS FEHB) plan instituted cutbacks in its coverage for outpatient mental health care as of January 1, 1981, resulting in a 50% increase in out-of-pocket expenses for persons receiving such care. (Further, BCBS FEBH cutbacks are threatened for the near future and may have already been instituted by the time of publication of this paper.†) This is especially significant for two reasons: (1) It followed major past

*Health Maintenance Organization Act, Title XIII, Section 1302 (1) (D) of the Public Health Service Act.

†Subsequent to the completion of this paper, Blue Cross/Blue Shield, in conjunction with the Office of Personnel Management (OPM) of the U.S. government, announced their intention to institute the following drastic reductions in benefits for mental health care coverage afforded federal employees under the BCBS FEHB (high option) program: (1) Benefits for inpatient mental health care are reduced to a maximum of 60 days per year (a reduction from 365 days per year). (2) Benefits for outpatient mental health care are reduced to 70% coverage of a maximum of 50 treatment visits per year to a mental health professional. Actually, under the newly revised coverage, an enrollee is allowed a maximum of 50 visits per annum for virtually all of his or her outpatient care, including treatment visits to physicians *of all kinds*, physical therapy, etc. In reality, therefore, mental health benefits for outpatient mental health care are reduced to a number well below 50 for most enrollees. It is certain that many patients who require extensive medical care for serious illnesses will be left in a given year(s) with *no* coverage for outpatient mental health care. (Of course, these patients especially can often utilize such care.)

It is possible that the reductions in benefits I have just described, announced in an OPM press release dated December 4, 1981, will be rescinded to one degree or another. (The entire health insurance program for federal employees is in a state of flux and massive reorganization.) Nevertheless, these reductions, as they currently stand, effectively result in the dismantlement of an insurance program for mental health care that served, as I have noted in the text, as an exemplary model plan. The reductions set the trend for and "justify" limited coverage for mental health care in other federally subsidized and private plans. Further, the reductions, arbitrarily arrived at, underline the perilous and precarious position of persons who suffer mental illness/emotional problems insofar as their being able to afford mental health care is concerned.

I should note that in early 1982 the U.S. Senate will hold hearings on the entire health insurance program for federal employees, *including* the status of mental health care under that program. It is possible that as a result of these hearings, the Congress *may* pass legislation that will mandate that coverage for mental health care under that program must be on a par with coverage for all other types of medical care. If such legislation is passed, it would be a monu-

cutbacks by other private carriers in their insurance packages for government employees and coincided with the announcement of major and minor cutbacks by still more carriers; and (2) the BCBS FEHB plan, up until now, has served as an exemplary model health insurance plan in terms of providing mental health care benefits—especially for outpatient care. In view of this and taking into consideration the fact that the BCBS FEHB plan is the largest plan (by membership) currently serving more than 9,000,000 federal employees and their dependents, the future for mental health care benefits under other health insurance plans would seem to be in more immediate jeopardy.

Of course, it should be apparent that as long as government-sponsored insurance benefits for mental health care remain, with few exceptions, inadequate or marginal at best, the private sector will be disinclined to provide anything more than fringe benefits for such care. In theory, government-sponsored health care programs such as Medicare and Medicaid should serve as pacesetters in terms of providing mental health care benefits. They should set standards for such care to which the private sector should be expected to conform—by regulation if necessary. The private sector's philosophy toward and approach to insurance benefits for mental health care is becoming ever more crucial. This is because it appears that the private sector will be responsible for providing a large portion of those mental health care benefits that will be available under NHI.

Mental health care coverage under Medicare deserves further discussion in view of the general model Medicare presents of the government's approach to mental health care and in view of the potential model Medicare presents for NHI. Medicare unfairly and unwisely limits inpatient care (in psychiatric hospitals) for mental illness/emotional problems. However, its major restrictions are directed at outpatient care. The current upper limits of coverage it provides for outpatient mental health care ($250) are grossly insufficient for the overwhelming majority of older persons who suffer mental illness/emotional problems. This is especially the case because the Medicare recipient is often a person whose financial means are extremely limited. He or she is, at

---

mental step forward by the federal government as regards its attitude and policies toward mental health care; it would constitute a dramatic reversal of the government's present stance toward mental health care. Until and unless such legislation is passed (and to me it seems highly unlikely that it will come "to pass"), BCBS FEHB plan members, as well as members of other health insurance plans for federal workers that feature more than *minimal* mental health care coverage, must now always feel in some jeopardy of losing additional benefits for mental health care, perhaps at a time when they are receiving treatment for mental illness/emotional problems and that treatment is in a particularly crucial phase.

I should also note here that persons who suffer mental illness/emotional problems are often extremely reluctant to step forward and argue for their legitimate rights to mental health care. Such persons are justifiably afraid of being stigmatized and subsequently discriminated against for admitting to receiving or wanting such care. Therefore, it is fallacious, if not insensitive and manipulative, for insurance companies, or for that matter the U.S. government (vis-à-vis Medicare, Medicaid, etc.), to cut back mental health care coverage, or to justify limited benefits, on the basis that there is little patient-consumer interest in it.

the same time, extremely susceptible to such symptoms as depression and anxiety due to the personal and social stresses older age imposes. The older citizen is likewise likely to suffer mental illness/emotional problems as a reaction to organic (physical) illness. Untreated or improperly treated, this only prolongs organic illness and leads to further physical deterioration.

In fact, the current Medicare limits for outpatient mental health care are hardly sufficient even for a proper diagnostic evaluation, much less for proper treatment. The result has been that many elderly persons who could benefit greatly from mental health care have been denied such treatment. Some who are not physically ill develop either physical symptoms or organic (physical) illness, extremely costly to diagnose and treat, as a secondary complication of the primary mental illness/emotional problems they suffer. Others who only *appear* senile or incapable of independent or semi-independent living are condemned to long-term stays in nursing homes and similar institutions. Such care is much more costly than full and proper evaluation and treatment of overt and underlying mental illness/emotional problems.

Medicare, therefore, has potentially catastrophic consequences for older persons who suffer mental illness/emotional problems—and for their families and society, which often bear all or a substantial portion of the older person's health care costs. Indeed, the very existence of severe limits for mental health care coverage under Medicare, supposedly a "compassionate" plan, demonstrates how easily inadequate health insurance can be legislated and instituted—in terms of any illness and any health care services. Unfortunately, criticism of limits on mental health care under Medicare has been largely ineffective in terms of increasing benefits for such care under that program.*
From both the humanistic viewpoint and the practical rationale of controlling the costs of health care, the inadequate coverage for mental health care under Medicare must be corrected.

Extreme care must be exercised in planning NHI to insure that inadequate limits for mental health care similar to those instituted under both Medicare and Medicaid are not enacted. Indeed, Medicaid, in the words of the Report of the President's Commission on Mental Health (1978),[2]

> reveals problems [with regard to coverage for mental health care] even more complex than those found with Medicare. . . . Mental health services under Medicaid are extremely limited. Medicaid provides federal matching funds for only a limited array of mental health services. Those that are covered are restricted in ways that services for the physically ill are not. . . . States are also free to define the amount, scope, and duration of services—including federally mandated services—they will cover. Medicaid permits States to reduce services by manipulating reimbursement rates. States may not deny services to a beneficiary on the basis of the patient's

---

*Legislation pending before the Congress would *theoretically* increase outpatient mental health care benefits under Medicare, though it would still legalize severe and discriminating limits on such care. In fact, even if such legislation is passed into law, the definition of "mental health care" under it may be so restricted as to effectively further limit outpatient mental health care under Medicare.

diagnosis, but they can influence the availability of care through their ability to
determine rates of compensation. In some States, Community Mental Health Centers are reimbursed for as little as 25 percent of their cost. In other States, psychiatrists are reimbursed for as little as $6.00 per hour-long visit. This rate is equivalent
to that paid other physicians for a routine office visit, which often lasts only five to
ten minutes. As a result, many health care providers refuse to participate in Medicaid, and many people eligible for Medicaid are denied access to needed services. A
person who needs care cannot receive assistance if the State plan includes health
and mental health benefits, but the reimbursement rate is so low that the services
are not provided.

The Report of the President's Commission on Mental Health goes on to
state that "Medicaid favors institutional care. Almost seventy percent of the
mental health care reimbursed under Medicaid in fiscal year 1977 was for
institutional services—these include State and County hospitals, private mental institutions, and nursing homes. Indeed, over half of all Medicaid funds
expended for mental health services went to nursing homes."

Of course, it is extremely unfortunate that Medicaid (as well as Medicare)
effectively encourages more costly inpatient care as opposed to less costly (by
a large degree) outpatient care. However, the real tragedy as regards the
Medicaid policy toward mental health care concerns the large numbers of
financially disadvantaged persons who are effectively denied such care. Because of the severe personal and social stresses generated by their financial
situations (including the stress of the struggle for basic survival), persons
eligible for Medicaid are more likely to suffer mental illness/emotional problems. Further, without proper treatment, such mental illness/emotional problems will often lead to organic (physical) illness or psychosomatic illness. I
believe that the overall cost for both the Medicaid and Medicare programs will
be decreased by making available full and complete mental health care services under those programs. Nevertheless, health planners and legislators
today take a more isolated view of the cost of the treatment of mental illness/
emotional problems *per se,* neglecting the reductions such treatment delivered
on a medically appropriate basis may produce in the total cost of health care.

The planned cutbacks in mental health care under NHI are based almost
exclusively on an economic (cost control) rationale derived from a narrow
conception and definition of illness and health care. Such a rationale yields a
policy that attempts mainly to control the specific cost of specific health care
services and, unfortunately, does not adequately anticipate, measure, or encourage the savings in complete health care costs to be derived from complete, if expensive, health care delivery. This presents a situation that has
implications for all medical practitioners and patients. Thus, although the
practice of psychiatry differs in certain respects from the practice of other
medical specialities, it is conceivable that rigid external controls and restrictions similar to those planned for mental health care under NHI could, in
the future, be proposed and implemented for care delivered by other medical
specialists. This could occur whenever the immediate and long-term benefits
and applications of a specific medical procedure or general modality of care

are neither recognized nor appreciated. Thus, the physician could be administratively denied under NHI the prerogative to utilize a particular diagnostic procedure (e.g., CAT scan X rays), monies for which might be excessively curtailed. Treatment modalities for various conditions (e.g., coronary bypass operation) might not be funded due to a premature determination of their questionable effectiveness. In addition, the physician's—the psychiatrist's and the nonpsychiatrist's—domain of practice might be excessively and unwisely limited or restricted in favor of an overly expanded role for paraprofessionals.

I hope most administrative and legislative decisions affecting the practice of medicine under NHI will be appropriate ones, but the proposed and already instituted limitations on mental health care (proposed for NHI, currently in effect under Medicare and Medicaid) demonstrate a danger that they may be based to a disproportionate extent on judgments relating to cost of service rather than need for service. This, in turn, may compromise medical care for the individual patient. In addition, it may result in a rigid, monolithic clinical approach to most patients in contrast to a more diversified approach where each patient is treated according to his or her unique, specific needs. This is not to sound a death knell or to hysterically overdramatize the current and potential dangers medical practice, including psychiatry, faces with the coming of NHI. Rather, I seek to emphasize the need for awareness, forethought, and vigorous action on the part of the entire health care community in order to insure (figuratively and literally) high-quality, appropriate medical care of all kinds under NHI.

Arbitrary limitations on mental health care, extant and planned, have serious implications for physicians of all specialities, for all patients, and for all potential users of mental health services. Obviously, the patients of psychiatrists and other mental health professionals (MHPs) will be the first to suffer from discriminatory limits on treatment. Blind, artificial limitations on the scope of mental health care, however, will be detrimental to the welfare of patients of nonpsychiatrists as well. In this respect, the interrelationship between organic (physical) illness and mental illness/emotional problems is well documented.

It should be realized that potential restrictions on mental health care under NHI pose no substantial personal threat to the psychiatrist himself. [The same cannot be said for other mental health professionals, such as clinical psychologists (Ph.D.s) and social workers (M.S.W.s), whose range of clinical expertise and function is considerably more narrow than the psychiatrist's. The nonpsychiatrist MHP, for example, cannot prescribe medication for patients.] The psychiatrist, as a physician, will always be needed in one capacity or another. It is the patient who will suffer the consequences of curtailment of mental health care. For example, if NHI is enacted as it is currently conceptualized, many persons who do not suffer "illness" in the classical sense will be deprived of the opportunity to receive and benefit from appropriate mental health care. (I do not know exactly what "illness" is! Is someone who has a silent single malignant cell, but who does not suffer symptoms, "ill"? On the other hand, is a person who suffers emotional problems, but who exhibits no demonstrable cellular pathology, "not ill"? It seems to me we must modify our concept of what constitutes "illness.") Here I am referring to persons who, though functional, exhibit maladaptive coping patterns and life-styles that leave them symptomatic (depressed, anxious)— sometimes to an extreme degree—and coincidentally frustrated and un-fulfilled in terms of personal goals, work, and relationships with others. Such persons can be said to suffer "chronic symptomatic maladjustment" (see Chapter 3). The psychiatrist and other MHPs must vigorously pursue the right to treatment under NHI for them. In so doing, however, the psychiatrist is calling for access to treatment that is often prolonged and costly. Politically speaking, it would be more advantageous for him to advocate only short-term treatment of mental illness/emotional problems under NHI; within this frame-work, he could urge slightly more liberal "set limits" on treatment visits than are currently planned. However, the psychiatrist (and other MHPs) cannot adopt an essentially expedient philosophy under which he would "sacrifice" any patient who requires long-term, expensive treatment to promote the adoption of broader limits under NHI for care of patients who require only short-term treatment. This would abrogate his responsibility as a physician.

In any case, when the psychiatrist or other MHP argues for broad cover-age of mental health care under NHI, he must be careful to be clinical and not metaphysical in his definition of "treatment." He must confine himself to mean by it (1) symptom cure, amelioration, or control—as for the person who suffers persistent depression; (2) remission maintenance, prevention of symptoms from recurring—as for the schizophrenic who has been stabilized and/or rehabilitated; and (3) symptom prophylaxis—as in the case of a rape or accident victim where early treatment intervention prevents hard-core symptoms from setting in. In the latter case, the individual is symptomatic to begin with but his (or her) symptoms relate to the acute stress of his situation. With treatment, then, he will not go on to develop chronic mental illness/ emotional problems.

The psychiatrist and other MHPs cannot mean by treatment "a process to enhance the quality of life." The psychiatrist cannot justify expenditures of health care monies under NHI for this cause, noble as it is. For one thing, it is too vague; for another, it is not in the strict province of psychiatry; finally, the psychiatrist is viewed as presumptuous when he pictures himself, or is per-ceived to picture himself, as the savior or moral benefactor of mankind and humanity. Though the psychiatrist (and other MHPs) may be able to contrib-ute to the general welfare of man and woman, this is not his primary direct task as a health care provider. Rather, he must concern himself with treating patients along the lines presented above.

Further clarification is necessary, however: The goal of psychiatric treat-ment and of mental health care in general is to relieve the patient's (client's) emotional suffering, whatever form it takes. The psychiatrist, in order to facilitate symptom relief, seeks to promote his patient's self-esteem; he also seeks to point his patient in the direction of achieving satisfaction and fulfillment in terms of the way he (or she) leads his life. In such respects, then, mental health care concerns itself with a person's general welfare and quality of life—but only as a product of a treatment process that aims in the first instance at the triad of (1) symptom cure, amelioration, or control; (2) remission maintenance, prevention of symptoms from recurring; and (3) symptom prophylaxis. I must note here that one clear and common object of all medical-surgical care is to promote the general welfare of the patient and to enhance the quality of his life as a product of the treatment process that aims to restore for him a condition of relative or absolute health. It seems to me that without such purpose, there is little rationale for either medical care or mental health care. This does not negate the principle that for either category of care (and they are often intertwined) symptoms are treated in the first instance strictly for their own sake. Nevertheless, it recognizes the fact that *all* health care does not operate in a vacuum; rather it takes into account and is employed to promote the potential to be gained by the patient in all spheres of his life from the modification or resolution of his symptoms.

This paper proceeds to address the specific questions and issues that National Health Insurance poses vis-à-vis mental health care. The scope of the problem of mental illness/emotional problems is described, followed by a discussion of what conditions (mental illness/emotional problems) should be covered, what the extent of coverage should be, and who should provide treatment and care. In this discussion, the cost of mental health care is considered in depth. The cost factor must be clarified, for it is an overriding issue, the major stumbling block upon which hinges full coverage for mental health care under NHI. I attempt to show that broad coverage is affordable and that comprehensive mental health care will actually reduce the overall cost of medical care.

On the surface, certain aspects of my presentation here may appear to be "basic" to the psychiatrist or MHP. However, the extremely precarious present-day status of mental health care mandates a comprehensive review of the topic from A to Z. It must include an analysis of the most primary and fundamental concepts, assumptions, and hypotheses concerning mental health care. In addition, mental illness/emotional problems and mental health care must be clearly defined and their scope illuminated in a way that will enable the entire health care community to understand the subject to the maximum extent possible. The health care community must recognize the magnitude and the specific nature of the problem mental illness/emotional problems pose for society. This is a prerequisite for the establishment of adequate coverage for mental health care under NHI.

This paper neither attempts to justify nor presents a plan for separate, special preventive mental health care services. I do call for the provision of such services through the public sector, but I have chosen to focus in this paper on the immediate, pressing issue of securing adequate treatment services for mental illness/emotional problems under NHI. (Of course, to the extent such treatment ameliorates and interrupts illness, and to the extent it forestalls further illness, it constitutes preventive mental health care.) Certainly we should make all possible efforts to promote mental health through preventive methods; this makes much more sense and is, of course, much less costly than treating mental illness/emotional problems. In this connection, it is very important that we teach persons (e.g., through education courses) psychological principles and so-called coping strategems that enable one to lead a healthy emotional life. Similarly, it is important that we teach parents the psychology of parenting as well as the psychology of childhood and adolescence so as to help parents foster emotional health in their children. Nevertheless, it can be argued that the best preventive mental health care consists of early identification and early treatment of mental illness/emotional problems. Of course, it is a maxim in medicine that the earlier symptoms can be detected and classified, the more successfully they can be treated. This is especially the case as regards (many types of) mental illness/emotional problems. This is because a person tends to develop rigid and inflexible "psychological defenses" (loosely considered, "coping patterns") over time that are often highly resistant to modification.

Mental Health Care and National Health Insurance complements and augments the recently published Report of the President's Commission on Mental Health.[2] Unfortunately, though the report is useful in many respects, it leaves unanswered key questions as to what directions mental health care should take under NHI. The report, for example, is vague in terms of setting forth specific, hard-core proposals for coverage of mental health care services. Though it calls for coverage based on "the appropriateness of care, not the discipline of the provider," it goes on to state that there is "inadequate information and little agreement about the most appropriate activity that can be provided by the various categories of personnel, both professional and paraprofessional." In sum, the commission's report does not define who should provide what and how much under NHI. Although it does call for considerable expansion of Community Mental Health Centers (CMHCs), it does not propose balanced guidelines as to how we as a nation shall meet the mental health care needs of the nation under NHI.

This paper goes beyond the Report of the President's Commission on Mental Health.[2] Where the report recommends *"appropriate* [italics added] coverage for mental health care" under NHI, I call for *full and complete* coverage for mental health care under NHI, though with the establishment of standards for such care by professional peer review committees and the monitoring of care by them. Of course, the issue of imposing limits on psychoanalysis or long-term intensive psychotherapy, which I deal with herein, is extremely complex and controversial. Professional organizations, such as the American Psychiatric Association, have been largely unwilling to openly consider or to advocate such limits, even in the broadest sense, in part for fear of alienating segments of their membership. (Still, the efforts of these organizations to insure the availability of intensive psychotherapy and psychoanalysis, as medically appropriate, for any individual patient are justifiable and, indeed, mandatory. Though we may and should dispute clinical methods, we cannot impose blanket limits in a blind fashion on the extent of legitimate care available to a patient—whether that be medical care or mental health care. Each patient's health care needs must be judged on an individual basis and his health care dispensed accordingly.)

This paper also calls for the preservation under NHI of the existing dualistic public and private mental health care delivery systems—each system providing the services for which it is best suited and designed. I do believe, though, and I shall attempt to demonstrate herein that private "fee-for-service" mental health care often constitutes better care than that delivered in the public sector. For example, the freedom of the patient-consumer to choose and to be treated by the specific individual provider of his choice can be a determinant of treatment outcome in mental illness/emotional problems, more so than for any other medical condition. In terms of mental health care, such choice of provider is most often, if not strictly, a feature of the private sector and does not exist, by and large, in the public sector. In addition, it is mainly in the private sector that the patient (client)* and the psychiatrist (or other MHP) can embark upon a total, comprehensive course of treatment that takes into account and responds freely to both the patient's complete treatment goals and the psychiatrist's judgment as to what constitutes the ideal, complete treatment plan. (Unfortunately, this is not always the case even in the private sector. The HMO, for example, often acts like the public sector to limit both the choice of provider and the extent of care available to the patient.)

In this connection, health planners and legislators who are formulating NHI must recognize and understand that mental health care differs significantly from other categories of health care. As will be made clear, mental health care can be significantly altered and shaped and facilitated or compromised by economic factors operating on the provider—more so than any other form of health care. Therefore, any NHI policy that would affect the currently existing mental health care delivery system—by limiting private

---

*Typically, when a person receives mental health care from a psychiatrist, and in some cases a psychiatric nurse, he (or she) is known as a "patient"; when he receives such care from other mental health professionals, he is known as a "client." Of course, it does not matter so much what the person is called as that he receives the care he needs. In this connection, many nonpsychiatrist MHPs do not view their clients as "ill." Indeed, many persons who suffer emotional distress may not be ill in the strict sense by which some define "illness." On the other hand, many such persons do require *medical* care for specific symptoms, such as depression and anxiety, or mental illness (classically defined), such as schizophrenia, "manic-depressive illness," and certain states of severe depression. Some may view it as patronizing to refer to persons who enter into treatment for emotional distress as "patients"; however, it can be a serious mistake, with profound consequences, to think of many of them and to treat them only as "clients."

sector fee-for-service care, for example—must be thoroughly evaluated in terms of the type and quality of mental health care it is likely to foster.

I must stress that in taking specific positions on mental health care and NHI and in making proposals to implement them, the psychiatrist (and other MHPs) must justify his viewpoints and "policy." A thorough, rational evaluation and explanation of the complexities involved in providing mental health care under NHI or under our existing health care system is imperative. If the psychiatrist is to call for full and complete coverage for mental health care, then he must define what constitutes "proper amounts" of mental health care; he must delineate the benefits to the patient of providing such care as well as the consequences of not providing it. Psychiatrists (as well as other MHPs) must be careful to avoid professional, chauvinistic bias and pejorative arguments in establishing and arguing their positions. Professional organizations such as the American Psychiatric Association and the American Psychoanalytic Association have long made strong and commendable efforts to obtain full and complete coverage for mental health care under NHI. Nevertheless, such organizations are often perceived as acting in their own self-interest as much as in the interest of the patient-consumer. Unfortunately, they do exactly that to a certain extent, creating an awkward credibility gap.

For example, there is a need to clarify the blurring of provider roles that has developed among the various mental health professionals. This must be accomplished if mental health care is to be provided on a cost-effective basis under NHI. In this connection, the psychiatrist cannot make the statement that he practices "pure psychotherapy" better than any group of equally highly trained clinical psychotherapists. [By "pure psychotherapy" I mean psychotherapy in which the psychotherapist does not utilize medication as a part of the treatment process; psychotherapy that relies solely for its efficacy on (1) the "therapeutic relationship" (see Appendix) and the interaction it fosters between the psychotherapist and his or her patient (client) and (2) a carefully devised nonmedical therapeutic regimen that often (a) promotes the understanding and "working through" by the patient of the way he thinks, feels, and behaves, and (b) includes the direct or indirect suggestion to the patient of alternative, more adaptive ways of thinking, feeling, and behaving, leading to the gradual and incremental acceptance by the patient of such alternatives and his subsequent "practicing" of them both within and without the psychotherapeutic setting.] The psychiatrist, supported by his professional organizations, has sometimes claimed a special skill or expertise as regards the practice of "pure psychotherapy," while the psychologist and other MHPs have attempted to prove themselves to be providers of mental health care equal to or better than the psychiatrist. In my opinion, such an approach by the psychiatrist can only compromise his basic recommendations on mental health care under NHI. To set the record straight, I attempt to define in this paper exactly who the psychiatrist is and how he differs from other mental health professionals. I suggest herein an organizational schema for providing mental health care under NHI that places the psychiatrist at the helm of the mental health care delivery system but at the same time includes rather than excludes various other mental health professionals as treatment providers.

I have tried not to be political in this white paper; I have, however, taken "positions" that must involve politics. This is because the issue of coverage for mental health care under National Health Insurance involves broad social, cultural, and financial considerations for the society as a whole as well as medical consequences for the individual patient (client). In any case, I have attempted to marshal and demonstrate evidence for the positions I take.

In connection with the key position I take in these pages—a call for full coverage for complete evaluation and treatment of mental illness/emotional problems under NHI—I want to stress that I am calling for coverage for treatment that is safe and efficacious. Furthermore, I am in general an advocate of the least costly treatment that is maximally safe and efficacious. (We should allow the patient some reasonable choice of treatment method, even when one form of treatment is more expensive than another.) I am not proposing here coverage for *isolated* education, advice, or emotional support for persons who do not suffer classifiable mental illness/emotional problems. I am proposing, rather, coverage for the *clinical evaluation* and *clinical treatment* of persons who do. Of course, if the psychiatrist or other MHP is to justify full coverage for mental health care under NHI, he must define exactly what he means by evaluation and treatment and he must attempt to prove his treatment techniques to be safe and efficacious. In the same sense, physicians of other specialties must be expected to demonstrate the value of the therapeutic modalities they employ. However, proof of the safety and efficacy of medical care, especially mental health care, is complicated. The end results of all medical care must be viewed and evaluated from multiple directions and perspectives. Often it is not the immediate treatment result but the long-term result measured across multiple indices that is most significant and meaningful.

I should also point out here that although National Health Insurance does pose a crisis for mental health care, mental health care will benefit in the end. It is a maxim in psychotherapy that when a patient encounters a crisis in his life, he has an opportunity to resolve his conflicts and actually to function at a higher level. In this sense, the field of mental health care must squarely face the crisis posed by National Health Insurance, deal with the dilemmas and challenges it presents, and hope to enhance in the process its total role in the health field. In any case, National Health Insurance should certainly not be seen as an enemy of psychiatry or an enemy of medicine in general. NHI ultimately presents psychiatry (and medicine) with the opportunity to review its function and purpose. (Psychiatry should be viewed by NHI planners and legislators not as the pariah of medicine but rather as one medical field of many that should properly review its function and purpose.) To this end, I present in this paper a review of the current-day status of mental health care.

This includes a view of the layperson's thoughts and feelings about mental illness/emotional problems and mental health care. Such a perspective is essential for any valid formulation of mental health care coverage under NHI.

Any broad restructuring of medical care, as NHI entails, should encompass a review of the philosophy of health care. Health care is extremely expensive and this factor complicates our concern for the ill person. It forces us as a society to define how we feel about health, illness, and treatment of illness. I cannot comment in this paper on a general and complete philosophy toward health care. I will say, however, that we must now recognize the all-pervasive impact of psychological factors on individual and collective human functioning. In this connection, we must acknowledge that it is our thoughts and feelings that often hold the key to our health in both the emotional and physical sense—not to diminish the importance and influence of other factors in this regard or to minimize the effects of organic (physical) illness itself on emotional health. I hope we shall soon realize and accept the verity that it is the mind, and the brain that encompasses it, that is at the heart of the body. (Indeed, messages from the brain conducted through the autonomic nervous system, a system highly sensitive to the emotions, control to a large extent the function of the heart.) In my opinion, health care delivery in the future will be based on this precept. And the future should start now.

No matter what form of health insurance we as a nation ultimately evolve, discrimination against persons who suffer mental illness/emotional problems and against mental health care must cease. Full and complete coverage for legitimate mental health care must be instituted. It is the psychiatrist's greatest and most compelling modern-day task to insure that such a revolution in mental health care comes about. We can no longer deny any person access to the best available evaluation and treatment for mental illness/emotional problems. Special attention must be devoted to the mental health care needs of the financially and socially disadvantaged, a group that has been largely denied such care under our present system. Still this group does not have a monopoly on mental illness/emotional problems. No health insurance program should provide one group with mental health care, or any medical care, at the expense of another. Thus, the psychiatrist and other MHPs must work to insure access for all persons to the highest caliber of mental health care—care based solely on emotional, not financial need.

2

Mental Illness/Emotional Problems
The Prevalence and the Cost

The cost of mental illness/emotional problems is both calculable and incalculable. We cannot affix a cost to the plight of millions of Americans who suffer from mental illness/emotional problems. We can, however, state how much it costs to care for these Americans. In terms of health and of cost, mental illness/emotional problems are probably the single greatest health problem of the American people. The Alcohol, Drug Abuse, and Mental Health Administration (ADAMHA) reports in its National Data Book (1980)[3] that in 1978 national health expenditures were estimated to be $192.4 billion, representing 9.1% of the gross national product. Of this total, it was estimated that approximately $19 billion, or 9%, were expended for direct care (evaluation and treatment) of the "mentally ill."

The ADAMHA National Data Book[3] provides a specific breakdown of mental health treatment expenditures (direct care) for 1975, when it was estimated that $12.3 billion were spent on such care. Significantly, at least 60 to 70% of the total cost for direct care in 1975 was accounted for by care and treatment of patients in hospitals, nursing homes, halfway houses, and other inpatient settings; only 11% resulted from psychiatrists' and psychologists' charges for treatment. These data clearly demonstrate that the bulk of the cost for the treatment of mental illness/emotional problems is for hospitalization and/or extended care (see Table 1 for an estimated breakdown of mental health expenditures, 1975).

The NIMH calculated the total cost of mental illness to be approximately $31 billion in 1975,[3] counting both direct care costs and indirect costs (as well as other expenditures—i.e., management expenses, facilities development costs, research funding, and training and fellowship costs). The indirect costs were judged to be approximately $16.9 billion. Indeed, this is a very low estimate: Indirect costs are actually much greater because the NIMH figure, in describing actual disability—that is, time lost from work—does not specifically take into account decreased work productivity arising from mental illness/emotional problems. In fact, there is no way of estimating the loss of work productivity resulting from mental illness/emotional problems. Undoubtedly, though, it is exceedingly high. Work productivity is bound to be affected by any degree of emotional impairment. In addition, many persons afflicted by

Table 1. Mental Health Treatment Expenditures by Provider, 1975 (in millions of $)[a,b]

Provider or cost category	1975 expenditures[c]
MH[d] specialty sector	$9,053
State and county mental hospitals	(3,080)
General hospitals (separate psychiatric units)	(1,792)
Private practice psychiatrists	(989)
Freestanding outpatient clinics	(798)
Community mental health centers (CMHCs)	(778)
Private mental hospitals	(438)
Private practice psychologists	(372)
Other public mental hospitals	(206)
Other mental health facilities	(600)
General health care sector *et al.*	$3,269
Nursing homes	(992)
General hospitals (no separate psychiatric units)	(780)
Psychoactive drugs	(728)
Children's educational programs	(541)
Private practice nonpsychiatric M.D.s	(160)
HMOs and BCHS-assisted programs	(68)
Total	$12,322

[a] Source: Derived from Cost of mental illness, NIMH/Biometry and Epidemiology, 1979, an unpublished NIMH working paper drawing its data from a wide range of published and unpublished NIMH and other federal data.
[b] Table taken from the Alcohol, Drug Abuse, and Mental Health National Data Book. Washington, D.C., U.S. Department of Health, Education and Welfare, Public Health Service, Alcohol, Drug Abuse, and Mental Health Administration, 1980, p 103.
[c] The table does not provide a total breakdown of treatment costs for alcohol abuse and drug abuse. For the year 1975, these were estimated by ADAMHA at $843 million and $518 million, respectively (see reference 3).
[d] MH = mental health, HMO = Health Maintenance Organization, and BCHS = Bureau of Community Health Services.

mental illness/emotional problems are unable to sustain themselves without financial assistance from the state.

We should supplement the preceding statistics with ADAMHA data[3] regarding the total economic cost to society of alcohol abuse, drug abuse, and mental illness disorders. The following figures for 1975 include both direct costs (for treatment and treatment-related functions) and indirect costs (lost productivity and others). The total economic cost of alcohol abuse was judged by ADAMHA to be approximately $3 billion, of drug abuse approximately $10.4 billion, and of mental illness approximately $31 billion. In addition, ADAMHA has set forth its best estimates as to total expenditures for *actual treatment* of alcohol abuse, drug abuse, and mental illness disorders.[3] For alcohol abuse, this was judged to be $843 million (1975); for drug abuse, $518 million (1978); and for mental illness, $12.3 billion (1975).[3]

As regards the prevalence of mental illness/emotional problems in the general population, it was estimated in 1975 that approximately 32 million

Americans suffered from mental illness—including alcoholism and alcohol "problems."[3] (This figure reflects only "concrete" mental illness/emotional problems such as depression, anxiety, schizophrenia, etc. It does not reflect the prevalence of mental illness/emotional problems that essentially manifests itself in the patient (client) by the expression of physical symptoms.) Further, we can estimate on an extremely conservative basis that at least 2.5% of the American people receive specialized mental health care each year—that is, treatment delivered by trained mental health professionals (psychiatrists, psychologists, social workers, nurses).[4] As long ago as 1973, when mental health care was even more stigmatized and less accepted by both patients and physicians as a legitimate form of health care, 0.5% of the population (1 out of every 200 Americans) received specialized inpatient treatment for mental illness/emotional problems and 1.8% (approximately 2 out of every 100 Americans) received specialized outpatient treatment. Thus, a total of 2.3% of the population received specialized treatment for mental illness/emotional problems in 1973. This figure is probably considerable higher today. However, even if we accept it as currently valid, it does not paint an accurate portrait of the incidence of treatment of mental illness/emotional problems within the population. In the first place, the data, as stated, refer only to "specialized" treatment, i.e., treatment delivered by professionals and other personnel trained specifically in the mental health field. It does not record the large number of visits to nonpsychiatrist physicians—which in essence constitute mental health care—because the physician prescribes only tranquilizers or antidepressants for the patient during these visits. In this connection, Regier and his associates at the National Institute of Mental Health (NIMH) cite data[5] that reveal that while 3% of the population receive *specialized* mental health care services in a given year, over 9% of the population receive *nonspecialized* "mental health care" from the primary care/outpatient medical sector. Further, it has been estimated[4] that 50% of all visits to physicians in health maintenance organizations (HMOs) are for emotional or psychosocial reasons—even though the patient may manifest and complain exclusively of physical symptoms. This figure may be high. The NIMH reports a separate study in which it is estimated more conservatively that 15% of patients who seek and receive medical care from nonpsychiatrist physicians suffer primarily from "psychiatric disorders."[4] Whatever the exact statistics, the importance of these data can be understood by considering that the physician (with the help of the psychiatrist or other MHP) can best treat a large percentage of his patients by treating their underlying emotional problems, the real cause of their physical complaints (e.g., fatigue, headaches, stomachaches, backaches).

We must also note as regards the prevalence and cost of mental illness/emotional problems that a wide spectrum of major organic (physical) illnesses are intimately connected with the patient's personality and/or emotional state. Personality and emotional state can predispose a person to illness, precipitate its onset, exacerbate it, or do all of the above. (See also "Psychosomatic Illness" in Chapter 3.) (This is not to exclude the role of other factors such as heredity, environmental toxins, and nutritional state in the pathogenesis and course of disease.) Of course, illnesses precipitated or contributed to by personality or emotional state frequently necessitate repeated expensive hospitalizations for the patient—or at a minimum, expensive outpatient care. There is another way in which the condition of mental illness/ emotional problems reflects itself in costly medical-surgical health care. Many patients are hospitalized on medical services of general hospitals for the syndrome of "exhaustion." Though they may display physical symptoms, their primary symptom is often emotional distress manifested by extreme fatigue. Their hospital treatment consists essentially of rest and a respite from emotional stresses operant in their lives. Often, they would be more appropriately treated by a psychiatrist or other mental health professional on an outpatient basis.

In tabulating the cost of mental illness/emotional problems, we must keep in mind the fact that alcohol and drug abuse, especially alcohol abuse, is a cause of or contributes to many diseases and recurring illnesses. In 1975, for example, fully 19% of all patients discharged from Veterans Administration (VA) hospitals were diagnosed as suffering from either alcoholism or alcohol-related diseases (e.g., delirium tremens (DTs), liver failure, bleeding ulcers, inflammation of the pancreas).[6] Clearly the VA hospital system differs from our domestic nonfederal hospital system, as does its population base, but the VA data may well reflect the incidence of admissions to private and public hospitals due to alcoholism or alcohol-related illnesses, population differences notwithstanding. Our society "hides" alcohol- and drug-related illnesses as well as other expressions of mental illness/emotional problems (e.g., states of exhaustion referred to above) due to the stigmata attached to them. Alcohol and drug abuse, of course, often result in the first instance, at least in part, from primary emotional problems that must be treated if we are to prevent expensive alcohol/drug-related illness. Most significantly, it has recently been estimated that the direct cost of care for alcohol abuse alone in 1976 was $11.6 billion (including detoxification itself and care for secondary, related medical-surgical illness).[7] The cost of lost production and wages (1976) because of alcoholism was estimated at $20.6 billion.[7]

The Report of the President's Commission on Mental Health (1978)[2] presents statistics that further qualify mental illness/emotional problems as the nation's number one health problem. The report states that although the prevalence of mental illness/emotional problems in the population has in recent years been estimated at 10%, the more proper figure is probably 15%. The report further states that at any one time as many as 25% of the population are estimated to suffer from "mild to moderate depression, anxiety, and other indicators of emotional disorders." As the report correctly points out, many of this group wind up receiving medical-surgical health care.* Finally,

---

*For an in-depth discussion of the prevalence rates of mental disorder as determined on the basis of multiple epidemiological studies, see the report by Regier.[5]

Brodie[8] notes statistics that indicate that "the prevalence of mental illness varies with the 'health care model'" in which patients receive their health care. Thus, he notes a range of prevalence rates of 4 to 39.6% as measured in 18 studies of fee-for-service settings; a range of 1.2 to 14.6% as measured in 12 studies of prepaid practices (such as HMOs); and a range of 15.6 to 50% as measured in studies of community health centers. As can be seen, the lowest prevalence rates occur among patients who are treated in prepaid practices. Although there are several factors that could account for these low rates, I believe they primarily reflect the tendency of prepaid practices (such as HMOs) *not* to diagnose mental illness/emotional problems and *not* to provide treatment for such—due in large part to the financial disincentives to provide mental health care under which such practices operate. (See Chapter 5 for a further discussion of incentives and disincentives, financial and otherwise, for the provision of mental health care.)

The impact of the problem of mental illness/emotional problems becomes much clearer and perhaps more tangible when we add to the above data the following hard numbers from the Report of the President's Commission on Mental Health[2]: At any one time more than two million Americans are estimated to suffer from schizophrenia, another two million Americans suffer from profound depressive disorders, and over one million Americans suffer from toxic psychoses (resulting, for example, from alcohol and drug abuse) or permanently disabling mental conditions. Finally, handicapping mental

Table 2. Estimated Prevalence of Selected Mental Health Disorders (Including Alcoholism and Drug Dependence)[a,b]

Age category/disorder	Point prevalence rate
Children (under 18)	8–10%
Adults (18–65)	10–15%
Depression and affective disorders	4.5–8%
Anxiety, phobia, and other neuroses	4–7%
Alcoholism and alcohol problems	2.5–8%
Drug dependence	0.5–1%
Schizophrenia	0.5–1%
Aged (over 65)	10%

[a] Source: Professional judgment of ADAMHA staff based upon multiple research studies.

   Caveat: A definitive epidemiological survey based upon a national probability sample has yet to be done. The current body of literature derives from a fair number of epidemiological surveys within particular communities over the past 25 years. These surveys have tended to include only noninstitutionalized populations and thus likely underestimated the prevalence of mental disorders requiring institutionalized treatment.

[b] Table and *caveat* taken from the Alcohol, Drug Abuse, and Mental Health National Data Book. Washington, D.C., U.S. Department of Health, Education and Welfare, Public Health Service, Alcohol, Drug Abuse, and Mental Health Administration, 1980, p 19.

health problems among children ages 3 to 15 range from 5 to 15% of that population (see Table 2).

The President's Commission on Mental Health assesses the situation correctly when it reports that although 12% of this nation's general health care expenditures are for mental health care,* this figure is hardly commensurate with the immensity of the problem of mental illness/emotional problems. The commission recommends an allotment of health care monies "commensurate with the magnitude of mental health problems facing the nation."[2] However, National Health Insurance in its present form will probably decrease total expenditures for mental health care. In fact, full and complete benefits for mental health care must be provided under NHI if the cost of health care in general is to be contained.

*Slightly different figure from the corresponding one just presented.

3

What Conditions Should Be Covered?

Throughout this paper, I use the term *mental illness/emotional problems* rather than *mental illness, psychiatric disorder, emotional disturbance,* and so forth. I have chosen this specific terminology to dispel the false idea that it is only people with "serious mental illness" who require mental health care. In fact, the vast majority of persons who now receive and who should seek such care suffer from emotional problems rather than from distinct "mental illness." NHI must provide full coverage for care for these persons. Thus, a recently divorced person suffering excessive *clinical* depression or anxiety as a reaction to his (or her) divorce should be entitled to full and complete treatment from a psychiatrist or other mental health professional to help him in the first instance to resolve these symptoms. In order to effect such a resolution, treatment may partially focus on helping the person to understand "what" happened to him and "why." This in turn enables the person to engage in future relationships in such a way that he avoids the psychological "mistakes" he has made in his previous relationship(s). Of course, I most definitely do not imply by advocating broad coverage for mental health care that the psychiatrist or other MHP should or can treat everyone—that he can or should offer blanket emotional support to all persons who suffer emotional "upset" or that he can solve all problems for all persons. I am advocating coverage strictly for mental illness/emotional problems as clinically defined. How do we define mental illness/emotional problems more exactly? First, I should point out that we as a society are reluctant to accept the reality of mental illness/emotional problems. Most of us have either a family member or a friend or acquaintance who at one time or another has suffered major or minor mental illness/emotional problems. In spite of this, we deny the high incidence of mental illness/emotional problems and diminish in our own minds their significance. We do so in part because we are actually aware, if only at an unconscious level, that mental illness/emotional problems (as defined below) can afflict each of us. In fact, the likelihood is that sometime during our lives it will—in the same sense that we are likely to suffer organic (physical) symptoms and illness. (We can accept without much difficulty the probability of the latter occurring, yet we deny the possibility of the former.) Beyond this unpleasant prospect, the onset of mental illness/emotional problems represents the unknown; it is mysterious and frightening to those who are not professionally trained to deal with it, especially since it involves the mind, the core and essence of our being. [When an organic (physical) illness strikes, we perceive that it affects a "part" of us—our stomach, kidneys, liver, heart, etc. On the other hand, when a condition such as mental illness/ emotional problems strikes, we perceive an attack on our total selves.] The resulting tendency is not to acknowledge the reality of mental illness/emotional problems. The next step is to ridicule those who suffer mental illness/ emotional problems. We are in fact deeply and irrationally prejudiced against such persons. We attach social stigmata to mental illness/emotional problems; worse, we deny the need for or requirements of treatment for those who suffer the condition. We feel, and too often we demand, that such persons should be responsible for getting well themselves. (Although we admit that we are not always in total control of the state of health of our body organs, we are extremely reluctant, at best, to admit that we are not always in control of our minds—the way we think, feel, and behave.) The fact, however, is that a person's mental illness/emotional problems are as real as any medical-surgical illness and require, for resolution or control, full and complete health care intervention—as opposed to "will power" on the part of the afflicted person. Given the proper resources, the psychiatrist or other MHP can effectively treat most categories of mental illness/emotional problems, although improvement will often be limited (sometimes very limited) for persons who suffer chronic illnesses or conditions.

Before delineating specific categories of mental illness/emotional problems, I should make clear that it is solely the responsibility of the individual person to choose or reject mental health care for himself for any given condition. No person should be treated, no matter how bizarre his behavior, if he does not feel "bad" and if he does not want treatment. The exception occurs and treatment is mandatory if a person is a threat to himself or to society or its members, or if he is unable to care for himself. However, psychiatrists and other mental health professionals must be extremely careful in defining and applying the terms *threat* and *unable to care* so as not to deprive any person of his civil rights insofar as his choice of health care is concerned.

The main purpose of the following survey is to provide some idea of the broad scope of mental illness/emotional problems in terms understandable to the layperson. Although the survey may seem somewhat simplistic to the mental health professional, it represents an attempt to spell out the general categories of mental illness/emotional problems for which mental health care should be made available under NHI. Without such a delineation, any discussion of coverage for mental health care can be only vague and imprecise at best. The mental health professional should be willing and eager to debate the feasibility and value of mental health care for each of the categories described. Finally, the survey below does not constitute a formal or complete classification of mental illness/emotional problems. For this, the reader should refer to DSM III: Diagnostic and Statistical Manual of Mental Disorders, published by the American Psychiatric Association (APA).[9]

3.1.1. Categories of Mental Illness/Emotional Problems

3.1.1.1. Category I: Psychiatric Syndromes. These are syndromes for which specific medication is generally accepted to be a primary and effective treatment. *Psychotherapy* (defined below) may be equally important in the treatment of these syndromes, e.g., manic depressive illness, schizophrenia, and many severe, unrelenting depressions, all of which frequently reach psychotic proportion. For purposes of this discussion, a "psychosis" may be defined as a condition in which a person loses touch with reality. His "thought processes" and "thought content" are abnormal. For example, he may suffer hallucinations and/or delusions; he may "see things," "hear voices," be convinced people are plotting against him, and so forth. Others define the psychotic state more broadly as a condition in which a person can no longer care for himself due to mental illness/emotional problems.

The psychiatric syndromes, whether or not they are manifested by psychosis, are quite often dramatic. They "cry out for help" and the patient frequently requires hospitalization. No doubt, care for the psychiatric syndromes will be covered under NHI—although not necessarily in full measure. However, it is important to emphasize that the majority of persons who require and can benefit from specialized mental health care do not suffer from these syndromes. Their mental illness/emotional problems are less dramatic. They may be functional or appear to be functional, but they suffer emotional pain that disrupts their lives more than the outsider would ever know or suspect.

3.1.1.2. Category II: Mental Illness/Emotional Problems Caused by Organic (Physical) Disease. Organic (physical) diseases can produce profound, severe emotional symptoms in affected persons ranging from depression to psychosis to personality change. In addition, these diseases may affect the person's ability to think, remember, learn, and recognize. "Senile dementia" ("senility") is an example.

Many organic (physical) diseases affect a person's nervous system mainly or exclusively, whereas others affect the nervous system only secondarily. Brain tumors, Huntington's chorea, and "senile dementia" belong to the first group; thyroid, liver, and kidney disease belong to the second. The distinction is somewhat artificial since the resulting mental illness/emotional problems can be quite similar.

Within this category of mental illness/emotional problems, a further separation should be made between "reversible disease" and "irreversible disease." With the former, a return to normal mental functioning and a normal emotional state is possible; with the latter, impairment is permanent to one degree or another. A common example of reversible disease would be thyroid deficiency, in which treatment with thyroid hormone is often curative. An example of irreversible disease would be, again, many cases of "senile dementia."

The psychiatrist works in tandem with other physician specialists to diagnose and treat the multiple aspects of organic disease. An extremely crucial task for the psychiatrist is to determine if the patient's disease process, as it affects his mental functioning, is reversible, and if it is, to institute proper treatment immediately. However, even when the disease process is irreversible, the psychiatrist works with the patient to help him adjust emotionally to his condition as fully and as painlessly as possible. Thus, of the many elderly citizens who suffer "senile dementia," a significant number can improve with treatment (experience a greater sense of well-being), even when the disease process has left them with mental impairment. NHI must not forget or neglect the emotional well-being of such patients with chronic illness.

Finally, it should be stressed that every organic (physical) illness, from the common cold to the most serious of disorders, has its emotional effects and complications, and the patient's rate of improvement may well be dependent upon the psychological attitude he develops and maintains toward his illness. Depression or anxiety about illness may retard the healing process, whereas a positive attitude toward getting well may speed up healing. Mental health care, even in the smallest of doses, may be extremely useful in helping the patient to develp such an attitude.

3.1.1.3. Category III: Psychosomatic Illnesses.
There can be no dichotomy between organic (physical) illness and mental illness/emotional problems. (Therefore all illnesses are in the purest sense "psychosomatic" or "somatopsychic" illnesses.) As Descartes said, "I think, therefore, I am." I would go beyond Descartes to say, "I think and *feel*. Therefore, I am sometimes ill." Thoughts and feelings exert a major influence on multiple brain functions such as the autonomic nervous system, which is intimately connected to and exerts a major influence on every tissue and organ in the body. The brain also manufactures and distributes regulating hormones to the various body tissues and organs. The biochemistry and physiology of this system, too, are highly sensitive to and are under some control(to what extent it has not been determined) of the emotions.

The most common symptoms from which patients suffer—headaches, backaches, stomachaches—are often of a psychosomatic nature. They are caused by anxiety and/or depression or by conflicting emotions and the major "tension states" they produce. (I do not mean by suggesting that a person's symptoms are "psychosomatic" to imply that they are not "real." Indeed, they are as painful and distressing as any symptoms caused by "purely organic" disease.) In addition, psychological factors frequently play a major role in the etiology and pathogenesis of many disease processes that manifest themselves as asthma, allergies, colitis, ulcers, high blood pressure, and heart disease—among many other illnesses. By treatment of the patient's personality and emotional state, the course of the disease process and, therefore, the patient's overall prognosis can often be favorably affected.

Recent research[10] has established beyond question the connection between psychological stress (such as death of a family member, divorce, loss of job) and illness. Given a particular personality and a stress that impinges upon it, a person is liable to become sick or die. The most obvious example is illness or death of a surviving spouse following the death of the other. Indeed, at some point in the future, we will likely find that illnesses of all kinds, including perhaps cancer, are psychosomatic—that is, they are under at least some control of the mind and emotions. Indeed, in a recent study of female patients who had undergone surgery for early breast cancer it was reported that "recurrence free survival was significantly [more] common among patients who had initially reacted to cancer by denial or who had a fighting spirit than among patients who had responded with stoic acceptance or feelings of helplessness and fear."[11]

By affording complete mental health care to persons under psychic stress, we may often prevent the very onset of disease or prevent the exacerbation of existing disease.

3.1.1.4. Category IV: Transient Situational Disturbances.

Many persons suffer mental illness/emotional problems as a reaction to stressful situations. As the term implies, *transient* situational disturbances are not of a permanent nature. Though they may include severe symptoms, they usually resolve in short order. They may, however, progress to chronic mental illness/emotional problems unless they are fully treated at their onset. Transient situational disturbances, or "adjustment reactions" as they are often called, are as common as there are stresses in life. Examples are the excessively disturbed and prolonged emotional reaction of a person to an accident, of a woman to rape, of a person to illness or loss of job. A person's emotional distress following a divorce would be included in this category. Further examples would be adjustment reactions to life phase changes: mid-life crisis, retirement syndrome, etc. Of course, not all persons experiencing such stresses will react with symptoms severe enough to warrant treatment.

3.1.1.5. Category V. Alcohol and Drug Abuse.

This category may well constitute the single most common illness afflicting Americans, especially if we include the medical - surgical illnesses that result secondarily from alcohol/drug abuse and the overuse and abuse of tranquilizers, sedatives, and hypnotics. The "disease" of alcohol and drug abuse accounts directly or indirectly for a high portion of our total national expenditures for health. Of course, alcohol and drug abuse reflect underlying mental illness/emotional problems and/or lead to them so that effective treatment is often complex and extended.

3.1.1.6. Category VI: Chronic Symptomatic Maladjustment (CSM)— "The Neuroses."

For purposes of our discussion here, "chronic symptomatic maladjustment" (CSM) will replace the concept of neurosis as a category of mental illness/emotional problems. The American Psychiatric Association has effectively downgraded the term *neurosis*. It no longer holds a primary and exclusive position in the preferred, official nomenclature of mental illness/ emotional problems. This is probably a good thing, because "neurosis" has become extremely difficult to define. It is a vague construct—subjective rather than objective—variously interpreted by various psychiatrists.

Chronic symptomatic maladjustment is manifested by symptoms such as depression and anxiety of a chronic, unrelenting nature. In this respect, then, CSM differs from "transient situational disturbances" wherein symptoms are limited in duration. By our definition, CSM does not refer to symptoms suffered as a residual of a "psychiatric syndrome." Further, it refers only to a *nonpsychotic* maladjustment. The person who suffers CSM does not usually experience any loss of contact with reality—as occurs in psychosis. Hallucinations, delusions, and other disorders of "thought content" are usually conspicuously absent. "Thought processes" are usually normal.

The person who suffers chronic symptomatic maladjustment is often able to function for long periods of time on an adequate and sometimes even on a superior level. Thus, he may appear "normal" to the outside observer. Nevertheless, he suffers moderate to severe symptoms (such as depression and anxiety) on a consistent basis. These symptoms lead to frustration and lack of fulfillment in terms of personal goals, work, and relationships with others. This in turn further exacerbates the person's symptoms in the manner of a feedback loop. (This is an appropriate place to point out carefully that we must never deny a person mental health care merely because he or she is capable of "functioning" and does not behave unusually or bizarrely in public—i.e., the person appears normal. We should prescribe and deliver mental health care for any person based on the *subjective internal emotional distress* he or she experiences and reports.)

Chronic symptomatic maladjustment does not result from any distinct, classifiable illness or abnormality *per se*. Rather, it stems from a self-destructive, self-defeating pattern of thinking, feeling, and behaving that a person repeats over and over again. The pattern and the reasons for it are beyond the person's recognition, or if he is aware of the pattern, he perceives himself to be and is relatively helpless without treatment to do anything about it—in spite of his best intentions and efforts. An example of the person who suffers CSM would be the ostensibly successful professional who nevertheless judges himself a failure. He suffers frequent periods of intense depression and anxiety. Still, he usually perseveres; he compulsively works long, long hours at his job to gain the approval, acceptance, and love of others (especially his superiors), even if he does not realize he is seeking it. His efforts to win approval are eternal failures. Even when others praise him, it is never enough. His persistent, painful efforts to "succeed" doom him to failure with his family—which he infrequently sees because of his work habits. His family life deteriorates, and though it is strictly not his "fault," his wife and children develop emotional problems of their own (see "Family and Marital Discord" below). He may proceed to abuse alcohol and drugs or to develop serious organic illness.

Such a person as described here is really not that atypical. Persons afflicted by CSM are found throughout the mainstream of American life. Furthermore, I am not just talking about "unhappy people" here. CSM goes beyond "common" unhappiness derived from "common" problems. Its symptoms stem mainly from discrete but complex and pervasive internal psychological defenses that a person uses "to cope," rather than from specific external problems that can be simply solved, removed, or "lived with." This is an exceedingly important distinction; it is at the core of the justification for providing mental health care to those who suffer CSM.

In treating the person who suffers CSM, the psychiatrist's first task is to point out the distorted patterns of thinking, feeling, and behaving that rule and regulate the person's life. Next, the psychiatrist must help him (or her) to *gradually* learn a different, more adaptive way "to be," a way that, when practiced, will lead to the moderation, control, or resolution of his symptoms. Treatment unshackles the person from the pathological bonds of his psychological past, allowing him the emotional "freedom" to think, feel, and behave in a positive, gratifying manner instead of in the psychologically predetermined, emotionally painful manner in which he has conducted his life up to that point. The treatment of CSM is often long and drawn out—and therefore expensive—because the person who suffers CSM must "unlearn" ways of thinking, feeling, and behaving that he has used to survive and cope since childhood. Though ultimately self-defeating, they have been adaptive. They have enabled him to get by as best he could, given his own unique psychological constellation.

I should stress here that the treatment of the person who suffers CSM is not designed to improve the quality of his life. Rather, it is directed at the management of his symptoms. Ideally, of course, the quality of life of the person who suffers CSM will be enhanced as a consequence of the successful management of his symptoms. [See my comments in Chapter 1 on the aims of mental health care as they do and do not relate to improving the quality of the patient's (client's) life.]

Treatment of CSM will often involve the utilization of psychotropic medication in addition to or separate from psychotherapy. Though CSM sometimes resolves or quiesces spontaneously, it will frequently worsen without appropriate treatment. In some cases, the person's symptoms become so incapacitating that the quality of his work is greatly affected or he cannot function at all. Therefore, treatment of CSM at the earliest possible moment can be construed to be preventive medicine in the best sense.

The above description of treatment as it applies to CSM serves as a good, though extremely simplistic definition of "psychotherapy" as it is referred to herein, provided we add the following: (1) Psychotherapy may also be "supportive," that is, it may serve partly or exclusively to provide comfort and sustenance; (2) psychotherapy may be combined with the utilization of psychotropic medication and/or social services and/or rehabilitation services as a part of a total treatment plan; (3) psychotherapy may be conducted on an individual basis for the individual patient (client). Alternatively or conjointly, it may take the form of couples (marital), family, or group psychotherapy. (See also my definition of "pure psychotherapy" in Chapter 1, and Chapter 7 on the poor image of psychotherapy.)

3.1.1.7. Category VII: The Personality Disorders.

The personality disorders include the antisocial personality—as manifested by persons who owe no allegiance to any group and feel no sense of morality in the usual sense, e.g., many white-collar criminals and "hardened" criminals. Many persons who display the antisocial personality can be helped by mental health care; their behavior can be controlled.* In this connection, we must decide what amount of mental health care resources we should devote under NHI to the rehabilitation of criminals (including persons who suffer from "psychosexual disorders," e.g., exhibitionism, sexual sadism.) Treatment for this group has only been minimally available up until now.†

---

*Dr. Lebensohn in his commentary strongly disagrees with my contention that many persons who display the "antisocial personality" can benefit from mental health care. He indicates that he is rather pessimistic as to how effective the psychiatrist can be in coping with this malignant problem (i.e., the antisocial personality). I must agree with Dr. Lebensohn that when the psychiatrist attempts to treat persons who suffer a *true* antisocial personality disorder, he will be unsuccessful in the vast majority of cases. He will most likely be unable to help most such persons to control their antisocial behavior to any great extent, given the current state of the art of mental health care. I would have been more correct to state in the text that "some" or "many" (depending upon how we define these modifiers) persons who display antisocial *behavior* and *elements* of the antisocial personality, without suffering from a full-blown antisocial personality disorder *per se*, can be helped by mental health care combined with appropriate social, support, and rehabilitation services. I should also make the point that many persons who display antisocial behavior are *misdiagnosed* as suffering from a *true* antisocial personality. It is this group that the psychiatrist can in my opinion sometimes expect to help. (I am not implying here that we should not make an effort to provide some form of mental health care to persons who suffer from a true antisocial personality disorder. If they are genuinely desirous of receiving such care, they may benefit to some extent from it—even if they cannot be rehabilitated.)

†In my opinion, we should increase mental health care and associated social and rehabilitation services for persons confined in the correctional system. Here I am referring not only to persons confined in "hospitals for the criminally insane" but to persons confined in all penal institutions. Perhaps, under NHI, a special agency should be set up, adequately funded, to administer a mental health care delivery system specifically designed to meet the mental health needs of this population—just as NHI shall fund the Community Mental Health Center (CMHC) to meet the mental health needs of the population it serves. (Alternatively the function could be assumed by the CMHC.)

To date, it seems to me, the dealings of mental health professionals with so-called criminals have been largely confined to the courts, with prosecutors and defense attorneys hiring and engaging "their own" MHP to serve their own side of an adversary proceeding—i.e., to work to convict the defendant or to acquit him. The ease and, in fact, the routine with which contrary evaluations of the defendant are rendered by psychiatrists and other MHPs damages the credibility of the mental health professional and, indeed, the mental health professions.

The personality disorders also encompass the so-called paranoid person-ality and the passive-aggressive personality. The former exhibits a high de-gree of jealousy, envy, and suspiciousness accompanied by a marked degree of hostility. Although the sufferer often feels he is well adapted and he does not usually desire treatment of any kind, these characteristics of his person-ality interfere markedly with his ability to function both in interpersonal relationships and at work. He is often discharged from his job and receives compensation for a "psychiatric disability." The same holds true for persons who suffer from the passive-aggressive personality. These persons express a high degree of hostility in a covert and disruptive manner. However, like persons who display the paranoid personality, they often feel they are well adjusted, and they resent treatment intervention. (The psychiatrist and other MHPs must be very careful not to label any person who simply does not "get along on the job or get along with others" as suffering from a "personality disorder.")

3.1.1.8. Category VIII: Mental Retardation. Treatment of some kind is often beneficial, even if it is mainly supportive rather than curative. Of course, persons suffering from mental retardation can be afflicted by a wide range of mental illness/emotional problems separate from that condition.

3.1.1.9. Category IX: Mental Illness/Emotional Problems of Children and Adolescents. There are many discrete emotional disorders of childhood and adolescence. In addition, children and adolescents may suffer from many of the same categories of mental illness/emotional problems from which adults suffer. It is especially important that NHI provide full coverage for mental health care for children and adolescents: It is preventive medicine in the best sense. Unless fully treated, the mental illness/emotional problems children or adolescents experience will often develop into chronic illness of adulthood. By that point, their symptoms have often become more difficult and more expensive to treat.

My own view is that the psychiatrist or other MHP should not be involved in the actual process of determining the guilt or innocence of the defendant. Rather, a panel of mental health professionals should convene only after a formal trial and conviction to determine the mental state of the convicted party and to recommend what mental health care, if any, is indicated—and at what location. The court could then act on the panel's recommendation. (The convicted party, of course, would have the right to representation on the panel by one or more mental health professionals of his choosing.) Perhaps panels of mental health professionals should be at least partially staffed and funded under NHI through a special agency such as I have suggested.

Remembering that many hardened criminals will not benefit from mental health care, I still maintain that the potential cost savings to society deriving from appropriate and adequate mental health care for the criminal is substantial—in terms of preventing recidivistic crime and in so doing preventing the experiencing of emotional trauma and its consequences by those victims who would suffer it.

3.1.1.10. Category X: Family and Marital Discord. Families or marital partners may experience severe difficulties and upset "relating" to one another. Quite often this reflects underlying mental illness/emotional problems in a family member(s) or spouse(s), and this person will require appropriate treatment. In addition, the family or couple is a unit: How one member feels and behaves affects all others. Therefore, it is frequently necessary to treat the whole family (or the couple together) to resolve whatever mental illness/emotional problems an individual family member exhibits. A mentally healthy family has the greatest chance of rearing mentally healthy children who will grow up to be mentally healthy adults. Therefore, preventive medicine dictates that NHI provide mental health care to promote the emotional well-being of marital partners and families.

4

Extent of Coverage; Liabilities of Limited Coverage

However insightful health planners and legislators are in recognizing the need for mental health care for all the diverse segments of the population, in recommending the establishment of the kinds of facilities needed for such care, and in calling for the prerequisite ancillary social services, the successful treatment of the individual person suffering mental illness/emotional problems will ultimately depend upon the quantity and quality of mental health care provided him. NHI must be structured so that mental health care will be available and accessible to the maximum number of persons requiring such care, but at the same time NHI must provide as much care as is needed to each individual recipient.

The extent of coverage that should be allowed for care of mental illness/emotional problems is a most controversial issue facing national health insurance planners and legislators. In fact, all NHI proposals currently before the U.S. Congress effectively restrict mental health care on a general basis. This must be corrected: We cannot under any circumstances limit or spare appropriate medical care (of any variety) under NHI if we are to insure the recovery or rehabilitation of the patient. To do so would be unfair at best and immoral at worst, whether the condition being treated is physical or mental.

We must not discriminate against mental health care under NHI; to do so would imply that a case of mental illness/emotional problems is not that "serious," that it is something a person should be able to manage himself/herself. The person with mental illness/emotional problems should have the right to full treatment for his condition on an equal basis with the medical or surgical patient for whom treatment is often far more expensive. Indeed, it is a myth that mental health care is more expensive than other forms of medical care. The cost of mental health care is hardly exorbitant: For example, in 1977 total benefits for mental illness/emotional problems paid out under the Federal Employee's Health Benefits (FEHB) program for federal workers amounted only to approximately $24 per year—including $14 for inpatient care and $7 for outpatient care.*[12] (Actually, these benefits comprise those

---

*The author of the study that reports these benefits observes that it is more accurate to report costs for a particular service or benefit on a "per capita" or "per enrollee" basis rather than as a

paid out under eight plans enrolling two-thirds of all members insured under the FEHB program.)

It is medical care, not mental health care *per se*, that is expensive. It is curious, then, why mental health care has been singled out as being too costly for society, why arbitrary limits for coverage of mental health care alone have been proposed under NHI. Admittedly, the positive results of mental health care may sometimes appear rather intangible. In general, however, the results of treatment of patients who suffer mental illness/emotional problems mirror the results of medical-surgical treatment of any type. Some patients are cured, some improve, and some become chronically ill. There is no more chronic mental illness/emotional problem than there is chronic illness of any kind. The majority of monies for medical care of all kinds is spent on illnesses that are either unremitting or chronic in nature, illnesses for which there are no cures but which the physician attempts to contain and control as best he can. Such health care is costly and, if not always ambiguous in method, frequently ambiguous in result.

In this connection, the Office of Technology Assessment (OTA) of the U.S. Congress states in a report[13] that "only ten to twenty percent of all procedures used in present medical practice have been shown to be of benefit by controlled clinical trials; many of the other procedures may not be efficacious."* The OTA's report goes on to state that "in fact, many technologies in use have had their efficacy and safety questioned, including oral drug treatment for diabetes, respiratory therapy, oral decongestants, thermography for diagnosing breast cancer, ergotamine for migraine headaches, immune serum globulin for preventing hepatitis, intensive care for pulmonary edema, coronary care units, and radical mastectomy. Such widely used technologies as tonsillectomy, appendectomy, and the Pap smear have not been completely assessed for efficacy. . . . Others such as electrical fetal monitoring (EFM) and coronary bypass surgery have been defused rapidly before careful evaluation. . . . Concern about risks has led to questions regarding the use of mammography and skull x-ray." These examples presented by the OTA are only a few of the many medical technologies that have not been proven efficacious and safe. Yet these medical technologies are highly utilized and they are extremely costly. Obviously they *appear* to cure or ameliorate the symptoms and illnesses of a great many patients. However, there is some question as to whether the benefits to the patient result from the specific

---

"percentage of total benefits." One reason this is the case, he notes, is that if the *total* benefits paid out by a given plan in any one year decrease or increase, the cost of a *particular* benefit that in fact has remained cost-stable will *appear* to increase (using the "percentage of total benefits" calculation) in the former case and decrease in the latter case. Such pseudochanges can be extremely misleading and can lead to false assumptions about the cost of care for a particular service.

*These data appearing in the OTA Report are culled from K. L. White, "International Comparisons of Health Services Systems," *Milbank Memorial Fund Quarterly* (1968): 117.

medical technology employed or from other nonspecific factors (e.g., the concerned and caring demeanor of the physician) or from both.

Let me be quick to point out that I am not maintaining that the technologies listed above are ineffective—although some may be. It is just that they cannot be unequivocably proven to be effective. The fact is that it is exceedingly difficult to prove on an absolute basis the value of most medical-surgical technology. It is even more difficult to prove the positive effects of mental health care because the judgment as to the effectiveness of mental health care must depend to a great extent on subjective factors. We cannot take X rays or perform laboratory tests to measure the positive results of mental health care. (It is probable that in the not too distant future, the psychiatrist will sometimes utilize newly developed or newly applied laboratory tests—e.g., the dexamethasone suppression test—to detect illness and measure treatment outcome in a limited way. Ultimately, however, it is the patient (client) who must tell the clinician *how he feels*.) Psychological tests may be of some value in evaluating mental health care. However, they can be imprecise and often do not measure the important variables.

The main point I am making here is that we cannot discriminate against mental health care (by denying coverage under NHI for mental health care) on the basis that it comprises a health care technology that is less proven than other forms of health care technology that relate to the medical-surgical field. I do not maintain that all forms of mental health care practiced by all breeds of mental health care practitioners on all patients work. Rather, I propose that the psychiatrist and other mental health professionals must carefully scrutinize the efficacy and safety of mental health care. Similarly, all practitioners of health care must do the same as regards the technology of their own fields. Certainly the challenge of all health care practitioners is to develop and prove safe and efficacious diagnostic and treatment methods that provide the full range of required evaluation and therapeutic services at the least cost to the individual patient and to society.

Some critics would distinguish between mental health care and general medical care by labeling the former as basically passive and supportive in nature in contrast to the latter, which they view as active intervention on behalf of the patient. Although mental health care, especially psychotherapy, is much more than a "supportive" process for the patient, it is nevertheless difficult to criticize, downgrade, or limit mental health care on such a basis. Critics would argue that it is wasteful and exorbitant to spend monies for "supportive" mental health care, but the reality is that a large percentage of all medical care is basically supportive in nature. Most physicians would agree that often it is the visit to the doctor itself, with the physical "laying on of hands," or the nonmedical personal interaction between the physician and the patient during the visit (the physical yet metaphysical "laying on of hands") that is curative. They would most likely admit, as well, that for a large percentage of illnesses from which patients suffer, the only medicine the physician has to offer is reassurance. This is not to demean the advanced technology of modern medicine. Nevertheless, the role of the physician is first to care and offer emotional support—whether the condition being treated is a heart attack or a divorce, a medical- surgical problem or mental illness/ emotional problems. The physician's involvement in this respect is as potent as instrument as any in his armamentarium of healing.

One possible difference between general medical-surgical practice and psychiatric practice consists of the following: For general medical-surgical care, the patient can often be transferred from one physician to another during the course of an illness without seriously affecting continuity of care or the prognosis for the patient. This is not the case for psychiatric care, however, because such care is largely dependent upon the *specific relationship* that develops between the psychiatrist and his patient, as well as the knowledge the psychiatrist develops about his patient. Although permanent transfer of patients can be successfully accomplished from one psychiatrist to another (though not without consequences), the psychiatrist, because of his *exclusive therapeutic relationship* with his patient (see Appendix), cannot temporarily transfer his patient to another psychiatrist for any interval of time without confining the patient to a holding pattern in his course of treatment. (The above paradigm for psychiatric care holds true as well for all mental health care delivered by any and all mental health professionals.) Nevertheless, it should be noted that the personal relationship between any physician and his patient is vitally important to the success of the patient's treatment. Long-term continuity of care between the individual patient and his physician provides the patient with the best possible care. This goes beyond the knowledge about his patient and the clinical sensitivity toward him that the physician develops over time. It involves the emotional relationship between the two of them, notably the trust and confidence the patient develops in his doctor. The patient grows to rely on his physician, and the good physician accepts this reliance and actively uses it in his treatment of the patient. He allows his patient to "lean on" him to an appropriate degree. This is a further example of the routinely "supportive" nature of general medical care.

In terms of supportive mental health care, I myself would be the first to acknowledge that when such care is the primary, exclusive order for the patient, the services of a highly trained mental health professional—psychiatrist or otherwise—are often not mandatory. Less highly trained mental health workers can definitely deliver a large portion of such care. In addition, the mental health community and society as a whole should and must encourage and foster the development of alternatives to mental health care *per se* for persons who do not require the latter modality of care. These might take the form of emotional "support" services, associations, or "self-help" groups designed to meet the emotional needs of those persons who suffer a particular dilemma or problem (e.g., Parents Without Partners, Alcoholics Anonymous, "Stop Smoking" groups, weight "watching" or "modification" groups, groups of people who suffer the same medical problem—cancer, pain, arthritis, etc.). Many persons, of course, will require some psychotherapy, at least at certain times, to supplement the support they receive from such services, associations, or groups. I should stress here, although it should be obvious from this paper, that I am hardly a "minimalist" (an advocate of the least) when it comes to the provision of mental health care. Rather, I think that by carefully defining mental health care, especially psychotherapy, we can provide such care more appropriately and more cost-effectively; we will be able to properly match specific categories of providers of mental health care to patients (clients) of specific categories. (See my further comments on this subject in Chapter 5.)

In connection with the concept of psychiatric care versus other forms of mental health care, I should point out this phenomenon: The "authority" of the physician-psychiatrist can often carry in and of itself a great deal of reassurance and comfort for the patient. (In some cases, this would hold true for other highly trained MHPs as well.) For many patients, therefore, a single visit with a psychiatrist may suffice to alleviate a great deal of anxiety and/or depression. We must not overlook this phenomenon. By affording patients access to a psychiatrist—even when the services of a psychiatrist are not strictly required—we may alleviate the need for further, extended mental health care. The same paradigm holds true for medical care in general. Often, a visit by the patient to a physician *per se* is not strictly necessary; paraprofessionals can successfully manage many patients who seek treatment from a physician. Nevertheless, the "laying on of hands" by the physician himself will often suffice to cut short the necessity for further medical care. We must be attuned to psychological and emotional factors operative in patients as we plan for medical care, including mental health care, under NHI. Such factors determine to a large extent the care-seeking patterns of patients. (Although we may be able to educate and train patients to accept their health care in many instances from the nonphysician, when this is appropriate, I believe the individual patient will always look to the physician—i.e., the most highly trained health care provider—to oversee and to be directly involved in his health care. Such an attitude on the part of the patient is certainly justifiable, although in the realm of mental health care, the patient-client would do well to learn that under many circumstances he can receive care from the nonpsychiatrist MHP that matches in quality the care he can receive from a psychiatrist.)

Finally, it must be realized that supportive mental health care (psychotherapy) is usually not indicated for the patient-client or employed by the psychiatrist (or other MHP) on an isolated basis.* The patient, most often, will require and benefit from "reconstructive" mental health care as well— that is, psychotherapy that aims to alter and reshape the way he reacts and responds to various external circumstances as well as the way he views himself in both his inner and his outer world.†

---

*Except in the initial phases of treatment for some persons, during some crises that occur in the course of psychotherapy, and in maintenance psychotherapy for some chronic patients.
†The term *reconstruction* is often used by the mental health professional to refer to the process of ascertaining the patient's personal and psychological "past." As should be evident from the

It is important to point out that if monies for medical treatment of any kind are arbitrarily limited under NHI, the development of more effective treatment methods will be slowed and in some cases halted. We cannot, in other words, afford to be too cost-effective.

Further, it should be realized that much medical technology is extremely expensive at its inception and initial deployment. However, as such technology is applied and refined, it often becomes less costly. Further, even technology that remains expensive may result in overall cost savings if it attenuates illness (on the acute or chronic level) or replaces other more complicated and expensive technology. (Such is the case for the initially much maligned CAT scanner, which is only now beginning to realize its potential as a medical-surgical cost-saver as well as a life-saver.)

As far as mental health care is concerned, NHI, as currently conceived, sets severe limits on outpatient visits to private sector psychiatrists and other mental health professionals. Actually, primary efforts at cost containment should be directed not at outpatient care but rather at inpatient care—for this is where the great expense occurs. If we limit outpatient coverage, the result will be to encourage inpatient care. This will create rather than solve cost-containment problems. The largest national health system we currently operate, the Veterans' Administration (VA) Hospital System, serves as an example. The VA funds mental health care largely upon the basis of care provided to inpatients in its psychiatric hospitals rather than on the basis of outpatient care delivered. Therefore, in the VA, there is a great tendency—in fact an economic imperative—to hospitalize patients rather than to treat them as outpatients. The individual VA hospital finds it necessary to do this in order to preserve its own level of funding (which is based on bed occupancy). The result of the VA budgeting philosophy has been to create a psychiatric hospital system that is a vast, expensive psychosocial caretaking system. The National Academy of Sciences[14] states that 40–50% of patients now in VA psychiatric hospitals do not require hospitalization. These patients reside in the hospital because the development of VA outpatient treatment facilities and other alternatives to hospitalization have not been financially encouraged by the system. (The VA has recently begun to encourage outpatient mental health care and to make such care more available and accessible than in the past.)

If NHI limits coverage for outpatient mental health care, the VA pattern of mental health care will repeat itself in other settings, leading to expensive, wasteful admissions of patients to hospitals. For example, if a psychiatrist knows that he has relatively unlimited resources to treat a patient on an outpatient basis, he will do so. However, if outpatient care is limited and the patient, because of restrictions on outpatient visits, cannot afford proper evaluation and treatment, the psychiatrist will have no choice but to hospitalize

---

text, I do not use it here in that sense at all. Rather, I use the term to refer to the process of "reshaping" the patient's psychological perspective and altering his psychological set and his pattern of emotional response.

the patient to effect successful treatment. Such a pattern of unnecessary hospital care has evolved under Medicare and Medicaid, under which provisions for outpatient mental health care are, as I have already documented (see Chapter 1), extremely limited and inadequate. (The same pattern generally repeats itself with regard to all medical-surgical care. As one prominent medical school dean has stated, "all of us [physicians] have had patients whom we've hospitalized because of the reimbursement paid them—not because *you* [the physician] get the money or I get more money, but because the patient's [financial] burden is relieved by hospitalization. Of course, there are some physicians who reap unjustified profits from third-party largess, but I think it's safe to say most do not.")[15] I should add a *caveat* here: Hospitalizing a patient for mental health care may be medically justifiable if it is the only way to get the patient the acute, intensive care he needs. However, this is a two-edged sword. Hospitalizing a patient when he does not strictly require hospital care, or if he could be managed with outpatient care if it were available in sufficient amounts, can lead to chronicity of illness with its suffering for the patient (as well as attendant high cost). Thus, we see the medical hazards of a health care policy that allows only partial and limited coverage of mental health care. (If health planners and legislators were held legally responsible for the medical consequences to the patient of their health care policy, just as physicians are held liable for providing the patient with responsible medical care, perhaps that policy would develop along more responsible medical lines.)

The primary goal of any health care delivery system must be to provide the full range of treatment and rehabilitation services that will allow a person to feel better and to function better. However, cost is a factor we must deal with in planning NHI. Let us show further, then, how a system that does not set arbitrary limits on mental health care services can provide a cost saving over one that does. Limits on coverage may only prolong treatment for some patients and thus increase overall cost. For example, a patient limited to 50 outpatient visits per year to a psychiatrist might then require further treatment—perhaps 5 years of treatment, using the maximum visits allowable per annum, for a total of 250 visits. On the other hand, if visits are not limited, a single continuous treatment of 100 visits in a single year might well "cure" the patient. The simple reality is that if a patient is left with little or no entitlement to care after an initial phase of treatment, and he requires additional care, he is very likely to regress to his pretreatment "sick state." The whole process of evaluation and treatment will have to begin again. A similar situation will ensue for many patients if inpatient psychiatric treatment is limited under NHI. In this connection, the most recent Kennedy NHI proposal calls for an upper limit of 45 days for "psychiatric" hospitalization. In fact, even under one of the most liberal of health insurance programs, the BCBS FEHB Plan, 90% of all patients hospitalized for the treatment of mental disorders are discharged within 45 days.[4] However, the patient who needs to be hospitalized for a longer period of time must not be penalized. In addition to being discriminatory—NHI will not set absolute limits on hospitalization for "physical" illnesses—such limits are liable to increase the total cost of inpatient mental health care. (They may also add to the cost of outpatient care.) If any patient is discharged prematurely, he will quickly deteriorate and will require further hospitalization. The cost, therefore, of one relatively longer hospitalization will be less than the cost of multiple short hospitalizations following one upon the other due to insufficient treatment sentence. Disregarding costs, the patient undergoes needless suffering.

I must also point out that limits on mental health care, especially on the extent of coverage available for outpatient care, pose the danger for the patient of severe misapplication of psychotropic medication. (I use the term *psychotropic* here in the etymological sense to refer to all medicines used to treat mental illness/emotional problems. This would include antianxiety, antidepressant, antimanic, and antipsychotic agents.) This liability of limited coverage for mental health care (under NHI or any other form of health insurance) deserves extended, comprehensive elaboration; it stands as a supreme example of the dangerously unhealthy consequences of a policy toward mental health care that is directed more at financial concerns than at the health care requirements of persons who suffer mental illness/emotional problems. In view of this, I shall devote a considerable portion of this section of my paper to an analysis of the uses of psychotropic medication and to a discussion of the correct and incorrect manner in which they are prescribed and used. I hope by this means to highlight the serious hazards of a myopic policy toward mental health care that imposes limits on the extent of such care available to the patient without regard to the deleterious consequences to the patient inherent in such limits and without regard to the way in which health care, in this case mental health care, works. (As I shall also discuss herein, a policy toward mental health care that extends independent provider status to nonpsychiatrist MHPs, although this is, I believe, justifiable, given certain restrictions, also poses a danger: namely, that psychotropic medications will be underused and not prescribed when they should be.) I believe that the improper utilization of psychotropic medication constitutes a "problem" of mental health care that arouses the greatest anxiety and concern on the part of the *consumers* of mental health care. This problem is in large part a direct result of limits on mental health care.

Indeed, psychotropic medication as a specific treatment modality for mental illness/emotional problems can be easily misused and abused. Clearly, the introduction of such medication has advanced the state of the art of mental health care dramatically. Nevertheless, there is often a tendency for the inexperienced clinician to utilize medicines for the treatment of mental illness/emotional problems when it is really not appropriate to do so. Too many persons, as a result, do not benefit from treatment. Some manage to achieve a form of pseudorelief, but this is usually temporary. Others are, unfortunately, overmedicated. (This is a danger especially for the psychotic patient whose psychosis is either active or in a state of remission.) Further, all psychotropic medicines can produce severe, even fatal, side effects. Thus, phenothiazines, often used to treat psychosis, can cause a serious and permanent neurological syndrome (tardive dyskinesia). We are also beginning to see pathology produced by the long-term use of lithium (irreversible renal damage). In sum, psychotropic medication is not to be dispensed lightly or casually. The clinician must realize that the mental illness/emotional problems of many persons stem from confused and errant views of their own (internal) personal worlds and the (external) world around them. They live their lives as a response to a series of long-ingrained psychic myths and constructs that relate to their own particular life experience. These myths and constructs govern the way they think, feel, and behave. Many persons also suffer from the practice and application of errant psychological "principles," such as "I must sacrifice myself to others," "I cannot be whole or successful until and unless I am loved," "If I express anger I will destroy myself or others," "It is dangerous to reveal how I feel." For the most part, long-standing *psychological misconceptions* and *distortions,* as opposed to symptoms *per se,* cannot be altered solely by psychotropic medication (whether these misconceptions and distortions relate to psychic myths and constructs or psychological principles). It is true that when a person's symptoms are relieved by such medication, he will often alter his view of himself and the world around him. It should also be noted that sometimes, psychological misconceptions and distortions, especially when suffered in the short run, constitute, as opposed to lead to, symptoms. (Thus, a person's sudden, intense view of himself as being "bad" or "worthless" may be symptomatic of a severe depression that will respond to psychotropic medication.) The point is that a combined pharmacological and psychological approach (psychotherapy) to treatment is mandatory for many persons who suffer mental illness/emotional problems. Many other persons will require and will benefit from psychotherapy alone. I fear, though, that with severe limits on mental health care, the psychological approach to treatment will take a definite backseat to the pharmacological approach and, too often, will be entirely excluded from the therapeutic vehicle to fall by the roadside.

The nonpsychiatrist physician, especially, will have a tendency to overuse and misuse psychotropic medications. He will always have a relative lack of training in the field of psychiatry, and frequently this will be severe. In these days when we are emphasizing patient's rights, and properly so, we have the obligation to provide the patient with a properly and thoroughly trained health care provider. We must protect the patient against the erroneous prescription of medication. It has been said that the good surgeon is the surgeon who knows when not to operate. Similarly, we can say that the good psychiatrist knows when not to prescribe medication. This is something that is very difficult to teach to the nonpsychiatrist physician. It is important to realize this because the nonpsychiatrist physician will, by default, treat a large share, if not the majority, of patients who suffer mental illness/emotional problems if severe limits on mental health care are imposed under NHI.

The internist, family practitioner, and general practitioner will become entrenched as the primary physician and functioning "psychiatrist" for most persons who suffer mental illness/emotional problems. (This misapplication of medical manpower is encountered in Great Britain under the national health program administered by that nation, although this situation is due in large part to the logistical operation of the program. In fact, the same situation already exists in this country today, given the extremely limited benefits for mental health care that are available to most persons and a shortage of psychiatrists as well.) Certainly, every physician must become involved in treating his patients' emotional problems, but he is not the "best physician" to prescribe and regulate psychotropic medications for any particular patient. This, of course, would necessitate a *precise* diagnosis by the physician of the particular mental illness/emotional problem from which the patient suffers. The fact is that the precise diagnosis of mental illness/emotional problems and the art of prescribing psychotropic medication is becoming increasingly more complex and subtle.

To further illustrate the potential negative consequences of the nonpsychiatrist physician's prescribing psychotropic medication, as opposed to the psychiatrist's performing this function, let us examine the decision-making process of the psychiatrist in terms of his prescription of psychotropic medication. For each and every individual patient, the psychiatrist must decide (1) whether or not to prescribe psychotropic medication—as opposed to prescribing "pure psychotherapy," (2) which specific medication(s) to prescribe, (3) what dosage he should prescribe, (4) when and if he should switch medications and/or change dosages, and (5) at what point in the patient's treatment he should discontinue psychotropic medication. Point 5 involves the determination as to whether the particular individual patient should remain on psychotropic medication for a considerable period of time or even for a lifetime. Indeed, there are some patients who must remain on psychotropic medication for extremely long periods of time, notably manic-depressive patients whose manic episodes can be prevented with the use of lithum, and many schizophrenic patients whose psychotic episodes can be prevented by the proper use of antipsychotic medication. Nevertheless, the long-term benefits of psychotropic medication must be continuously weighed against the possible side effects (known and unknown). This involves a crucial and exceedingly difficult determination for each individual patient based on the psychiatrist's critical judgment as to the future course of the patient's illness—a judgment that depends in large part on the psychiatrist's in-depth understanding of the patient's unique personal history.

Of course, the nonpsychiatrist physician goes through a specialized hierarchy that resembles the above decision sequence in determining when, how, and if to prescribe medication for the various symptoms or diseases from which his patients suffer. My point here is to emphasize that the mechanics of the prescription of any medication ideally require the expertise of a specialist. The nonpsychiatrist physician too often simply concludes, when treating persons who suffer mental illness/emotional problems, "My patient is depressed and/or anxious so I will prescribe for him an antidepressant or a tranquilizer." Indeed, this is likely to be a counterproductive, if not a contraindicated, approach to treatment. The last reason a psychiatrist prescribes psychotropic medication is because his patient is depressed or anxious. Rather, these symptoms only lead the psychiatrist to an analysis of the *type* of depression and/or anxiety from which his patient suffers. The psychiatrist will prescribe psychotropic medication only if the patient displays a *specific presentation and constellation* of such symptoms. Psychotropic medication must be prescribed with the same considered care and expertise with which, for example, an immunologist or "transplant specialist" will prescribe medication to counteract a patient's tendency to reject or his actual rejection of a transplanted organ. This example may seem dramatic; nevertheless, I am attempting to illustrate here the absolute precision with which any physician, including the psychiatrist, must operate in determining the indications for and the best use of psychotropic medications. Our willingness to ascribe an expertise to any physician who prescribes psychotropic medication partly results from our unwillingness to recognize the primary validity and the complicated nature of mental illness/emotional problems and the requirement, as logistically possible, for *specialized treatment* for this group of disorders.

I do not wish to disparage the pragmatic approach to mental health care of the nonpsychiatrist physician. Still, this approach is often too rudimentary. It operates on the principle that "the patient is 'generically' upset, depressed, and/or worried so he (or she) needs a little or a lot of medicine and requires a little or a lot of listening to his problems as well as some advice." The nonpsychiatrist physician in fact does not provide his patients with psychotherapy so much as he provides them with "emotional support." Of course, this therapeutic dimension is extremely valuable in and of itself. However, practiced exclusively, it is separate from psychotherapy. Psychotherapy, as I shall describe in depth later in this paper, is a unique and complicated process that must be dispensed with the same skill and precautions that any medical specialist observes in treating his patients.

In reality, most psychotropic medication employed by the psychiatrist is for the treatment of depression and/or anxiety in patients the psychiatrist has engaged in psychotherapy (whether on a frequent or an infrequent basis). The psychiatrist prescribes medication to enhance the patient's cognitive function and to improve his affective state (mood) to the point where he can truly benefit from psychotherapy. Although some patients will require a prolonged course of medication, the psychiatrist most often discontinues the patient's medication—at least on a regular basis—when his symptoms have been reduced in intensity to the point where he can effectively utilize the intellectual and emotional knowledge, insight, and experience that psychotherapy can afford him. (There are, of course, some patients who will mainly benefit from psychotropic medication and for whom psychotherapy will not be of substantial help.) By contrast, when the nonpsychiatrist physician employs psychotropic medication, he often does so on an isolated and exclusive basis; he does not do so as an adjunct to psychotherapy, which he neither is trained to perform nor, realistically, has the time in which to engage his patients. Therefore, the nonpsychiatrist physician has the tendency to utilize psychotropic medication on an exclusive basis for the treatment of patients who suffer mental illness/emotional problems, a use of medication that is most certainly not indicated for most persons and that may yield serious negative therapeutic effects. For too many patients the well-meaning but insufficiently trained nonpsychiatrist physician prescribes potentially hazardous medication on a blanket basis for vague systems of depression and/or anxiety. The situation is analogous to the "old days" (to some extent still current) of medicine when penicillin was prescribed on a blanket basis for colds or flulike syndromes. Clearly, we must avoid such a therapeutic plague.

The problem with nonpsychiatrist physicians prescribing psychotropic medicines can be put in additional perspective by considering the prospect of the psychiatrist diagnosing and treating the patient who suffers coronary heart disease, complicated, as it often is, by hypertension. Many psychiatrists, with their medical backgrounds, perhaps supplemented by "continuing education courses," could certainly read the patient's electrocardiogram, monitor his blood pressure, and prescribe a combination of antiarrhythmic and antihypertensive medication. (Indeed, as an intern in internal medicine not so many years ago, I did just this.) However, any patient "in his right mind" would not seek out a psychiatrist on a primary basis to treat his coronary heart disease and/or hypertension (although he might do well to consult a psychiatrist on a secondary basis so as to partially or completely control his illness through resolving those psychological factors attendant to it). The patient recognizes the obvious: It takes a highly skilled clinician with much experience and expertise to correctly diagnose the specific condition(s) from which the individual patient suffers and then to determine the best single medication or combination of medicines and the correct dosage(s) to treat it. This is why medical specialization has evolved! And although medical care has probably suffered overspecialization, and although we probably can and should reassign certain elements of medical care to the generalist or to the new "general specialist," the family practitioner, the continuing need for the specialist is beyond question. (This does not negate the principle that the patient gets the best care when he has a single physician coordinating his care, treating him appropriately, and referring him to the specialist as necessary.) Still, we have difficulty accepting the specialist role of the psychiatrist. Yet, if it is ideal for the cardiologist to read the patient's electrocardiogram and institute appropriate medical treatment, then it is ideal for the psychiatrist to read the patient's emotional state and institute appropriate medical treatment. Of course, what is ideal is not always practical with respect to the logistics of medical care. There are not enough psychiatrists to treat all patients who require psychiatric care and there probably never will be. In fact, it is estimated that today 60% of all patients who receive "mental health care" get that care on a nonspecialized basis from the primary care/outpatient medical sector.[5] This, I believe, is not strictly due to a shortage of psychiatrists; rather, it reflects in part a predisposition on the part of both physicians and patients against referral of the patient for specialized psychiatric care. In fact, the mental health care delivery system, with appropriate triage of patients into the various components of the system, can provide care for many more patients than it does now. Nevertheless, it is simply not possible for the psychiatrist personally to treat on an ongoing basis all patients who require psychotropic medication—that is, patients who require a medical approach, at least in part, to their mental illness/emotional problems. Thus, now and in the future, the psychiatrist will have to devote much of his professional efforts to consultation with nonpsychiatrist physicians on the care of their patients who suffer mental illness/emotional problems. (Such consultation takes place now, but not often enough; too many patients who suffer mental illness/emotional problems are treated "in isolation" by their primary physicians.) Often this will take the following form: A patient's primary physician will refer him to a psychiatrist for direct consultation. The psychiatrist, after seeing the patient, will recommend to the referring primary physician the type and course of psychotropic medication he should prescribe for his patient. The primary physician will then periodically discuss the patient's clinical course with the psychiatrist, who will see the patient in "follow-up" consultation as necessary. In many cases, of course, the psychiatrist will advise a nonpsychiatrist physician against prescribing psychotropic medication for a particular patient; he will recommend that the patient be referred for "pure psychotherapy." I must make a very important point here. There is, as I have just described, a definite and proper role for the nonpsychiatrist physician with regard to his providing some mental health care for his patients himself—ideally through the auspices of a close liaison between the physician and a psychiatrist. However, most patients who suffer from *distinct, classifiable* mental illness/emotional problems will require *at least some* formal psychotherapy from a mental health professional (or paraprofessional, etc.), as opposed to "emotional support" from their physicians. This will be the case whether or not psychotropic medication is prescribed for the patient. The physician can perform an extremely valuable and medical cost-saving service by providing "emotional support" during isolated periods where the patient suffers nondistinct emotional distress. However, we simply cannot substitute the nonpsychiatrist physician for the psychiatrist (or other MHP) any more than we can substitute the psychiatrist for other medical specialists—although the psychiatrist can play a major role in evaluating and managing the physical symptoms of his patients. Under NHI, we must provide a person with full and complete *specialized* mental health care services—even while we encourage coordinated care for the patient under one primary physician (which in some cases may be the psychiatrist).

As I maintain throughout this book, psychotropic medication has now and will continue to have a very important role to play in the treatment of mental illness/emotional problems. However, in addition to the danger that such medication may be overused by the nonpsychiatrist physician, there is also the danger that it will be severely underused (or underrecommended) by the nonpsychiatrist mental health professional. It is not surprising that the physician has a tendency to use medication to treat symptoms. It is the nature of his trade and training. On the other end of the spectrum, the nonpsychiatrist MHP often has an extreme bias against the use of psychotropic medication, a bias that is just as dangerous as the predisposition to utilize medication. The bias of the nonpsychiatrist MHP against medication derives to some extent from his (or her) training, which frequently fails to expose him to the proper utilization of psychotropic medication and fails to educate him regarding its potential. (In addition, since the MHP cannot prescribe such medication, he may sometimes see it, if only unconsciously, as a threat to his trade.) The general prejudice against psychotropic medication extends beyond the nonpsychiatrist MHP to include the general public as well.

The point is that for the patient's benefit, we must guard against both the *overuse* and *underuse* of psychotropic medication. To do so we must educate the nonpsychiatrist physician as to the proper uses of psychotropic medication. We must also educate the nonpsychiatrist mental health professional and the layperson as to how such medicines work. In this connection, we should seek to dispel the alarmist notion that they act as "mind-control agents." (In fact, these medicines only facilitate the normal transmission of chemically mediated electrical impulses within the brain. They act more like hormones than like "medicines.") Indeed, the psychiatrist cannot neglect the total mind-set of both the mental health professional and the layperson if he is to promote proper and responsible mental health care. The mind-set of the layperson often includes the notion that psychotropic medication, if not psychotherapy as well, strips a person of his ability "to think and feel." The mind is a person's most private possession—it is the sanctum sanctorum—and any therapeutic efforts directed at it are bound to elicit anxiety.) Psychological factors play a very prominent role in both providers' and consumers' acceptance or rejection of various forms of mental health care and of medical (surgical) care as well. As for the consumer, a certain apprehension regarding all forms of health care is not ill-grounded. Medical (surgical) and mental health care have not been sufficiently monitored in the past. Although the vast majority of patients receive responsible care from responsible physicians, medicines have been overused and misused by physicians of all specialties, surgery has been performed too often, and with regard to mental health care, chemical and electrical (electroconvulsive) modalities of treatment have been improperly employed. The psychiatric profession must continue its efforts to develop and refine general standards, as exacting as possible, for the employment of chemical and electrical treatments so as to insure their proper utilization.

As I have demonstrated in this section, there are good reasons why we should not place artificial, arbitrary limits on inpatient or outpatient mental health care under NHI. At the same time, we must also establish an effective form of professional peer review—acceptable and fair to both the provider and the consumer—so that the patient receives the best available treatment and so that society does not incur needless costs for extraneous treatment. Peer review, however, must not be limited to oversight of the specialist in mental health care—specifically the psychiatrist. (There are disturbing trends in this direction in the name of cost control.) Psychiatrists do not need to be "watched" any more or less than surgeons or internists.

Though physicians may regard peer review as a nuisance—and, in fact, it is a nuisance to those who already practice in a responsible fashion—it can be an effective means for monitoring patient care and insuring fiscal oversight of all categories of medical care delivered under NHI. The exact mechanics of peer review will have to be carefully worked out. It must not be over-employed any more than it is underemployed. It must perform its function while eschewing excessive control. Peer review must be structured in such a way so as not to encumber the physician with regulations. Rather, it should facilitate the physician's efforts to practice effectively and productively and to expand his skills and knowledge in a creative fashion.* With specific regard to mental health care, peer review panels must be well balanced with psychiatrists of different psychological/medical persuasions so as to regulate patient care fairly and to avoid the injection of psychological politics and extraneous professional prejudice into decisions affecting patient care. Finally, again with specific regard to mental health care, evaluation and review of the clinical work of nonpsychiatrists as well as psychiatrists [e.g., clinical psychologists and social workers (M.S.W.s)] must be given high priority. I am of the opinion that to date, mental health care delivered by the nonpsychiatrist MHP has been poorly monitored and reviewed, even more so than is the case for care delivered by the psychiatrist. This has led, in too many instances, to the practice of "wild" psychotherapy that incorporates dangerous (for the patient) theories and practices.

I must emphasize here that excessive or inappropriate control or regulation of any system, from within or without, will produce morale problems. If severe enough, it will encourage defection from the system. In fact, many "socialized" health care delivery systems—including the VA hospital system—encounter difficulty retaining their physician personnel because they compromise the freedom of the physician to practice in accordance with his own standards—which are *higher* than those the system sets. In this connec-

---

*The question as to how best to regulate the quality and cost of medical care is indeed a difficult one. In many states, current requirements for physician relicensure involve mandatory attendance by the physician at a certain number of so-called continuing education conferences. The physician, to renew his license, must prove that he has attended x hours of what amounts to structured, approved "class." The physician, however, need not demonstrate that he has *learned* anything in those classes. Some have suggested formal (recertification) examinations as an alternative to continuing education requirements. However, such a policy could actually impede the physician in his quest for theoretical and clinical knowledge. In addition, forcing the physician to continually face and pass a series of examinations could be quite demoralizing for him.

tion, it must be realized that placing limits on coverage for mental health care under NHI may have a drastic effect on manpower potentially available to provide such care. The conscientious physician will not be willing to practice medicine under conditions where arbitrary, artificial constraints are placed upon what he can and cannot do therapeutically, regardless of what the patient requires. The net result will be to discourage physicians from entering the specialty of psychiatry. This will exacerbate the already existing shortage of psychiatrists (see Section 5.4). Of course, there are many factors that in theory could be deterring the medical school graduate from entering the specialty of psychiatry. For example, psychiatry has now become one of the lowest paying specialties of all the medical specialties. Furthermore, new medical specialties (notably family practice and emergency medicine) have recently emerged that are attracting many medical school graduates who might have otherwise chosen to become psychiatrists. Nevertheless, I believe that the drain of manpower away from the specialty of psychiatry reflects in part the denial of legitimacy to the field of psychiatry by national health policy in general.

Obviously, cost-control programs for health care can have serious consequences far beyond deleterious effects on the "provider pool." Programs and policies aiming at cost-effective mental health care have often led, in the past, to compromise in the quality of care delivered by a provider. This presents the striking possibility that when cost of care becomes a *primary* consideration, providers become primarily "cost-control-conscious" rather than "care-conscious." (The government has fallen victim to such an attitude in its policy under Medicare and Medicaid.) Safeguards against such a phenomenon must be built into NHI.

Additional arguments for establishing broad unlimited coverage for mental health care services under NHI are found in Chapter 5. Realistically, the extent of coverage that can be allowed must be linked to a certain extent to the cost of such coverage. The linkage, however, in addition to being *fiscally responsible,* must reflect a commitment to provide *medically responsible* mental health care.

I should like to close this chapter with one final admonition: Unless and until we as a society recognize the legitimacy of mental illness/emotional problems on a par with illnesses of any and every other sort, we shall continue to shortchange mental health care and in the process shortchange those persons who require such care. Another way of stating this would be that unless and until we recognize the validity of mental health care on a par with health care of other varieties, those persons who manifest mental illness/emotional problems will be relegated to borderline and insufficient treatment of the symptoms and illnesses from which they suffer. The extent of coverage available for mental health care now and in the future under NHI will always reflect our psychological attitude toward such care as well as our concern with fiscal constraints.

Who Should Provide Mental Health Care?

5.1. Public and Private Outpatient Care

The terms *public* and *private* may be somewhat of a misnomer when applied to the concept of medical care under NHI. NHI, after all, will ostensibly provide equal access to medical care for all persons, so that "public" and "private" care could cease to exist *per se*. In reality, this will probably not happen under NHI. The public health care section will be maintained even though its size may be somewhat diminished. In this connection, it is of interest to note that two-thirds of all mental health care costs are accounted for today by the public sector.[16] Under NHI, there may be some redistribution of public sector functions to the private sector as that (latter) sector is better financed and is able to expand the scope as well as the quality of the services it delivers. In any case, a distinct division of mental health care services has developed within the public and private sectors under our current health care system, and the different services will need to be continued under NHI, no matter who provides them. For purposes of discussion, the terms *public* and *private* will be used herein to refer to those services and the institutions/providers that have come into being to furnish them.

If NHI does evolve as a full and comprehensive partnership between the private sector and government, the public sector will continue to fill in the gaps between those mental health care services the private sector provides to the population it serves and the complete requirements for mental health care services by the population at large. Logistically speaking, it is probably wise at this point to preserve the currently existing amalgamated mental health care delivery system under NHI in order to provide well-balanced and inclusive outpatient treatment for mental illness/emotional problems. Community Mental Health Centers (CMHCs) and their cousin agencies—the public sector—and private providers of mental health care should exist and function side by side, each performing the functions they are best suited to perform. This is not a unique perspective; it is the recommendation of the NIMH and multiple professional groups.

It is important to ask how the public and private sectors differ in terms of providing mental health care? Certain segments of the private sector function in many respects like the public sector. However, the private practitioner of psychiatry and other private-based MHPs, although they often work hand in hand with the CMHC and other public agencies, are oriented more exclusively toward meeting the treatment needs of the individual patient, couples, and families where such treatment can be accomplished in a limited setting—most often within "the office" or within a single inpatient facility. In contrast, CMHCs, by way of their organization, can usually provide a much broader range of care and services than can the solo private practitioner. CHMCs are especially well conceived and designed to implement the "team approach" to the patient (client)—to coordinate with schools, the courts, and various social agencies (welfare, protective, etc.) to provide evaluation, treatment, and rehabilitation of the patient. CMHCs are also well suited to provide, by themselves, certain services such as day care, hospital aftercare, and comprehensive rehabilitation that the solo private practitioner would have difficulty providing in his own setting. Further, the CMHC, in order to meet the special needs of the population it serves, is often actively tied into a vast psychosocial network (day treatment centers, half-way houses, etc.) that can facilitate the return of hospital patients to the community and can keep marginal patients functioning. (The private practitioner can be, but is usually not, tied into this network to any great extent.)

CMHCs are also crucial for implementing "outreach" programs within the community—bringing care to the patient who cannot come to the source of care—and for establishing broad, organized programs of preventive mental health care. They are well staffed by mental health professionals, paraprofessionals, and "aides" and "workers" capable of treating those patients who do not require the services of a psychiatrist. Significantly, now and in the past, the CMHC has played an important role in providing mental health care for those patients who could not afford private-based treatment. Perhaps this has been its major function, although it is a function that may change under NHI—to a greater or lesser degree, depending upon the nature and extent of the government–private sector partnership that develops under NHI.

There are marked differences in the patient population now treated at the CMHC compared to the population treated by the private practitioner. The private practitioner generally treats patients who come from a higher socioeconomic class.[17] The private practitioner also treats a relatively higher proportion of patients whose prognosis is better.[17] (There is some debate as to this point.) However, the latter (prognosis) is undoubtedly related to the former (financial status) on multiple accounts. It must be clearly recognized that the differences in the patient populations—CMHC versus private practitioner—are to a large extent the result of or a reflection of financial barriers. If these are eliminated, the populations will shift to approximate one another much more closely. So-called poor prognosis patients will become financially entitled to treatment in the private sector, which, one can predict, many of them will seek. Ideally, NHI will allow people who have been previously unable to afford private-based mental health care the choice and opportunity to receive it rather than disenfranchise people who up to now have been able to afford private-based care through their own health insurance.

However, as currently envisioned, NHI does severely limit outpatient visits to private providers (i.e., private practitioners) of mental health care, whereas there are no limitations on such visits to CMHCs or other prepaid "health clinics" such as Health Maintenance Organizations (HMOs). If such differential limits are allowed under NHI, the effect will be to deprive many patients of the "right" to seek mental health care from the private practitioner. The patient will simply not be able to afford private care, as he would not be able to afford surgical care on a private basis if unrealistic limits were placed on surgeons' fees covered. Of course, "rights" are relative, but if NHI allows the patient to be treated by a private internist or surgeon of his choosing (by covering such care), it should also allow him to be treated by a psychiatrist or other MHP of his choosing. Especially with regard to psychiatric treatment, the relationship between the physician and the patient is paramount: It must embody a strong rapport and deep trust if the patient is to benefit from treatment. Thus, the patient should be free to carefully select the individual psychiatrist (or other MHP) who is best for him or her.

Most persons, if they can afford it, seek treatment in the private sector when they suffer mental illness/emotional problems. They believe they will receive better care on a private basis. Just because they believe this, of course, doesn't make it so, but there is rationale to back up their point of view.

As a preface to the following remarks, I should state that I do not wish to engage here in a theoretical discussion of the financial abuses and inefficiency that may occur under and flaw either a private sector or a public sector health care delivery system. Indeed, I am concerned by the tendency of health care delivery systems within both sectors to take certain advantage (even if frequently unintended) of the special privileges which their structure and status grant them with the result that they often fail to fully meet their obligations and responsibilities to the patients (clients) they serve. I shall leave the final debate as to the total merits and flaws and efficiency and inefficiency of private sector versus public sector systems to the economic and political theorists. Nevertheless, I do wish to catalog here my concept of the ways in which the private sector and public sector mental health care delivery systems differ from each other.

The individual patient (client) is more likely to receive in-depth treatment from the private practitioner—whether he or she be a psychiatrist or other MHP. Even though NHI may not impose upper limits on outpatient visits to CMHCs—and HMO mental hygiene clinics—patient visits will be severely limited by these providers themselves. To understand why, we must take a closer look at the way in which CMHCs (and HMO mental hygiene clinics) operate. For multiple reasons, especially mode of funding, CMHCs are highly oriented toward treating the patient in a brief number of visits. The CMHC operates under a set of economic principles that for the most part do not take into account the length or depth of treatment provided to the individual patient. Consequently, the CMHC's treatment goals for the patient will often differ from the patient's own goals—the CMHC focusing on rapid resolution of a particular crisis in the patient's life, the patient desirous of broader changes in himself that require a longer period of treatment to effect. Statistics bear out the differences in treatment the patient receives from the CMHC versus the private practitioner. The average patient of the CMHC is seen for only 5.3 treatment visits.[17] Compare this with an average of 38 treatment visits (per year) for patients who receive their care from psychiatrists in private practice.[18](The latter figure excludes psychoanalysts. If psychoanalysts are included, the average number of visits per patient per year to all psychiatrists in private practice is 46.[18]) It should be noted that these statistics for public versus private treatment visits *partially* reflect the different patient populations treated in the two sectors and the different missions of the two sectors. Clearly, however, only very superficial mental health care can be delivered when a patient is treated only five times. An acute crisis can perhaps be resolved during the course of such care, but the patient's basic personality and behavior pattern can hardly be altered. One could predict another acute crisis for the patient—or two or three or ten—during his or her lifetime. Of course, some patients, though less than would be expected, require only minimal mental health care, and many more patients do not desire anything more than short-term treatment, no matter what they may "need" in the way of care. For these patients, the CMHC, with its treatment orientation toward very short-term care, may suffice. However, for most patients (clients), such an orientation, in my opinion, leads to insufficient care. (The HMO clinic, like the CMHC, is mainly predisposed to provide its patients short-term care. An analysis of one HMO plan (the Health Insurance Plan of Greater New York) reveals that this treatment philosophy proves to be a potential handicap for providing quality care.[19] I believe this finding can be extended to the CMHC.

It can be hypothesized that more long-term treatment is practiced in the private sector because, in part, MHPs who are oriented toward this form of treatment gravitate to the private sector (private practice), where they can practice in accord with their own treatment philosophies, not under the aegis of a system that limits the degree and extent to which they can treat a patient. As stated, most clinics' orientation toward treatment is, expressed or unexpressed, strictly short-term. (The exception is the clinic in the teaching or research setting.) The MHP who does not wish to stop treatment at a point that is *satisfactory* but not *ideal* for his patient may find it difficult to work in the clinic setting, which too often ignores the importance of intensive long-term care and essentially discriminates against it.

In contrast to the situation at the CMHC (and at many HMOs), the psychiatrist (or other MHP) who is engaged in private practice in the private sector is able to work with his patient (client) until both feel that a "cure" or the optimal possible resolution of symptoms has been attained. (This presupposes, of course, that financial resources are available to support such treatment.) The psychiatrist (or other MHP) and the patient can work together without constraints so that not only is the acute presenting problem alleviated but the patient changes as to personality, and his crises do not repeat themselves ad infinitum.* The whole iceberg of the patient's emotional disorder is eliminated, therefore, not just the part sticking out.

It is very difficult to assess the comparative cost of mental health care at CMHCs versus such care in the private sector because of the differences in the patient populations and services provided. Surprisingly, however, an NIMH report reveals that the unit cost per psychiatrist treatment hour is actually higher at the CMHC than it is in the private sector ($45 vs. $37).[17] (These dollar figures were calculated several years ago. They should be adjusted for inflation.) This oddity—the reverse of what we would expect—exists because 30% of the salary of the CMHC psychiatrist is attributable to administrative overhead. In the CMHC, psychiatrists and many psychologists (Ph.D.s) spend much, if not most, of their working time in activities other than direct patient care. They administer, coordinate, conduct training conferences, and supervise patient evaluation and treatment being carried out by mental health paraprofessionals and "workers" less well qualified than themselves. (These personnel in fact perform the bulk of the treatment delivered by the CMHC.) It is certainly legitimate and necessary for the CMHC psychiatrist or psychologist to supervise a social worker or psychiatric aide who is treating a patient; nevertheless, well-trained psychiatrists and psychologists who spend their time in this and other administrative fashions—rather than in direct patient care—deprive (even if not of their own accord) many patients of the optimal, specialized mental health care they deserve.

The private practitioner is motivated to spend the majority of his time actually providing treatment to his patients (clients) because he is paid exclusively for this. On the other hand, it must be emphasized that since the psychiatrist or psychologist working at the CMHC (or HMO in the private sector) receives a fixed salary, there is little personal *economic* incentive for him to involve himself directly in patient care. As a partial consequence of this, the

---

*As Dr. Lebensohn implies in his commentary, it is a difficult matter to effect a "personality change" in the patient (client) during the course of psychotherapy, especially in the complete sense. I use the term *personality* here and elsewhere in this paper only in the lay sense (except with regard to the definition of the "personality disorders" in Chapter 3). What I am really referring to by "personality change" here and elsewhere are changes in the way the patient (client) thinks, feels, and behaves (the latter obviously includes the way the patient relates to others) as perceived by the patient and by others. I do maintain that such changes do result from the practice of psychotherapy, to a greater or lesser extent depending upon the success of the psychotherapy (or not at all, if the psychotherapy fails). Of course, no matter how successful psychotherapy is and no matter how profound the "changes" that a patient experiences, he (or she) always retains a large part of his "old personality." It is just that he is now better able to control those aspects of his "old personality" that previously caused him pathological emotional distress. In addition, he has developed new and more adaptive modes of behaving, as well as thinking and feeling.

mental health professional employed by the CMHC (or other similarly styled clinic) often avoids delivering direct patient (client) care himself! This phenomenon does not reflect negatively on the integrity of the professional; rather, it underscores the fact that the practice of mental health care (psychotherapy) is extremely difficult—for the patient, of course, but for the mental health professional as well. It is simply emotionally consuming and exhausting for the professional to be sympathetic, empathic, and understanding while at the same time remaining objective—i.e., somewhat emotionally "distant" or psychologically "removed" from his patient. Yet he must do so if he is to effect a successful treatment for his patient (client). In this sense, the practice of mental health care differs from all other medical care, where the physician can be more strictly "clinical" in his involvement with his patient even while he cares for him. This is not to say that the nonpsychiatrist physician, or any other person working at any job, does not face among other things anxiety, frustration, and deprivation, often to an extreme, as a part of his daily work. Still, the requirements of the psychiatrist's (or other MHP's) job expose him to unusually severe emotional and psychological demands. The psychiatrist, for example, is routinely forced to face and accept, without retaliating, his patient's anger toward him. (The psychiatrist must not discourage his patient's anger—often a difficult thing to do. Most often, he must encourage, if only in a passive manner, his patient's negative feelings toward him. And he must not take his patient's attacks on him personally.) The psychiatrist must also resist the patient's wishes or demands to be taken care of. (The psychiatrist will at times comfort or provide emotional support to his patients, but ultimately he must partially or wholly restrain himself in this connection in favor of teaching the patient to be self-sufficient.) Much, if not most, of the time, the psychiatrist must keep his personal feelings toward his patient to himself. He must carefully monitor his emotional reactions to his patient and control his responses to him if he is to help him to "get better." It is important to point out here that the patient does not visit the psychiatrist (or other MHP) to meet or satisfy in any way, shape, or form his (the psychiatrist's) emotional needs—except insofar as the psychiatrist receives pleasure from engaging himself in the creative process of psychotherapy and is gratified when the patient improves. (Even the latter normal response on the part of the psychiatrist, if too openly displayed, can retard or defeat the patient's progress—if, for example, the patient is engaged in a struggle, conscious or unconscious, to defeat the psychiatrist in his efforts. See also in this connection the Appendix.)

Though we might want to view our health care providers in a more idealistic way, the simple reality is that financial recompense to the practitioner of mental health care serves as part of his "reward" for his work. Without appropriate compensation for direct patient care, the mental health care provider is to some extent discouraged from practicing such care because of the heavy emotional toll the work extracts. This proposition points out the need for a *psychological analysis* of *provider systems* by planners of National

Health Insurance. The creation of the final provider systems must take into account not only the needs and desires of patients and the cost of services, but also the emotional needs, ambitions, and goals of health care providers of all varieties. A physician of any speciality, frustrated by the system within which he works, will perform at a lower level of efficiency, and the quality of his work will suffer. (The same will hold true, of course, for any person working at any job.) Ultimately, the system itself will work extremely inefficiently or it will fail.

One recent study[20] confirms my remarks above about the nature and extent of practitioner involvement in direct patient care in the clinic setting. The study focused on mental health care delivery in a prepaid health care plan in the private sector, but as I have previously indicated, private sector mental health clinics operate in many respects in much the same fashion as does the CMHC. (Although the types of patients they treat may be quite different and the range of services they provide quite diverse, the quantity of treatment they deliver is often similar due to the manner in which they are funded.) First of all, the authors of the study described their experience that "staff often gravitate towards activities that are personally rewarding (e.g., staff conferences) and take time away from the primary task of the organization (direct patient care) unless . . . a monitoring mechanism is available." The authors then reported on professional staff productivity in one particular organization (the Group Health Association of Washington, D.C.); measurement of productivity, *after* the establishment of monitoring of the clinical case loads of the various MHPs and paraprofessionals was found "to support an expectation of 50–60% direct service in a program whose primary task is direct service but indicate the need for adjustments according to professional role differences; psychiatrists generally devoted over 65% of their work time to direct service, psychologists spent about 50%, and alcoholism counsellors spent less than 45%." This study also summarized the results of other studies that measured professional staff productivity rates in mental health settings, finding such rates to range from 11% to 45% (presumedly as a measurement of the percentage of a full-working day spent by staff in providing direct care). Indeed, the productivity rates found in the present study may reflect an optimal amount of time devoted to direct patient care by staff! From 5 to 5½ hours per day of direct patient care (the maximum level of productivity reported here) may constitute the maximum amount of clinical work that one should expect *in the ideal* of a mental health care practitioner, given the emotionally consuming nature of his work. (It may be that health care practitioners of all specialties operating in a prepaid or public health care clinic function at a similar rate of productivity. We should not examine the productivity rate of the practitioner of mental health care in isolation.) Nevertheless, the private practitioner of mental health care functions at a higher productivity rate than those described in this study. Since he does not receive a set salary, the private practitioner cannot afford to spend only 50 to 65% of his time delivering direct patient care because, as I have stated, he is paid only for this function. If we are looking toward designing a mental health care delivery system that meets the health care needs of its patients in the most economical manner, we should carefully examine productivity rates such as those I have presented here. Of course, whereas the private clinic and the private practitioner may serve much the same patients and provide much the same services, the public sector (CMHC) currently serves a different population whose treatment requires a broad range of services. Therefore, in the public sector, staff hours spent in direct patient care do not completely reflect the total picture of patient care—more so than for the private sector.

In the final analysis, the planning of provider systems and health care delivery systems in general under NHI must be based not only on the economic efficiencies of the systems but also on a careful evaluation of what the patient (client) actually receiving health care services "gets for his money." In comparing the patient's (client's) purchasing power at the CMHC versus the private sector, it is important to emphasize that when a person seeks his care from a private practitioner, he (or she) is not only able to contract for the type of treatment he desires but is able to enter into his health care with the specific provider of his choice. This is by no means the case at the CMHC (and private sector clinics that operate like it), where it is possible and even probable, as I have described, that there will be a certain disinclination on the part of the treating professional to furnish extensive, comprehensive care. In addition, the patient (client) who seeks his care at the CMHC faces a further problem. The decision at the CMHC as to exactly who shall treat a particular patient is largely an administrative one. It does not usually take into account the patient's choice as to who should treat him. Indeed, the likelihood of his being treated by a psychiatrist, as opposed to a psychologist, social worker, or paraprofessional, is almost nil. This situation will be only slightly ameliorated if CMHCs are expanded under NHI. The CMHC will still decide exactly what the patient's treatment needs are and who should provide his treatment. In contrast to this, I believe strongly that any person should have the opportunity to decide not only what type of treatment he should receive but also who should treat him—provided, of course, the treatment he desires is indicated and the services of a particular type of professional (e.g., a psychiatrist) are warranted. In any case, I believe that any person who suffers mental illness/emotional problems, or thinks he suffers them, deserves the right to consultation with a psychiatrist or other MHP of his choice. (This is especially justifiable, for one reason, because of the differing attitudes of the various mental health professionals toward the use of psychotropic medication. A person may desire treatment from a psychiatrist (an M.D.) because he has an inclination to treatment with medication as opposed to "talk"—even if his inclination is not justifiable.)

Besides its failure to respond to the desires, needs, and rightful predilections of its consumers, the CMHC has in other respects failed to meet the general expectations that have been held for it. It has not become independent of federal monies; it has not been able, as originally intended, to shift its financing to state, local, and private funding.[21] CMHCs have filled a much-needed gap as regards the provision of certain mental health care services not available in the private sector. In addition, the CMHC has successfully served many members of a population unable to afford mental health care services in the private sector. However, the CMHC has failed many members of that same population. Of particular note, the CMHC has not delivered adequate aftercare (posthospitalization) services to chronically ill patients—who constitute a large segment of those persons it serves. As a result, these patients are often trapped in a "revolving door" syndrome. Surely enough, they are admitted to the hospital for care when their symptoms require it, and with treatment, their symptoms remit to the point where they can be discharged. However, having returned to the community, they receive little or no aftercare, their symptoms return full force, and they must be readmitted to the hospital. This sequence repeats itself ad infinitum.

It is possible that with increased financing for CMHCs under NHI, such patients as I have just described will receive proper aftercare and rehabilitation, but we must consider the possibility that another system might have to be developed to replace or complement the CMHC in serving the chronically ill patient, and perhaps other categories of ill-served patients as well. For example, the CMHC functions for many patients as an agency that does not provide mental health care *per se* but rather facilitates the provision of social services. In other words, the CMHC now devotes much of its resources to patients who suffer "social" problems rather than discrete, distinct mental illness/emotional problems.[21] This is in contradistinction to the CMHC's primary mission to dispense mental health care. For many patients, of course, the provision of social services must come before, or at least at the same time as, the provision of mental health care. Adequate food, clothing, and shelter—along with employment opportunity—are a prerequisite for mental health for any individual person. However, it is not clear that the CMHC can survive and function both as a social service agency and as an agency whose mission is to provide mental health care. Reorganization of the CMHC—and the public sector mental health care delivery system in general—may be necessary or advisable under NHI to facilitate the provision of mental health care and social services. Public sector mental health care may have to be redefined, reoriented, and refinanced.

Some discussion of the Health Maintenance Organization (HMO) is warranted at this point in terms of the mental health care delivery system it administers. (I use the term *HMO* loosely here to include any prepaid comprehensive health care plan.) Because the HMO, like the CMHC, operates under significant economic disincentives regarding the provision of long-term comprehensive mental health care, it tends not to provide such care. Under some HMO health plans currently in operation, mental health care services are not even provided. When they are provided, they are most often limited to a minimal number of outpatient visits, with the focus on brief consultation and short-term care for acute problems. In this connection, Brodie[8] cites data from the Harvard Community Health Plan, a plan that provides health care services to approximately 75,000 members of the Harvard community. Approximately 20% of the enrollment carry diagnoses of mental illness; however, only 50% of patients with such diagnoses are referred for *specialized* mental health care. Further, fewer than 1% of these patients "require" treatment beyond the benefit limit of 20 psychotherapy sessions per year. I believe this is a gross distortion of the true requirements of Harvard plan members for specialized mental health care. Further, if a prepaid health plan administered by a premier academic institution provides such limited specialized mental health care, one can easily imagine the justification for and tendency of other prepaid plans to follow suit.

I should also point out that, as at the CMHC, patient selection of provider at the HMO is limited, if available at all, and may not include the option of treatment by a psychiatrist. Thus, at the Harvard Community Health Plan to which I have just referred,[8] 99% of those patients who carry a diagnosis of mental illness are seen initially by a health professional (not an MHP), who may or may not refer the patient to a mental health professional. (As I have stated, the patient is referred approximately 50% of the time.) The only patients who can see an MHP directly are those who present with psychiatric emergencies.

Finally, the case loads of the various mental health professionals (and paraprofessionals) at the HMO are subject to careful, if not severe, scrutiny as a part of the built-in health care review process conducted by the HMO. I am most certainly in favor of health care review as a means, first, to improve health care delivery for the individual patient and, second, to control the cost of health care. However, I am concerned that the review process at the HMO is subject to being geared more to the latter than to the former (for both mental health care and other forms of health care). The HMO, after all, operates on a fixed income, and it must be conscious of that fact as it schedules and dispenses health care. Therefore, it is possible, if not probable, that individual patients (clients) of MHPs working at the HMO are liable to have their mental health care terminated prematurely. Additionally, it is likely that such care will be offered only on an abridged basis, inadequate for many patients to begin with.

Currently, many HMOs that do provide mental health care services do so by contract with external "private" groups. The services are provided at a separate location from the HMO. In some HMOs, however, mental health care is provided "under the same roof" as the primary health care services the organization delivers. This model has one definite advantage: The complete care of the patient can be managed in a single setting. The emotional aspects, complications, and/or etiology (derivation) of the patient's physical symptoms or illness can be treated by a psychiatrist at the same time that an internist (surgeon, etc.) treats the symptoms or illness itself. The two physicians can closely coordinate their care of the patient. However, although such a total approach to medical care is to be desired, mental health care as delivered in the HMO is too often practiced merely as *an adjunct* to the medical treatment of the patient. It is short-term, and it is frequently not available when the patient does not have a "medical problem."

HMOs of the future must be reoriented to provide long-term comprehensive mental health care when such care is indicated. Treatment of the patient who does not suffer a medical problem *per se* must be emphasized, and full and complete mental health care must be available and encouraged for him. This can only be accomplished, I think, by specific legislation under NHI that mandates such responsible mental health care. Marginal and irresponsible care is actually encouraged now. As I have pointed out in Chapter 1, federal enabling legislation for HMOs requires only that the HMO provide a patient a *maximum* of 20 outpatient visits for mental health care per year. Furthermore, the federal "final regulations"[22] for HMOs do not specify how much, if any, inpatient mental health care a HMO must provide. Essentially, this opens the way for the HMO to greatly restrict, if not deny, both outpatient and inpatient mental health care to those persons it serves; it essentially legitimizes a situation wherein persons afflicted by mental illness/emotional problems are likely to suffer minor to catastrophic limitations in the levels of mental health care available to them. Although the legislation referred to here specifically affects only HMOs, it is likely that other health care systems will take their cue from it and provide their subscribers only the barest, minimal mental health care. They will realize and take advantage of what I have pointed out elsewhere in this paper—namely, that restrictions on levels of both inpatient and outpatient mental health care, as opposed to other forms of health care, are relatively easy to justify and thus relatively easy to effect.

Indeed, it is highly unlikely that many HMOs (or other health care provider systems) will go beyond federal legislation as regards the provision of mental health care services. As one major HMO plan states regarding its mental health care coverage,[23] "this benefit includes 20 private or 40 group outpatient visits per year at the health plan . . . for acute mental illness and mental disorders which, *in the judgement of the health plan providers are subject to significant improvement through short-term therapy. . .*" (italics added). Other HMO plans are quick to point out to the potential subscriber that they do not provide any substantial care for chronic conditions. It appears that HMO administrators, tacitly supported by health planners and legislators, are possessed of the unfortunate attitude that the individual patient (client) can "survive" with minimal mental health care—when, in fact, any such care is required. Most certainly, the HMO would appear to maintain, the patient (client) can do without any substantial care for chronic conditions. Such a view seems, to this author at least, to be out of synchronization with the primary mission of medical care—namely, to provide, to the maximum extent possible, for the physical and emotional health of each and every individual person who seeks health care. It also ignores the premise that a person's emotional health constitutes the essential underpinning of his (or her) physical health.

I have emphasized throughout this section the fact that the specific mental health care an individual person receives is partly dependent upon the economic incentives and disincentives that operate on the health care provider who is administering his care. (Unfortunately, these incentives and disincentives can compromise the primary responsibility of the psychiatrist or other MHP to his patient or client.) In fact, it is crucial to realize that economic factors can play a greater role in determining the extent of mental health care services afforded a patient (client) than is the case for any other form of medical care. Why? Because for the large percentage of medical care, exclusive of mental health care, the physician's medical approach to the patient should not, and in most cases will not, vary to any great extent—whether the care is delivered in the private or public sector. Set diagnostic and therapeutic regimens are mandated for a great many organic (physical) symptoms or clusters of physical symptoms, and the physician's task is simply to follow these regimens in order to effect the complete cure of the patient or to control his disease process to the maximum extent possible.* The picture, however, is very different as regards mental health care. Here, treatment goals for most, if not all, patients can be variously set, practiced, and defended, depending upon provider orientation and motivation—as well as on patient motivation, of course. We do not often speak of "cure" of mental illness/emotional problems, and control, rehabilitation, or improvement can be described in various ways. Thus, the patient in the clinic setting—public or private (CMHC or HMO)—can be mandated to receive short-term "supportive" care until his acute situation quiesces and reverts to chronic form because in the majority of cases there is no strict medical injunction to provide anything more. The practitioner (more specifically the institution that directs him) can "get away" with what in my opinion often constitutes poor medical care.

I do not, however, mean to suggest in any way that those MHPs who work in the public sector (or in HMOs) are not dedicated and capable. Neither do I wish to impugn their professional integrity, including their commitment to offer their patients (clients) the best possible care. I am only suggesting that the system in which they are employed too often works against them. This notwithstanding, many MHPs who work in the public sector (or in HMOs) manage to "defeat" the system in which they work and provide their patients the comprehensive and complete treatment they require. Further, there are obviously many factors involved in the MHP's decision to practice in the public sector or HMO. Thus, many professionals believe strongly in the "community approach" to mental health care and work in the public sector on this account. Further, many MHPs work in the public sector out of a desire to provide mental health care to those persons the private sector does not

---

*In fact, there will at times be significant variation in treatment offered for the same medical-surgical condition by the private physician, the HMO, and the public institution. The HMO and the public institution are more likely to provide the least costly care for the patient if the justification exists to do so. In my opinion, patients who elect to receive their medical care at the HMO can, under certain circumstances, compromise their total health care.

currently reach and/or adequately serve. This includes many persons who simply cannot afford private care.

Of course, if I am going to argue in this paper that mental health care as delivered in the public sector is often excessively abbreviated due to the system of economics under which that sector operates, I must also consider here whether mental health care as delivered in the private sector (by the private practitioner) is sometimes excessive in length (and cost) due to the particular economic structure that underlies that sector. The private practitioner, especially when he is not restricted by his patient's insurance coverage, or when his patient can afford to pay for some or all of his treatment, effectively operates under relatively fewer controls, compared to the public sector, as regards the specific amount of treatment he can provide his patients (clients). The question to ask is whether private practitioners (psychiatrists and other MHPs) appropriately and responsibly dispense their services in consonance with their patients' (clients') demands for such services; alternatively, does the available supply of professional services in the private sector, as provided by the private practitioner, create or exceed patient demands for such services? I believe the evidence points to the first postulate. The average patient treated by the private practitioner in the private sector appears to receive an amount of treatment that is not excessive and is consistent with a responsible professional approach to the treatment of mental illness/emotional problems. Nevertheless, mental health care in both the private and public sectors is undoubtedly delivered to some patients in excessive quantities. In this connection, it is probably true that although intermediate to long-term mental health care is clearly indicated for many patients (clients) who suffer mental illness/emotional problems, some mental health professionals have a tendency to overprescribe and practice such care because, in part, they feel comfortable with its technique and pace. On the other hand, let me be quick to point out that many mental health professionals may overutilize short-term mental health care for their patients because they feel more comfortable with this approach to treatment and do not possess the personality characteristics that are required for one to practice intermediate to long-term care.

For the most part, I believe it is fair and accurate to state that neither the physician (of any specialty) nor the average, emotionally healthy patient desires to extend the frequency or intensity of health care beyond the requirement for such care. Indeed, many patients engaged in treatment by physicians of all specialties seek to disengage themselves from care before they have received the *minimum* amount of care necessary to resolve or stabilize their condition. This is especially true for patients receiving mental health care—which often generates a high level of anxiety in the patient as a part of the treatment process.

To the extent that any patient seeks excessive quantities of diagnostic and/or theraupeutic health care, the physician, no matter what his specialty, must regard this as a symptom of the patient's excessive emotional dependency upon the health care delivery system—as personified by the treating physician. In such cases, the patient, in essence, seeks excessive health care from the physician as a way of dealing with his or her dependency needs and/ or various anxieties. The patient's symptoms persist despite adequate health care, for he is willing to give up "independent" living in a state of absolute or relative health for a modicum, no matter how modest, of emotional support and nurturing from his physician. (The fact that a patient must pay fully for his treatment often will not deter him from seeking excessive and inappropriate care. It may even allow him to feel more justified in doing so.)

The psychiatrist or other mental health professional is especially attuned to the patient's (client's) tendency to seek excessive health care in lieu of attempting to resolve his or her basic mental illness/emotional problems. The psychiatrist (or other MHP) seeks to wean such a patient (client) from his need to seek health care. To the extent that any physician (or MHP) engages his patient (client) in health care in lieu of separating the patient from such health care at the appropriate time, the physician performs a therapeutic misservice to his patient. He is simply practicing "bad medicine." It is the physician's (or the MHP's) professional obligation to his patient to be aware at all points during treatment of his patient when such treatment is no longer likely to be effective and when it may in fact be harmful for the patient from both the physical and the emotional point of view.

Ultimately, I believe it is the *professional orientation* on the part of the physician, rather than the amount of health care resources he does or does not have available to treat his patient, that is the major factor in his controlling the length, amount, and cost of his patient's treatment. I should add that although physicians (including psychiatrists) do sometimes extend unnecessary care to their patients, I believe this is most often a function of a lack of education on their part as regards the optimal level and type of care that they should administer for a given condition. (In some cases the physician delivers extra care as a precaution against malpractice suits.) Except in uncommon instances involving less than honorable physicians, I do not believe the extension of superfluous care to a patient stems from an effort by the physician to take advantage of or to misuse those health insurance benefits available to his patient.

It is true that the psychiatrist (and other MHPs) in particular must always be alert to the possibility that when free or substantially free mental health care (psychotherapy) is available to his patient (client), through either the public or the private sector, the patient may have difficulty "giving up" (terminating) such care because of its supportive and comforting nature— which is often more intense and sustained than for other forms of medical care. On the other hand, it is also true that mental health care may be more anxiety-provoking for the patient than other forms of health care, and because of this, as I have previously suggested, he may terminate his treatment abruptly and prematurely. In any case, the psychiatrist (and other MHPs) must be sure that treatment proceeds at a proper rate and in proper amount for any given patient if he is to insure that patient's ultimate well-being.

I have especially stressed in this section the differences between mental health care delivered by the private practitioner and mental health care delivered by the CMHC because most plans for NHI, as I have related, would provide unlimited mental health care for an individual person at the CMHC (public sector care), whereas there would be severe limitations on care delivered by the practitioner operating in the private sector. The decision of health planners and legislators to structure mental health care delivery in this way is preeminently based on financial considerations, their thinking being that care delivered by the private practitioner within the private sector is too costly. To the health planner and legislator, such a dichotomy in funding of care seems both economically desirable and responsive to patients' needs. However, the latter is only an illusion. In fact, as I have shown, the CMHC will ultimately provide only severely limited care for most persons. Further, even with increased staffs and monies devoted to them, the CMHC is likely in the future to become even more overtaxed and overburdened than it is today as the demand for mental health care services increases. (Currently in many CMHCs, the applicant for care, except in true emergencies, is subjected to exceedingly long waiting periods before he or she can be treated. This may not be harmful in all cases; however, most persons seeking care for mental illness/emotional problems should at least be evaluated immediately.) I feel strongly that health planners and legislators have an obligation to understand how a health care system works *in vivo* as opposed to *in vitro* ("in life" as opposed to "in the test-tube"). Certainly they must propose and enact legislation that is fiscally responsible, but they must realize the amount, the kinds, and the quality of mental health care they will legislate into existence through a mental health care delivery system that relies heavily, if not almost exclusively, on clinic-based care—CMHC or otherwise. Health planners and legislators should delude neither themselves nor the public.

Finally, an NHI philosophy toward mental health care that limits outpatient visits to private practitioners will not in any way mean the end of long-term, comprehensive private-based mental health care. The net effect, rather, will be to make such care accessible only to those persons financially able to purchase it. Such a situation currently exists in Great Britain, where the national health program offers mainly short-term clinic-style mental health care and where those persons who can afford it avail themselves, if they so choose, of long-term complete treatment from consultant psychiatrists. This type of preferential treatment is not what NHI was to be about.

5.2. Public and Private Inpatient Care

It is important to make the distinction that whereas for outpatient mental health care the public sector has a definite, contrasting role vis-à-vis the private sector (i.e., it provides certain unique services), the same "natural" division between the public and private sectors does not hold true for inpatient care. Here both sectors serve essentially the same function, and it is mainly the individual patient's personal finances that determine which system he uses. If he can afford private inpatient care, he utilizes it, and if he cannot, he utilizes the public system.

In terms of cost, some studies indicate that public hospitals (Public Health Service Hospitals) are more expensive to operate than private hospitals.[17] The reality, though, is that they are probably about 30% less expensive on a unit-cost basis.[17] Cost comparisons are difficult because public and private hospitals currently serve different kinds of patients. However, a simplistic model would be that private hospitals are often more active in caring for the acutely ill patient who has the financial means to pay for his care. They employ comprehensive, intensive mental health care to effect a successful treatment and thus to enable discharge of the patient as quickly as possible. By contrast, public hospitals, though frequently engaged in acute care and goal-oriented toward discharging the patient at the earliest possible date, operate in large part as vast psychosocial systems that care for indigent patients with chronic illnesses on a long-term or even an indefinite basis quite simply because the patients too often have no other place to go. They may or may not require continuing care of one degree or another, but often they do not require hospital care *per se*. [For example, a National Academy of Sciences (NAS) study cited earlier in this paper reveals that fully 50% of patients in VA psychiatric hospitals do not actually have a medical need to be in the hospital.[14] Of course, VA hospitals are, strictly speaking, "government hospitals," but they operate in many respects as public hospitals—in terms of mode of funding and with respect to much of the population they serve.] Since public hospitals are disproportionately involved in caring for patients with chronic illness, the cost per patient is generally less than in private hospitals, where patient illnesses are more acute and staff:patient ratios are higher because therapeutic efforts are more intense.

In fact, private hospitals exist largely to allow private sector psychiatrists, private sector clinics (such as HMOs), and in many cases "teaching" institutions to care for their patients when they require hospitalization. Such patients are usually well insured under individual or group health plans. (I should note here that many private hospitals devote a larger or smaller portion of their beds to public care.) Public hospitals, by contrast, exist largely to care for patients who cannot afford private care because they are either uninsured or inadequately insured. The same paradigm holds true for private versus public day care and extended-care facilities of all kinds. Thus, the "senile" patient who can afford private care will be placed in a private nursing home—until he or his family runs out of money. The "senile" person who canot afford private care will be placed in a public facility of some kind.

I believe that under NHI, the utilization of private inpatient care is likely to increase and the utilization of public inpatient care is likely to decrease in direct proportion to the extent persons are entitled to private-based mental health inpatient care (in hospitals or extended-care facilities). This model should hold true for all kinds of medical care in addition to mental health care, but of course, the model will be valid only so far as the individual patient perceives private-based care to be "better" than public-based care.

Some additional comments are warranted here on the cost and quality of care delivered in private and public hospitals (or in extended-care facilities). Although private psychiatric hospitals are generally more costly than public hospitals (with the exception of some public hospitals that function as teaching hospitals), this does not by any means constitute an indictment of private hospitals. Probably the major reason that the cost of care is less in public hospitals than in private hospitals is that professional staff levels are much lower in public hospitals. Indeed, it is questionable at best whether proper and effective care can be delivered in many public hospitals, given their extremely low staff levels. VA psychiatric hospitals have been severely criticized in this connection. The NAS found that in many VA hospitals, the staffing levels were so low as to prohibit virtually any mental health care and to permit only custodial care.[14] Such a serious finding by the NAS leads one to question the quality of care generally delivered in public hospitals. In fact, many public hospitals have probably not functioned at an adequate level over the past decade in terms of providing high-quality mental health care to the majority of their patients. Strictly speaking, this has not been their "fault" in most cases but rather has resulted from the great political pressures operating on them not only to reduce their patient censuses but to put themselves out of operation. The result has been a high flow of patients out of the public hospital and into the community, where they reside in relative or total anonymity, too often completely out of contact with any mental health care delivery system—or at best marginally in touch with one. Unfortunately, many of these patients were probably better served in the hospitals from which they were discharged—where at least they received adequate food, clothing, shelter, and protection, as well as minimal mental health care.

It is interesting to hypothesize why there is often a discrepancy between the professional staff levels (psychiatrists, psychologists, social workers, nurses, etc.) employed at private versus public hospitals—beyond that which can be accounted for by differences in patient populations. If anything, it would seem that a private nonprofit or a private for-profit hospital would tend to keep its professional staff levels down so as to reduce its operating costs. Apparently, though, minimizing professional staff levels is more of a concern within the public hospital system. The private hospital may have more financial leeway to maintain appropriate professional staff levels. This leads to the conclusion that public mental health care facilities need to be monitored, in terms of the quality of care they deliver, as much as, if not more than, private facilities. It seems that in the former, financial concerns and economic pressures may jeopardize patient care even more than in the latter.

In the final analysis, the cost of patient care in private hospitals may be more expensive than in public hospitals, but private care probably also equates with better care for most patients (unless the public hospital is a teaching hospital). Under NHI, funding of public hospitals will have to increase from present levels if these hospitals are to provide responsible patient care. (Their funding should be increased *now* if we are seriously concerned about providing public sector patients with responsible inpatient care.) Consequently, the cost differential currently observed between private and public hospitals will decrease under NHI. Finally, I would note that the majority of public funds devoted to mental health care are spent on inpatient care.[8] Due to the high cost of hospital care, it is important that at the same time as we provide public hospitals with adequate funds to meet their clinical responsibilities to their patients, we should embark upon a major program to provide alternatives to hospitalization (and hospital-based care) for the public hospital patient population, as well as for patients of private hospitals. Such alternatives, including outpatient care, day care, and halfway-house care, are less expensive on a unit basis than is hospital care and constitute appropriate care for many current inpatients who, as I have noted, do not require hospital care. Still, I must caution that if we are to provide hospital patients with alternatives to hospital care, these alternatives must be real; they must afford the patient complete and appropriate mental health care, and to do so, they must be well funded. In all good conscience, we can no longer deprive patients of hospital care on the basis of an empty and false promise that we will meet their mental health care needs with community-based care that is in reality nonexistent.

5.3. The Cost of Outpatient Private Care

As we have seen, private-based mental health care, especially that delivered by the private practitioner, differs from public-based mental health care in terms of actual treatment services provided and general orientation toward treatment, both being largely a function of economic incentives and disincentives operating on the respective sectors. In any case, for those health planners and legislators who would limit private-based mental health care under NHI, the key issue is the cost of such care. Ultimately, it would seem that their concern is not whether private-based care (mainly as delivered by the private practitioner) is better or worse than care delivered by the public sector; ultimately, their concern centers around whether or not the nation can afford to sponsor private-based mental health care. This is a most legitimate focus that cannot be ignored, although it should not be paramount or exclusive. It should not, as I have warned, obscure the differences between private and public care. Concerns over the costs of private versus public care must be balanced by careful consideration of the qualitative differences in the care provided in the two sectors.

In terms of cost alone, there are copious data to suggest that unlimited private-based mental health care is indeed affordable under NHI, that it will not "run away with itself" and precipitate financial disaster. Note, for exam-

Table 3. Federal Employee Health Benefit Program Blue Cross and Blue Shield: High Option
Covered Persons with Physicians' Charges for Outpatient Care of Mental Disorders under Supplemental Benefits: Distribution of Persons and Their Covered Charges by Expenses Incurred and Year, United States, 1971–1973[a]

Expenses (dollars)	1973			
	Persons		Covered charges	
	Number	Percent	Amount	Percent
Under 1,000	22,634	78.1	$6,685,580	30.3
1,000–1,999	3,694	12.8	5,161,024	23.8
2,000–3,999	1,772	6.1	4,946,042	22.8
4,000–5,999	547	1.9	2,668,491	12.3
6,000–9,999	315	1.1	2,212,239	10.2
10,000–14,999	2	0.2	21,159	0.1
15,000–19,999	—	—	—	—
20,000 or over	—	—	—	—

[a] Source: Blue Cross and Blue Shield: Federal Employee Health Benefit Program. Adapted from Appendix Table 3, *Draft Report* (see reference 4).

ple, the statistics I previously quoted regarding average patient visits to psychiatrists in private practice: 38 visits per annum excluding psychoanalysts, 47 including them.*[18]

To give further credence to the argument that we should provide unlimited coverage for private-based outpatient mental health care under NHI (or under existing health insurance programs), let us look at what happens when a population is allowed such coverage. Let us examine nationwide statistics[4] (see Table 3) as regards visits to private psychiatrists under the Blue Cross/Blue Shield Federal Employee Health Benefits (BCBS FEHB) High Option Plan, a plan that, at the time the statistics were tabulated, allowed the patient essentially unlimited treatment visits to private practitioners of mental health care since the insurance covered 80% of the cost of treatment after an annual $100 deductible fee (for *all* outpatient medical care) was paid by the patient. (As of January 1981, the BCBS FEHB plan changed its coverage of mental health care to reimburse the patient for 70% of the cost of his treatment after he had paid an annual deductible fee of $150. See footnote on p. 5.)

*Quoting "average numbers" and "mean numbers" of patient visits to psychiatrists (or to other MHPs) is revealing, but it may not portray a totally accurate picture of utilization of mental health care services by the individual patient. For example, if a psychiatrist sees 5 patients for 5 visits and 5 patients for 100 visits, the "average" number of visits per patient is 52.5 visits, which is obviously a distortion of the distribution of treatment. Similarly, the "mean number" of patient visits in this sample could be construed to be "5" if patient visits were tabulated by groups of "5 or less visits" and "more than 5 visits."

In 1973, under the BCBS FEHB high option plan, a total of only 29,000 persons (0.63% of all enrollees) sought outpatient treatment from private sector psychiatrists (or infrequently from nonpsychiatrist physicians), a surprisingly low figure considering the number of covered persons, the extremely broad coverage, and the minimal expense to the patient.* When we examine this patient group in greater detail, we see that 22,600 persons, or 78% of the 29,000-person cohort—by far the vast majority—incurred total treatment costs (charges covered by the insurance) of less than $1000. This amounts to only 20–30 physician visits or fewer per year for those persons receiving the full $1000 reimbursement. Furthermore, of the 29,000-person cohort, 26,300 persons, or 91% of all persons receiving treatment, incurred treatment costs of $2000 or less, equivalent to 50–60 visits per annum for those persons receiving the maximum reimbursement. Thus, it would appear that under a privately sponsored health insurance plan offering very inclusive, essentially unlimited coverage for private-based outpatient psychiatric treatment, the vast majority of patients who utilize the coverage are seen in treatment relatively few times in any given year.

To complement the data presented above and bring them up to date, let us look at results of the "Mental and Nervous Disorder Utilization and Cost Survey" (MANDUCS), which tabulated the utilization of and the costs for outpatient mental health care under the Blue Cross/Blue Shield Federal Employee program in 1977 in the Washington, D.C. area.[24] The MANDUCS for the plan studied revealed (see Table 4) that the average number of treatment visits per individual person receiving outpatient mental health care (1977) was 32.7; the median number of visits per individual treated person was 19.5. In terms of cost of treatment, the MANDUCS revealed $1299 average dollars claimed per individual person receiving treatment; the average dollars per visit claimed were $40. The MANDUCS also illustrated (see Tables 5 and 6) that 63.4% of all patients making claims for outpatient mental health care in 1977 were seen in treatment for 30 or fewer visits. Further, 80% of all patients making such claims were seen for 50 or fewer visits. These data are consistent with the previous experience of the BCBS FEHB plan as illustrated by the 1973 data presented above. The data confirm the contention that the vast majority of patients who utilize outpatient mental health care in the private sector are seen in treatment relatively few times per year—considering the nature of mental health care and the potential for high-intensity utilization. I should also point out that if we divide the total cost for outpatient mental health care as determined by the MANDUCS survey by the total number of persons enrolled in the plan studied by that survey (including those who did and did not utilize outpatient mental health care), it is determined that the cost per

*Any initial deductible fee and any requirement of a copayment by the patient can cause many persons not to seek treatment or to settle for minimum treatment. These costs can be financially prohibitive for many persons, even if they seem small in amount. Thus, BCBS FEHB plan data on the utilization and cost of psychiatric outpatient treatment as well as on the numbers of persons seeking such treatment may be skewed toward the low side.

Table 4. MANDUC Survey Data on the Utilization and Cost of Outpatient Services for Mental Disorders for 15,484 Individuals in 1977, by Type of Provider[a]

Measures of utilization and cost[b]	Board-eligible psychiatrists	Clinical psychologists	Psychiatric social workers	Psychiatric nurses	Nonpsychiatric physicians	All providers[b]
Individuals						
Number	11,232	3,760	2,459	126	91	15,484[c]
Percent	72.5	24.3	15.9	0.8	0.6	100[c]
Total visits	352,303	93,155	58,713	1,376	904	506,451
Average number of visits per individual	31.4	24.8	23.9	10.9	9.9	32.7
Median number of visits per individual	15.9	15.4	14.7	6.8	6.2	19.5
Total dollars claimed	14,788,492	3,504,803	1,760,327	27,861	33,826	20,115,309
Percent of total dollars claimed	73.5	17.4	8.8	0.1	0.2	100
Average dollars per individual claimed	1,317	932	716	221	372	1,299
Average dollars per visit claimed	42	38	30	20	37	40

[a] From Towery et al., reference 24.
[b] The first column and the last column list the data specifically referred to in the text.
[c] Not a row sum because some individuals were seen by more than one type of provider.

Table 5. MANDUC Survey Data on the Cumulative Percent of 15,484 Individuals with a Specified Number of Visits to Various Types of Providers in 1977

	Percent of individuals					
Number of visits	Board-eligible psychiatrists	Clinical psychologists	Psychiatric social workers	Psychiatric nurses	Nonpsychiatric physicians	All providers
1–5	24.7	21.9	20.0	42.9	44.0	17.0
1–10	39.0	37.2	37.1	66.7	72.5	31.5
1–20	55.9	57.8	60.3	87.3	86.8	50.8
1–30	66.2	70.9	75.1	92.1	92.3	63.4
1–40	74.9	80.3	84.3	96.8	96.7	73.4
1–50	80.5	87.4	89.0	98.4	97.8	80.2
1–60	83.9	90.5	91.5	98.4	100.0	84.0
1–80	89.6	95.1	95.4	99.2	100.0	90.2
1–100	93.5	98.1	98.0	100.0	100.0	94.2
1–150	97.4	99.7	99.3	100.0	100.0	97.8
1–200	99.5	99.9	99.7	100.0	100.0	99.6
1–200+	100.0	100.0	100.0	100.0	100.0	100.0

Table 6. MANDUC Survey Data on the Cumulative Percent of Dollars Claimed by 15,484 Individuals with a Specified Number of Visits to Various Types of Providers in 1977[a,b]

	Percent of dollars claimed					
Number of visits	Board-eligible psychiatrists	Clinical psychologists	Psychiatric social workers	Psychiatric nurses	Nonpsychiatric physicians	All providers
1–5	2.1	3.5	2.5	12.4	13.7	1.7
1–10	5.8	8.5	8.3	29.9	36.2	5.4
1–20	14.0	21.5	23.1	57.3	57.1	14.4
1–30	22.3	34.6	38.8	67.9	68.3	23.9
1–40	31.9	48.3	52.1	86.3	82.6	34.4
1–50	39.9	60.7	60.9	93.3	88.1	43.6
1–60	45.6	67.4	66.7	93.3	100.0	49.9
1–80	58.3	80.2	77.7	96.1	100.0	62.7
1–100	68.6	90.6	87.4	100.0	100.0	73.3
1–150	84.3	97.7	93.8	100.0	100.0	87.3
1–200	96.3	99.5	97.1	100.0	100.0	96.9
1–200+	100.0	100.0	100.0	100.0	100.0	100.0

[a] From Towery et al., reference 24.
[b] As is evident from Table 5, approximately 50% of all persons receiving treatment were seen for 20 visits (treatment sessions) or less, equivalent at the maximum to approximately 1 visit every other week. Approximately 80% of all persons receiving treatment were seen for 50 visits or less, equivalent at the maximum to approximately 1 visit per week. Such persons, as can be seen from Table 6, accounted for 43.6% of the cost of all treatment tabulated under the MANDUCS. It is noteworthy that approximately 6% of persons receiving treatment were seen for more than 100 visits, and this group accounted for over 25% of the cost of all treatment tabulated under the MANDUCS. The overall pattern of utilization of outpatient mental health care seen here confirms the data from other studies cited in the text and reemphasizes their implication: namely, outpatient mental health care (psychotherapy) seems to be a self-limiting process for most patients (clients), but a relatively small percentage of patients, most of whom we can assume are engaged in psychoanalysis (and some in intensive psychotherapy), account for a disproportionate degree of the cost of such care.

enrollee for outpatient mental health care is $26.50. (This figure includes charges for services provided by psychiatrists, clinical psychologists, psychiatric social workers, psychiatric nurses, and nonpsychiatric physicians for outpatient mental health care.) The average cost of outpatient mental health care per enrollee as reported for 1977 in the MANDUCS is higher than that reported in other studies. This may be largely accounted for by the fact that the MANDUCS, as stated, reports on utilization rates in the Washington, D.C., area only, which, because of the relatively high socioeconomic status of the insured population and the extremely high density of mental health professionals in the area, can be expected to be at a peak.[24] The 1977 MANDUCS data also reflect the fact that in 1975 there were severe cutbacks in mental health care benefits afforded by non-BCBS federal employee health insurance programs. These cutbacks were immediately followed by the transfer of many government employees into the BCBS FEHB plan. (Presumably, many of these persons were already utilizing or anticipated a need to utilize outpatient mental health care benefits and switched from one program into the other in order to be eligible for such benefits.) This resulted in a higher utilization rate of outpatient mental health care benefits for the BCBS FEHB plan than in previous years. The MANDUCS data, in sum, reveal a higher utilization rate of outpatient mental health care services and a higher cost for these services than one would encounter in an average population.

I should emphasize that the various sets of data regarding the utilization and cost of outpatient mental health care benefits often differ profoundly from one another, based upon the specific population being studied or the mental health benefits afforded by a particular insurance program or both. For example, a recent study[25] reports on the nationwide total of all benefits paid in 1977 for outpatient mental health care (psychiatrists' services) under the BCBS FEHB high option plan. The cost of such benefits in 1977, according to this study, amounted to only $7.93 per person enrolled in the plan (cost per enrollee), demonstrating once again that the cost of outpatient mental health care spread over the population at risk is extremely small. In 1973 the corresponding figure, as reported in the same study, was $4.81. In terms of "constant dollars" (dollars adjusted for the increase in cost of physician services; 1978 = 100%), the 1973 figure calculates to be $7.75. It is important to note that the data just cited refer to the BCBS FEHB *high option plan*. This plan does not portray a true picture of the cost of outpatient mental health care (psychiatrists' services). This is because the plan offers the most comprehensive mental health benefits of any insurance plans available to the federal employee. Therefore, as mentioned in terms of the MANDUCS, an employee anticipating the need for mental health care, or already receiving mental health care, is likely to transfer into the BEBS FEHB high option plan (which he can do without restriction at designated times of the year). Thus, let us examine the combined cost of all benefits paid for outpatient mental health care (psychiatrists' services) under eight health insurance plans that enroll approximately two-thirds of all federal employees.[25] In 1978 such benefits amounted to only $8.35 per person enrolled in these plans—in contrast to $5.07 in 1973. In terms of constant dollars, the 1973 figure equals only $8.17. It can be seen that between 1973 and 1978 the cost per enrollee of outpatient mental health care increased only 2.2%.*

It appears, therefore, that the cost of outpatient mental health care in the private sector is both affordable and containable. This would seem to hold true in terms of all the separate studies reported on above. Nevertheless, the data I have presented here should not obscure the fact that as mental health care is recognized by both patient and physician as a "legitimate" and "acceptable" form of health care, the utilization of mental health care benefits will most likely increase. The increase will be even greater if we expand the base of providers of mental health care to include various categories of "psychotherapists" whose clients are not now eligible for reimbursement under most health insurance plans. (Insurance plans today mainly cover the services of psychiatrists, in some cases clinical psychologists (Ph.D.s), and in even fewer cases social workers (M.S.W.s). We certainly need to utilize the skills of such psychotherapists—fully trained and qualified; we need to employ them in an appropriate capacity within the mental health care delivery system. Exactly how they should function and how they should be reimbursed for their services under NHI (and under present health insurance programs, for

---

*There is some debate as to this point. John Krizay, in an article published in the American Psychiatric Association's *Psychiatric News* 16, no. 18 (September 18, 1981) after the completion of my paper, notes, "It has frequently been argued that its broad coverage of treatment of mental and nervous disorders has attracted psychiatric users to Blue Cross-Blue Shield, while non-users have tended to leave Blue Cross-Blue Shield for less expensive plans offering more limited coverage of mental and nervous disorders. Neither the data presented here, nor earlier studies regarding psychiatric utilization by new Blue Cross-Blue Shield enrollees support such an argument. That the new enrollees who have been attracted to the minor plans evidently include many users of psychiatric services suggests that the Blues' more liberal psychiatric coverage has not been a major factor in the decision of those joining less expensive plans in recent years. These data, combined with previous studies showing that only a small percentage of new enrollees in Blue Cross-Blue Shield file claims for mental and nervous disorders, indicate that psychiatric coverage itself is probably a secondary consideration in accounting for the sizeable shifts in enrollment during recent open seasons."

Obviously, there are many reasons why subscribers shift from one health insurance plan to another. Of course, various benefits must be balanced against cost and the anticipated use of particular benefits. I would only point out that a person who is receiving mental health care on a very limited basis under the BCBS FEHB high option plan may well transfer into a minor and less expensive (as compared to the BCBS) plan under the following conditions: (1) Mental health care benefits under the minor plan are sufficient to cover the person's treatment needs, and at the same time, the premiums are less expensive; or (2) the savings in premiums from switching to a minor plan are in excess of the anticipated out-of-pocket dollars a person will have to spend on mental health care, i.e., care beyond that which the minor plan covers. As regards a person switching into the BCBS plan from a minor plan, it seems to me that if the mental health care benefits to be received and subsequently used by joining the BCBS plan far outweigh the additional cost of joining, a person will strongly consider transferring into that plan.

This particular discussion might be moot by the time of publication of this paper (see footnote on p. 5). Nevertheless, it would seem relevant on a general basis as regards the role of mental health care benefits as a factor in a person's choice of health insurance plans.

that matter) are questions we must answer with respect to both the demand and the cost for their services. (See Section 5.4 for an expanded discussion of the manpower issue in mental health care.)

Despite the fact that private-based outpatient mental health care seems affordable on the broader scale, we cannot call for unlimited coverage for such care under NHI without examining the cost of psychoanalysis, a generally open-ended form of treatment that much of the public erroneously considers typical of psychiatric care. Psychoanalytic treatment of mental illness/emotional problems is in the distinct minority; however, when employed, it is expensive. Additional data from the BCBS FEHB insurance plan for 1973 reveals that only 2% of the nationwide population receiving outpatient treatment for "mental disorders" incurred covered treatment charges of greater than $5000 per year.[18] However, this group of patients, most of whom we can assume were receiving psychoanalytic treatment, accounted for 17% of all outpatient psychiatric benefits paid out under the BCBS FEHB plan in 1973.[18] (This uneven cost distribution is confirmed for 1977 by the MANDUCS reported on above. See Tables 5 and 6, and the note to Table 6.) With regard to this finding, Judd Marmor, M.D., a prominent psychoanalyst and a past president of the American Psychiatric Association, has stated that "a heavy burden of responsibility rests on the advocates of such therapy [psychoanalysis] to justify so disproportionate a cost."[18] (Of course, any diagnostic or therapeutic medical care for any condition must be justified in terms of the benefit to the patient's health. Especially if it is expensive care, it must be shown to yield particular benefits to the patient that cannot be achieved through another method at a lesser cost. Again, mental health care must not be singled out for fiscal monitoring.)

Indeed, for the patients of psychoanalyst psychiatrists, the average number of treatment visits is high—140 visits per patient per year.[18] In this connection, it is necessary to point out that the validity of classical psychoanalysis as a treatment as opposed to an investigative method is certainly open to question. Many psychiatrists disagree as to its value compared to other treatment methods. Dr. Marmor[18] makes the following comment:

> I personally have long been convinced that even in terms of analytic objectives, for most patients the crucial determinant is not so much how frequently they are seen, but over how long a period. Putting this another way, seeing patients psychotherapeutically once or twice a week over a period of several years, in my belief, will often achieve the same therapeutic results as seeing them three to five times a week over the same period. Why? One reason is that attempts to change the coping patterns and intrapsychic percepts of a lifetime usually take a certain time span to achieve, and daily or four to five times weekly therapeutic interventions do not necessarily hasten that learning process. Indeed, Franz Alexander and others have argued that sometimes a high frequency of visits may even be anti-therapeutic in that it tends to enhance the patient's dependence on the therapist.

Dr. Marmor goes on to say that "probably few psychiatrists doubt that there are at least some patients who by reason of their high anxiety level and intense symptomatic distress do indeed require frequent, even daily, therapeutic visits at least from time to time. . . . Certainly such treatment [psychoanalysis or intensive psychotherapy] ought not to be denied to any patient if it is truly essential to his health."[18]

Dr. Marmor's remarks are to the point: NHI (and existing health insurance programs) must not discriminate against psychoanalysis or intensive psychotherapy *de novo*. (Such treatment has been unfairly scapegoated in the past.) However, psychiatrists themselves must develop the strictest peer review methods to insure that when psychoanalysis is the employed treatment method, there is no other treatment that is equally effective for the individual patient and less costly to both the patient and the insurance program that is sponsoring his care. (Obviously, peer review should not be limited to psychoanalysis. As I have stated elsewhere, it should be an instrument of oversight for all mental health care and for all medical-surgical care.)If a patient wishes to pursue psychoanalysis on an optional basis, then he should be expected to defray a fair portion of the cost of his treatment. However, to reemphasize: There will always be persons who will require long-term, costly treatment for mental illness/emotional problems—just as many medical-surgical patients will require long-term, costly treatment for their illnesses. NHI must not penalize these persons—any more than it should penalize medical-surgical patients. Outpatient mental health care, including psychoanalysis and intensive psychotherapy, must be made available under NHI (and under existing health insurance programs) strictly in accordance with what is medically appropriate.

I should add that in terms of the provision of long-term treatment, the psychoanalyst, in view of the extreme cost of his method, does have a special responsibility to show that the particular treatment he offers is more efficacious than other less costly modalities of long-term treatment. (No school of psychiatry should ever be averse to any legitimate professional debate of its treatment methods. Such debate, carried out with integrity and with a spirit of enlightenment, can only enhance the methods of mental health care.) This applies especially to the psychoanalyst who practices "classical, traditional" psychoanalysis, often involving four to five therapeutic sessions per week over a period of 4 to 6 years or longer. Indeed, I believe it is highly possible, if not probable, that in terms of long-term treatment, intensive psychotherapy may be more effective than psychoanalysis *per se*—in addition to being less expensive. In fact, both the terms *psychoanalysis* and *intensive psychotherapy* are in my opinion indistinct and at times confusing. In many respects, it is difficult to define the borderline between these treatments, especially when "intensive psychotherapy" follows a psychoanalytic orientation. Although the styles of these treatments may be quite divergent, their goals are often similar—namely, to effect *broad, comprehensive changes* in a person's manner or style of coping. (Many psychoanalysts would disagree with me on this point; they would claim that "the non-analyst is generally concerned, at least initially, with relieving symptoms and restoring homeostasis, while the analyst usually aims at modifying basic coping techniques and self-esteem."[18] I would note that the nonanalyst is more frequently, rather than less frequently, concerned with "modifying basic coping techniques and self-esteem.")

Space does not permit me to comment extensively here on the technical differences between psychoanalysis and intensive psychotherapy. In general, though, it can be stated that intensive psychotherapy employs a wide and flexible spectrum of treatment modalities. It applies many of the principles of psychoanalysis but features a reduced number of treatment sessions per week (usually one to three) and focuses on concluding treatment in a much shorter period of time (usually 1 to 3 years) for most patients. It incorporates non-analytic techniques to accelerate the treatment process. Where psycho-analysis is often a passive, time-unlimited process, intensive psychotherapy is more "active." It recognizes and is responsive to both the temporal and fiscal constraints that most patients face. In fact, many psychoanalysts now favor a clinical approach to the patient that departs from "classical, tradi-tional" psychoanalysis and begins to resemble intensive psychotherapy in certain respects. Among other things, they agree with their non-psychoanalyst colleagues that treatment can and should be speeded up. (For purposes of our discussion, we can very roughly define "classical, traditional psychoanalysis" as psychoanalysis practiced strictly in terms of the tech-niques and metapsychology developed by Sigmund Freud. Even here, though, it must be realized that some latter day "Freudian psychoanalysts" interpret and practice the Freudian psychology more strictly than did Freud himself. It must also be noted that there are many schools of psychoanalysis and that psychoanalytic theory can vary tremendously from one school to the other. Also, psychoanalytic theory is changing and evolving—to differing degrees, depending upon the particular school of psychoanalysis.)

In "analyzing" and evaluating psychoanalysis as a specific treatment technique, it must be remembered that many practitioners of psychoanalysis were trained 20 or 30 years ago (or more), when the wide variety of psycho-therapeutic tools now available to the practitioner were not yet developed. Many psychoanalysts still adhere to older treatment philosophies, in many cases exclusively applying the principles of "classical, traditional" psycho-analytic theory to their practice. On the other hand, the nonpsychoanalyst practitioner, in my opinion, has successfully incorporated and applied to his practice new techniques and treatment modalities as they have become avail-able—for example, he employs conjoint (marital), family, and group therapies, as appropriate and necessary, in the treatment of his patients. He also utilizes psychotropic medication in their treatment. It is true, in this connection, that some psychiatrists overprescribe such medication for their patients. On the other hand, only 14% of psychoanalysts, according to one large survey,[18] prescribe psychotropic medication for those persons they treat on an outpatient basis, even as an adjunct to psychoanalytic treatment. (None of the psychoanalysts employed electroshock therapy.) Such a philosophy

toward treatment, outdated in my opinion, results in an unnecessary prolongation of treatment for many persons who are undergoing psychoanalysis.
(By contrast, the nonpsychoanalyst psychiatrist prescribes psychotropic medication for 29% of his outpatients.)[18] Similarly, the practitioner of psychoanalysis is often reluctant to employ family therapy in order to involve the
patient's family in the patient's treatment. When the patient's primary problem involves marital or family discord, the psychoanalyst's refusal to involve
the spouse or family in the treatment process (at a minimum to facilitate
evaluation of the patient) will often result not only in prolonged treatment but
in ineffective treatment as well. Many psychoanalysts are also hesitant to
employ "group therapy" as an ancillary treatment for their patients. In fact,
group therapy, when it is appropriately employed, can complement and facilitate individual treatment as well as shorten the treatment process.

Of course, group therapy, family therapy, conjoint (marital) therapy, and
all treatment modalities, for that matter, have definite and specific limitations.
They can be easily misapplied. However, psychoanalysts in the same survey
reported on above[18] utilized group, family, and/or conjoint (marital) therapy
for only 2% of those persons they treated on an outpatient basis. In spite of
the fact that the goals of psychoanalytic treatment (and intensive psychotherapy) are often quite distinct from the goals of shorter forms of psychotherapy, this represents a severe underutilization of these specific treatment
techniques. Let me be quick to point out, however, that nonpsychoanalyst
psychiatrists also underemploy group, family, and conjoint (marital) therapy.
Only 8% did so for their outpatients in the aforementioned study.[18] (I believe
this figure is very much on the low side. It may be accounted for by the fact
that many patients of the nonpsychoanalyst psychiatrist are seen for only
brief evaluation and/or treatment or for "medication visits"—renewal of pre-
scriptions for psychotropic medication.) The use of these therapy methods
must be increased. In this connection, Marmor[18] points out:

> As we move towards a system of national health insurance with its inevitable focus
> on cost-benefits, it may well be that the system itself will put continuous pressure
> on psychiatrists to make greater and greater use of . . . less expensive (on a unit
> basis) and often more efficient techniques. It is strongly to be hoped that the mem-
> bers of our profession will be able to meet this challenge and loosen their current
> overdependence on the traditional one-to-one therapeutic model. . . . I am not
> implying by this that individual psychotherapy will or should disappear—I believe
> it will always be the cornerstone of psychiatric practice—but . . . technical flexibility
> will have to be the keynote of the future in our field.

I concur strongly with Dr. Marmor's remarks and emphasize the extreme
and often exclusive importance of individual psychotherapy as a specific
treatment technique. Virtually all patients who suffer mental illness/emo-
tional problems will require some and usually a substantial amount of individual psychotherapy. The psychiatrist, of course, must never shortchange
the patient by utilizing an inappropriate treatment technique so as to reduce
the cost of care. He must utilize individual psychotherapy as necessary and

appropriate for his patient. However, the psychiatrist must not "longchange" the patient either. He has a responsibility to utilize the treatment method that is most beneficial, but he also has a responsibility to be aware at all times of the cost of treatment so as to effect the best possible care for the patient at the least possible expense.

It must be emphasized that we can probably never establish absolute standards, rules, or regulations for treating a particular patient—whether the patient suffers from mental illness/emotional problems or any medical-surgical illness/problem. Indeed, the practice of both medical-surgical care and mental health care involves as much art as science. Any standards, rules, or regulations established with regard to either medical-surgical care or mental health care must not unduly confine the practitioner in terms of his ability to design and implement a unique treatment plan for each individual patient (client). Nevertheless, the psychiatrist and other physicians can take a more definite stand in terms of advocating treatment forms for their own specialties that are medically as well as fiscally responsible.* In this connection, the American Psychiatric Association (APA), through its Commission on Psychiatric Therapies (established 1977), has embarked upon a major review and evalua-

---

*It is my understanding that under the American Psychiatric Association's (APA's) peer review program, practiced in conjunction with case review by one large insurance company, preferential treatment is essentially given to psychoanalysts—as opposed to nonpsychoanalyst psychiatrists—in terms of review of psychoanalysts' long-term intensive outpatient treatment cases. Specifically, the patient cases of the psychoanalyst are often reviewed at greater time intervals than are the cases of the nonpsychoanalyst psychiatrist. Further, the patient of the psychoanalyst is often allowed more "visits" between reviews than is the patient of the nonpsychoanalyst psychiatrist. (It should be noted that it is ultimately up to the insurance company and not the APA peer reviewers to decide when a particular patient's care should be reviewed, how often it should be reviewed, and whether or not the patient should be allowed to continue his treatment. However, the insurance company often bases its decisions in these respects at least partially on the recommendations of the APA peer review process.)

In the first place, the policy I have just described discriminates against nonpsychoanalyst psychiatrists. In the second place, it is an extremely costly policy since it gives special privileges to psychoanalysis—the most expensive and often the least effective (in my opinion) of all long-term intensive outpatient treatments (because, in part, the psychoanalyst, when he practices in the classical manner at least, does not utilize the multimodal approach to the patient, including the use of medication, that is available to and often used by the practitioner of intensive psychotherapy). Patient cases of all psychiatrists, including psychoanalysts, should be reviewed by type of case, not treatment, at the same frequency, and reviews should be governed by the same constraints. In other words, the frequency of peer review should depend upon the type and level of the patient's (client's) pathology, not the specific kind of treatment he or she is receiving. Peer review should measure the patient's progress, no matter what system of treatment is being employed on his behalf. The APA and insurance companies make a mistake, I think, by effectively accommodating any subgroup of practitioners of mental health care—not to suggest that this is done intentionally. In the specific instance of psychoanalysis, the current peer review policy tends to promote extremely expensive care. Finally, I shall add that the APA's peer review policy for cases of psychoanalysis is designed in theory to disallow the unnecessary utilization of psychoanalysis. Even though the policy is flawed in design, the APA is to be commended for this effort.

tion of the various psychotherapies. According to the *American Psychiatric Association Operations Manual* (1980),[26]

> This Commission is to review the somatic, dyadic, group, familial and social therapies in current use by a thorough and critical examination of the literature (including reports of other APA components), as to techniques, duration, results, costs, and other characteristics; to correlate and analyze the findings for the purpose of eliciting the common vectors that are therapeutically effective as distinquished from procedures that are extraneous or counterproductive. The Commission will be naming therapies, describing therapies, evaluating outcome data, collecting data, interviewing patients and therapists, observing therapists, etc. When the largest common denominator is found, all material will be integrated for use in recommending standards and evaluating approaches.

In addition, the Commission on Psychiatric Therapies is in the process of preparing the *Psychiatric Treatment Manual I* (PTM-I). This manual, scheduled for completion circa 1985, will set forth the best and preferred courses and modes of treatment for the various diagnostic categories of mental illness/ emotional problems as delineated in the APA's *Diagnostic and Statistical Manual of Mental Disorders III* (DSM-III). It must be noted that the PTM-I will be an exceedingly difficult document to prepare because of the continuing controversy that exists regarding "the best" treatment for any given type of mental illness/emotional problem. Nevertheless, the APA's effort to compile PTM-I represents the most responsible approach to mental health care and should be emulated by other health care specialty organizations in terms of setting forth approaches to treatment for which the specialties they represent are responsible.*

Even before the publication of PTM-I, taking into account the current state of the art (science), organized psychiatry must be willing to air the possibility that psychoanalysis may be unnecessary, in addition to being cost-ineffective for many, but certainly not all, patients. To date, organized psychiatry has often chosen instead to present a "united view" regarding the viability of all forms of treatment methods currently practiced, including psychoanalysis. (Considering that a fair proportion of psychiatrists are psycho-

---

*With regard to the American Psychiatric Association's efforts to set standards for mental health care, it should be noted that since 1970 that organization, through specially constituted task forces, has issued 19 comprehensive, authoritative reports on psychiatric care and related issues. Many of these reports focus on the evaluation of specific therapeutic modalities and recommend, in many cases, guidelines for their usage. As examples of the broad scope of these reports, note the following: (1) Biofeedback (1981), (2) Tardive Dyskinesia (1980), (3) Electroconvulsive Therapy (1978), (4) Megavitamin and Orthomolecular Therapy in Psychiatry (1974), (5) Behavior Therapy in Psychiatry (1973), (6) Encounter Groups and Psychiatry (1970). Also, the APA frequently publishes in the *Journal of the American Psychiatric Association* major review articles on clinical topics. Of course, such articles (along with those appearing in other professional journals) do not offer formal diagnostic and therapeutic standards and guidelines, but they serve to establish informal standards and guidelines and to promote a recommended clinical approach to various categories of patients. They offer immense aid—if not a rigid protocol—to the individual practitioner in terms of helping him to establish his own regimen for the diagnosis and treatment of various conditions in accordance with state-of-the-art knowledge.

analysts, many of whom hold leading positions in organized psychiatry, this is not surprising.) Indeed, an open discussion by the psychiatric community of the merits of one form of psychiatric treatment versus another is imperative in order that appropriate treatment can be delineated. Under no circumstances can the psychiatrist—or any other physician—consider sacrificing quality of care to effect cost savings in care, but steps to reduce the cost of care without affecting the quality of care can and must be taken. With regard to long-term treatment such as psychoanalysis and intensive psychotherapy, this means an attempt must be made to set *general* standards regarding the optimal frequency of treatment sessions.

Here, though, it must be emphasized that treatment guidelines for mental health care are exceedingly difficult to set. The psychiatrist must proceed with extreme caution in formulating such guidelines. He must refuse to be rushed into setting standards or protocols for treatment that may or may not be valid. He must not promote treatment that yields a favorable result for the patient only in the short run and does not extend him meaningful and lasting benefits. Treatment guidelines for mental health care must be based upon long-term as well as short-term evaluation of treatment. (The evaluation of all medical care is based on longitudinal assessment that often extends to a decade or more.) The evaluation of the treatment of mental illness/emotional problems is highly complex; one cannot measure the success of such treatment merely by recording the patient's "happiness level" at the end of "x number" of treatment sessions. Mental health care, as is the case for all health care, must be evaluated beyond its capacity to provide symptom relief. It must be judged in terms of its effectiveness in resolving, or controlling as possible, underlying pathological processes operant in the patient. Because of the concrete (though by no means simplistic) nature of organic illness as manifested by physical signs and symptoms, it is much easier, as compared to mental health care, to determine how much medical-surgical treatment to deliver to a patient and when to interrupt or terminate such treatment. Mental health care, by contrast, must be judged in terms of an extremely wide and complicated set of psychological as opposed to physical measurements that can be exceedingly difficult to assess. It should also be noted that mental health care may (and often will) involve a temporary *increase* in the patient's (client's) level of symptoms. Further, this may last for a considerable period of time. This occurs because the patient, over the course of treatment, becomes conscious of the considerable underlying psychological conflicts that govern his total emotional state and his conduct of life. His awareness of these conflicts is likely to cause him considerable emotional pain—until he resolves or learns to control them. Of course, some medical - surgical care also involves a temporary increase in the patient's level of pain as a part of the treatment process. Surgery serves as an example.

The fact is that psychiatry today is in the midst of a profound state of change, which has repercussions for the evaluation of treatment methods and treatment results. It is difficult to formally define the best approach(es) to mental health care for various categories of patients because the proponents of various "psychological schools" often disagree with one another as regards general philosophy of treatment. Clearly, though, most psychiatrists would agree that mental health care is moving away from vague and interminable treatment of mental illness/emotional problems. The trend is toward shorter treatment for the majority of patients because of new treatment modalities and methods: for example, as I have previously specified, the use of psychotropic medication, involvement of family members in treatment, utilization of group psychotherapy, and conjoint (marital) psychotherapy. Freud himself anticipated such an evolution of mental health care—notably the evolution of the field of pharmacotherapy (the theory, science, and art of the utilization of psychotropic agents in the treatment of mental illness/emotional problems). In his last book, *An Outline of Psychoanalysis* (published posthumously in 1939), he stated, "The future may teach us how to exercise a direct influence, by means of particular chemical substances, upon the amounts of energy and their distribution in the apparatus of the mind [which, when "out of balance," Freud partially conceived of as the cause of mental symptoms]. It may be that there are other undreamt-of possibilities of therapy."[27]

In the near future, I believe, continuing research will lead to the development of even more effective psychotropic medicines and refinements in psychotherapy technique that will shorten treatment for many more patients. Long-term treatment is not now the rule, as evidenced by the data and statistics presented above.*

*In reviewing the cost and efficiency of insurance for mental health care in this section and other parts of my paper, I have attempted, by summarizing and analyzing certain key studies of health insurance, to demonstrate the feasibility of insuring mental health care and to debunk certain myths surrounding the insurance controversy over mental health care. Yet, although I have tried to show herein that mental health care can be fully insured on a cost-effective basis, and that it is practical as well as wise to insure mental health care, neither my White Paper, nor this book as a whole, has as its sole design or purpose to present a complete analysis of the complex intricacies involved in insuring mental health care—under NHI or under other insurance programs. Indeed, such an analysis would take a volume in itself. In any case, I have concerned myself in this paper as much with "why" mental health care should be insured as with "how" it can and should be insured.

For a concise, abbreviated analysis of the multiple factors involved in insuring mental health care, I refer the reader to an article published by Sharfstein and Taube after the completion of my paper. (Sharfstein SS, Taube CA: Reductions in insurance for mental disorders: adverse selection, moral hazard, and consumer demand. *Am J Psychiatry* 139: 1425–1430, 1982.)

Although I have already considered and discussed in my paper many of Sharfstein's and Taube's contentions, it would be useful here to highlight and comment upon several important points they make as regards the insurance of mental health care, especially outpatient mental health care.

1. Insurance programs (carriers) are generally averse to fully covering mental health care, especially outpatient mental health care, so long as mental health care is not considered a basic health care service. The assumption is that by fully covering mental health care, the insurance program (carrier) will "adversely select" (for subscribership) persons who suffer mental illness/emotional problems, thus making the program noncompetitive and

5.4. The Mental Health Professionals

The various mental health professionals view mental illness/emotional problems from different perspectives and approach mental health care from different bases. I shall discuss this below. However, I shall begin this section

---

even nonprofitable. (Of course, the same paradigm will hold true for any care that is not considered a basic health care service.)

2. Coverage for mental health care, especially unlimited outpatient mental health care, is seen by many health insurance carriers as a "moral hazard"—i.e., carriers see unlimited coverage for outpatient mental health care as granting the insuree the option of seeking mental health care not on the basis of his medical need for mental health care, but on his philosophical perception of the ultimate usefulness of such care to him. (The perception of the usefulness of mental health care by the insuree, insurers often contend, is not based on the insuree's concept of medical well-being, but rather on his concept of striving toward "self-actualization.") The assumption by insurers of health care here is that the utilization of "medical" care and the cost of treatment for "medical" illness is relatively constant, no matter what insurance a person has, but the utilization of mental health care, especially outpatient mental health care, and the subsequent cost of such care depends to a great extent on the whim, or more politely, preference for type and amount of care by both the recipient and the provider of mental health care. This is a false assumption. If unlimited care for many, if not most, medical conditions is available, both the recipient and the provider of care will often plan and utilize care in a different fashion than if only limited health care resources are available. Although "standard treatment" for many so-called "medical illnesses" is on the surface, at least, more objective than standard treatment for certain categories of mental illness/emotional problems (and there is no question that the psychiatrist must work diligently to objectify his treatment methods for any given mental illness/emotional problem), the physician who treats medical illness often has significant leeway in terms of the way he can manage his patient. For example, the physician often has the legitimate choice of treating his patient as an inpatient or outpatient, he (the physician) often has a legitimate choice in terms of the extent and frequency of tests he orders, and he oftentimes has a legitimate choice as well as to the specific treatment he employs (e.g., medical versus surgical management of the patient). There is a so-called "moral hazard" (I dislike the term) to most health care when such care is fully insured. The patient may request and be given too much care, he may have prescribed for him too much care without his requesting it, or he may receive too little care when the system under which he is "fully insured" overstrives to control costs. Further, there is a "moral hazard" involved in health care whenever a person is relatively health care uninsured. In such a case, a person may well deny himself appropriate health care no matter what illness he suffers from, including mental illness/emotional problems, on the basis that he must bear a small or large part of the cost of such care himself. In such a circumstance, can we say that a person is acting "immorally" toward himself? (Let us discard the use of the term "moral" as regards the utilization of health care and say, rather, that both the recipient and the provider of health care of all kinds have a responsibility to utilize appropriate amounts and types of health care whenever care is sought for any medical condition, including mental illness/emotional problems. The patient must receive "the most proper care" independent of the patient's financial access to care or the constraints, or lack thereof, placed on the physician by the provider system under which he operates.)

3. A small percentage of those persons who utilize mental health care, especially outpatient mental health care, account for a high percentage of the cost of such care. As Sharfstein

with a quotation[28] that focuses on one central issue (of many) that reflects a polarization of the therapeutic styles of the various MHPs and clearly divides them into separate classes of providers of mental health care.

> For twenty years there has been a tendency to consider pharmacotherapy and psychotherapy as antagonistic or competitive. There are many reasons for this. Among the most prominent are historical commitments to ideology; differences in

---

and Taube point out, this may well be the case, but the same situation holds true for other types of health care. Indeed, Sharfstein and Taube allude to studies that show that "the distribution in mental health (care costs) seems, if anything, to be less extreme" (than the distribution of health care costs in general.)

4. There is a lack of overt demand for mental health care on the part of health care consumers based on the reluctance of such consumers to "speak up" for such care and their lack of foresight in anticipating mental illness/emotional problems and the possible need for extensive mental health care. This influences the structuring of insurance plans by carriers. The implication here is that insurance carriers should structure their plans based not only on potential users' demands, but also on other factors. In other words, basic, if not extensive coverage for certain definable medical conditions, including mental illness/emotional problems, should always be included in insurance plans.

5. In connection with 4, the "Achilles' Heel" of the procompetitive approach to health insurance is that such an approach tends to select health insurance benefits on the basis of what are believed to be "popular benefits." As Sharfstein and Taube state, "the high risk or sick population finds it costly or impossible to purchase comprehensive coverage when insurers are competing on the basis of different levels of benefits." In relation to this phenomenon, since mental health care benefits, especially for outpatient care, are generally not now popular in the insurance population at large, these benefits tend to be "discriminated against" by insurance carriers even though, in the opinion of this author, they should be considered as basic as benefits for surgery. Mental health care should be considered as integral to the state of health of the individual person as any other form of usually covered health care. I hope, in presenting a philosophy of and an approach to mental health care for the future in my paper, that I have presented an adequate proof for this postulate.

6. Sharfstein and Taube state, "When psychotherapy is accessible and available, the poor make use of it with the same number of average visits as the rich." (In other words, it is a myth that psychotherapy is the "play-toy" of the well-to-do.) To dispute the notion that "for mental health care . . . health insurance represents 'a subsidy to the rich from the poor'," Sharfstein and Taube point out that "Public facilities, such as state hospitals and community mental health centers, serve the indigent disproportionately. If we take into account taxes paid and benefits received, these federal, state, and county programs redistribute . . . income toward the bottom of the socioeconomic ladder." One can hypothesize, therefore, that by instituting comprehensive coverage for mental health care, especially outpatient mental health care, in private insurance programs, we are providing mental health care benefits to those persons who can afford private coverage that the indigent are already in theory (and only in theory) eligible to receive. (As Sharfstein and Taube state, "Forty-two percent [of the cost of health care] is paid by federal, state, and local governments, . . . [while only] 26% [is paid] by private and other third-party insurance.") I make absolutely no pretense here that in most cases, the mental health care indigent persons receive is in reality equal in quantity or quality to the mental health care the generally more well-to-do person can avail himself of. Rather, my point is that the indigent, the wealthy, and the vast majority of persons in-between, should all have access to the highest quality mental health care.

theories of the etiology of mental illness; antiquated training which tends to per-
petuate ignorance of the principles, values and limitations of each form of treatment; differences in treatment goals; and legal restrictions on the use of drugs by
nonphysicians. The competition between psychotherapy and pharmacotherapy has
been attenuated in recent years because young psychiatrists, trained in both areas,
use both comfortably. . . .

Psychiatrists and nonpsychiatric physicians frequently prescribe psychotropic
drugs in an unthinking and unsystematic fashion without adequate follow-up,
safeguards or awareness of the hazards of behavioral toxicity. These drugs are
correctly used, underused, overused and misused.

Nonmedical mental health professionals, such as clinical psychologists and
social workers, have had no training in the indications for psychotropic drugs and
are legally restricted from using them. In consequence, they provide inappropriate
treatment for many of their patient-clients. This is also true for many psychiatrists
whose training did not include detailed instruction in the principles and practice of
psychopharmacology. Thus, older psychoanalytically trained psychiatrists tend to
view drugs with suspicion or alarm, while younger psychiatrists trained in both
forms of treatment frequently combine them, but without an adequate rationale.

The above quotation is taken from a report of the prestigious Group for
the Advancement of Psychiatry (GAP), *Pharmacotherapy and Psychotherapy:
Paradoxes, Problems and Progress*. The report was written in 1975 and therefore
does not take into account the advanced theoretical and practical training that
most psychiatrists now receive in the field of pharmacotherapy. I believe it
generally underestimates the psychiatrist's knowledge of the field and his
skill in prescribing psychotropic agents. Nevertheless, the quotation as a
whole defines certain "paradoxes" and "problems" that exist with regard to
mental health care delivery (as the title of the GAP report suggests). It also
correctly implies that every mental health professional, no matter what his
specialty, must carefully measure his professional "range"—i.e., he must
know when "to treat" and when "to refer" his patient (client) if he is to make
available responsible, balanced mental health care to every person who requires it. As such, the quotation serves as an insightful introduction to this
section of my paper.

In connection with point 6, above, I would note that in reality, the extent of utilization by a
patient (client) of outpatient mental health care (especially for nonacute conditions such as
"chronic symptomatic maladjustment"), provided open-ended resources are available to the
patient, will depend not on the socio-economic status of the patient so much as on his "psychological capacity." This is true because psychotherapy is to a great extent a method of treatment
that depends for its effectiveness on the communication of psychological concepts by the psychotherapist to his patient and the understanding of such concepts by the patient. Of course, the
extent of treatment a particular patient will require will also depend on how ill he is, how much
supportive care he requires, etc.

Finally, although I have based the points in this footnote and many of my corollary remarks
on the above cited paper by Sharfstein and Taube, I have also interpreted and expanded upon
their thesis here. The reader should not construe my remarks, for better or for worse, as an exact
replica of the meaning Sharfstein and Taube intended.

There has been much debate, extremely vitriolic at times, among the various mental health professionals on the very crucial and basic issue of who should treat persons who suffer from mental illness/emotional problems. Too often, psychiatrists, psychologists, and social workers, among others, have been at war with each other on this subject. To a great extent, this results from the fact that each professional group has a vested economic interest in being a self-advocate and advancing the special qualifications of its own lot. The current fighting among the groups is to a large extent a battle for the fee-basis dollars NHI (as well as current health insurance programs) will allow for mental health care services rendered by private providers. The strongest conflict exists between psychiatrists, represented by the American Psychiatric Association, and psychologists, represented by the American Psychological Association. Psychiatrists seek to limit the role of psychologists as providers, whereas psychologists essentially seek parity as providers of psychotherapy.* In fact, the question as to whether or not to limit outpatient visits to private sector mental health care practitioners under NHI might not arise if it were not for the existence of multiple professional groups "specializing" in mental health care, all adding to and forming a large provider pool. This situation, unique to our country, immensely complicates NHI financing. In Canada, for example, NHI provides for unlimited visits to psychiatrists practicing in the private sector, but there is a relatively small pool of non-M.D. mental health professionals providing mental health care in that sector.

---

*In what would appear to be a rather striking departure from the long-standing debate between the two, the American Psychiatric Association and the American Psychological Association (along with other groups) combined forces to present a united view in an April 4, 1979, letter to members of the U.S. Senate Finance Committee. This letter was in reference to various national health proposals before the committee, notably Senator Russell Long's (Democrat, Louisiana) bill for catastrophic national health insurance. In the letter, the two professional societies called for a broadening of the base of providers specified in Senator Long's bill to include, besides psychiatrists and other physicians, psychologists as independent providers of outpatient mental health care. In addition, the societies urged that nurses and social workers be included as providers with the provision that there be ongoing supervision of their work with patients by a physician. Besides the American Psychiatric Association and the American Psychological Association, the letter was signed and endorsed by the Association for the Advancement of Psychology, the Mental Health Association, the National Association of State Mental Health Program Directors, The National Council of Community Mental Health Centers, the National Association of Social Workers, and the American Mental Health Counselors Association.

Perhaps the above-mentioned letter signifies a genuine policy shift on the part of the American Psychiatric Association—namely, a positive attitude toward the inclusion of non-psychiatrists such as clinical psychologists as equal providers of outpatient mental health care under National Health Insurance. It remains to be seen whether this shall be the case and, if so, whether the majority of psychiatrists who make up the membership of the American Psychiatric Association will support this stance. Clearly, at the present time, debate continues between the American Psychiatric Association and the American Psychological Association (and others) as to who should be eligible under National Health Insurance and under existing insurance programs to receive independent reimbursement for the provision of mental health care on both an inpatient and an outpatient basis.

The fact is that no single professional group by itself can meet the treatment needs of all persons suffering mental illness/emotional problems. This is best illustrated by data the NIMH presented in a report to the United States Senate in June 1980.[29] The NIMH estimated in its report that there are currently about 29,000 practicing psychiatrists in the United States, of whom about 3000 specialize in child psychiatry. The number of full-time-equivalent (FTE) psychiatrists engaged in patient care was estimated to be less than 25,000. The NIMH further reported that in a sample of 1978 graduates of NIMH-supported psychiatric residency programs, "58% had their *principal employment* in organized care service settings (Community Mental Health Centers representing the largest component), only 10% were principally in private practice, and the remainder were pursuing advanced training in child psychiatry (11%) or were principally employed in medical schools or other academic settings (21%)." (From these data it would seem that the majority of psychiatrists are not primarily engaged in full-time private practice, where the cost of outpatient psychiatric care can be expected to be the greatest. Another source,[4] however, estimates that about 50% of psychiatrists practice their specialty in the private sector.) The NIMH remarked on the geographic distribution of psychiatrists in its report as well. It summarized 1974 data revealing that "the average number of FTE psychiatrists/100,000 catchment area population was 20.7 for urban mental health facilities as compared to only 4.0 for rural facilities." (Thus, it is evident that many areas of the country are poorly staffed by psychiatrists, if they are staffed at all.) Furthermore, the NIMH emphasized the decline in medical school graduates entering psychiatric training and the fact that of those physicians entering psychiatric residence training programs, foreign medical graduates are represented in highly disproportionate numbers. (In the 1974–1975 academic year, they constituted 39% of all first-year trainees.)

As far as nonpsychiatrist mental health professionals are concerned, the NIMH estimated that there are about 100,000 psychologists representing all fields of psychology at both master's and doctoral levels in the United States and that, of these, 26,000 at the doctoral level provide mental health care services (and are eligible for licensure for the independent practice of psychology). With regard to the work setting in which psychologists are employed, the NIMH stated that "among recent graduates of NIMH supported programs, 29.8% took positions in academic teaching or research settings; 62.3% in organized settings providing services, including the military; 2.7% entered private practice; and 3.7% continued training at the post doctoral level."

The NIMH also reported that in 1978 there were estimated to be about 80,000 master's level (M.S.W.) social workers in the United States. Of these, about 20,000 were identified as working in mental health facilities and programs, with others working in welfare or other human services agencies. Finally, the NIMH reported on numbers of "psychiatric nurses," defined as nurses holding a master's degree or above in psychiatric (mental health) nursing. According to the NIMH, nursing schools have graduated fewer than 9000 master's degree psychiatric nurses since 1950.

The NIMH concluded in its report that there is a clear and demonstrated need for increased numbers of psychiatrists, clinical psychologists (at the Ph.D. level), social workers (at the master's level—M.S.W.s), and "psychiatric nurses." The NIMH's conclusions are bolstered by a report of the Graduate Medical Education National Advisory Committee (GMENAC),[30] established by the Health Resources Administration, Department of Health and Human Services. In its report the GMENAC estimates that in 1990 there will be a need for 37,000 to 40,000 general psychiatrists and 8000 to 10,000 child psychiatrists. The GMENAC also estimates that there will be a greater shortage of general psychiatrists and child psychiatrists in the year 1990 than for any other medical specialty—with a total projected shortfall of approximately 13,000 general and child psychiatrists.

In connection with the NIMH and GMENAC manpower reports, I wish to caution here that unless mental health evaluation and care—and appropriate ancillary support and rehabilitation services—are fully recognized as necessary and legitimate health care services, the numbers of all mental health professionals are likely to remain at inadequate levels. It may well be, though, that even by attaching a full level of significance to mental health care and by devising a wide variety of incentives to attract persons to the mental health field, we shall never be able to attain the numbers of psychiatrists that we need to meet the mental health care needs of the nation. We shall therefore have to expand the roles of nonpsychiatrist mental health professionals and of mental health paraprofessionals and "workers" ("aides"). This will mean we will have to define very precisely exactly what mental health care these providers can deliver (or can be trained to deliver) and what care must be left exclusively to the province of the psychiatrist. It also means that we shall have to specify exactly what we mean by "mental health care" *per se*, as opposed to support, education, counseling, and rehabilitation services for persons who suffer mental illness/emotional problems. Both mental health care *per se* and such services should be made available as appropriate to the patient (client), but they are different. Both can be improved and provided on a broader, more cost-effective scope by applying a proper definition as to what they include.

Ultimately, health planners and legislators will also be faced with specifically deciding which mental health professionals should be authorized under NHI to provide mental health care. (This will obviously include a determination as to which mental health professionals should be eligible to receive payment for the care they render.) In this connection, NHI must seek to make available to the patient (client) the most comprehensive and responsible care; at the same time, such care must be made available on the most cost-efficient basis. With these concerns in mind, I would postulate that "psychiatric care" *per se* is both justified and desirable for most persons who suffer mental illness/emotional problems—although the extent of that care might most appropriately consist of a simple, brief consultation with the psychiatrist. In terms of facilitating both appropriate care and cost savings in care, psychiatric care has special relevance. For example, the prescription by the psychiatrist of psychotropic medication for a patient, as therapeutically indicated, may allow for a considerable decrease in the frequency of psychotherapy that patient will require, or it may shorten the process of psychotherapy entirely for him. I believe that psychiatric care *at some level* should be specifically encouraged for most patients under NHI on the same basis that many private insurance companies today encourage patients facing surgery to seek "second surgical opinions." The rationale in both cases would be, or should be, to provide the patient with the best care and, at the same time, the least costly care.

The final decision as to which mental health professionals should be entitled to deliver mental health care under NHI must be based not only upon the level and type of professional training the different categories of MHPs possess but also on the functions they perform. The various mental health professionals all serve different roles to a certain extent. However, one role they commonly share is that of providing "pure psychotherapy," as previously defined (see Chapter 1). When it comes to providing pure psychotherapy, it is difficult to judge one type of MHP as superior on an absolute basis to another—provided their theoretical and clinical training and experience in psychotherapy is equivalent. This is often not the case, but when it is, it is the *person* rather than the *profession* that makes the good psychotherapist. The fact is that we have as yet no precise measuring stick that will allow us to predict on an absolute basis the quality of psychotherapy an individual mental health professional can or will provide—whatever his particular profession. One thing that most MHPs do agree upon, however, is that in addition to having a thorough knowledge of the theory of psychology and psychotherapeutic technique, the good psychotherapist must be able to relate to his patient (client) in a warm, empathic, and compassionate manner. If the psychotherapist cannot do this, it does not matter if he is a psychiatrist, psychologist, social worker, or anyone else, insofar as his being able to help his patient (client) is concerned.

5.5. The Role of the Psychiatrist and Other Mental Health Professionals

The psychiatrist does not hold a patent on mental health care; he should not hold a monopoly on delivering it—under NHI or under our current mental health care delivery system. Nevertheless, there are definite reasons why the psychiatrist is especially well qualified to evaluate and treat persons with mental illness/emotional problems, why he should be at the hub of whatever system we devise to meet the mental health care needs of the nation. Psychologists, social workers, psychiatric nurses, and others should be included on the treatment wheel; they should play a full role in delivering mental health care.

The reality is that nonpsychiatrist MHPs (and paraprofessionals), along with nonpsychiatrist physicians, currently deliver the great majority of mental health care. They will continue to do so in the future; indeed, the role of the nonpsychiatrist MHP in delivering direct mental health care is bound to grow. In the ideal, however, the nonpsychiatrist MHP (as well as the non-psychiatrist physician) should coordinate the care he delivers his "client" with the psychiatrist; with certain exceptions (such as when a client only requires short-term psychotherapy), he should ideally treat his "client" in conjunction with the psychiatrist. This concept is especially valid during the period of a person's initial evaluation and (obviously) whenever his treatment entails the ongoing prescription of medication. In addition, when a non-psychiatrist MHP is providing treatment to a person that extends beyond the short term, that person should, ideally, be evaluated by a psychiatrist at regular intervals. This is desirable, if not imperative, because although a person may initially appear to be suffering from a "nonmedical" condition requiring only "pure psychotherapy" or counseling (delivered by a non-psychiatrist MHP or paraprofessional), he may in reality be suffering from a "medical" condition, a mental illness/emotional problem (such as "manic-depressive illness") that is best treated, at least in part, by medication as prescribed by a psychiatrist. In fact, the diagnosis of such "medical" conditions is often not made during an initial evaluation of a person; rather, the diagnosis only becomes obvious over time and after repeated observations.

The psychiatrist's training uniquely qualifies him to lead the "mental health team." The comprehensive 3- to 4-year psychiatry residency following 4 years of medical school and an internship provides the psychiatrist trainee (psychiatric resident) with an in-depth, closely supervised clinical experience. It involves him as well in detailed study of the field of psychology. Most important, the training program in psychiatry involves the future psychiatrist in working with the "whole person." The psychiatrist does not treat his patient's "mind" in isolation. He is trained to view his patient as a complex, integrated human organism whose thinking, feeling, and behavior must be viewed in the context of total physiological functioning. Thus, the psychiatrist is always supremely attentive to the complex interrelationship between state of mind (and nervous system) and state of body. The psychiatrist's bimodal attention set is a product of his specific training along the lines of the medical model as well as his nonmedical training in the field of psychology. This is in direct contrast to the unidimensional "psychological" training of most non-psychiatrist mental health professionals.

The psychiatrist, by nature of his training, is often in a position to be a quasi-"primary physician" for those patients he treats—to be their first line of contact for all their care. In such a role, the psychiatrist evaluates and monitors his patients' physical symptoms and refers them to other physician specialists for treatment as necessary. (The psychiatrist can best fill this role for the patient who suffers multiple "medical problems," many of which are of a psychosomatic nature. Such patients often have multiple physicians (specialists) who too often function independently of each other. The psychiatrist is the only physician who "sees" and deals with the total picture of the patient's illness. He can, therefore, coordinate and direct the patient's care in the complete sense.) I should also point out that the psychiatrist, in light of his medical background, is also supremely qualified to treat those patients who suffer "emotional complications" of organic (physical) illness and to treat those patients who suffer psychosomatic symptoms and illnesses, whereas most other mental health professionals are at a disadvantage in this respect.

The psychiatrist, of course, is trained to conduct psychotherapy of various modalities and frequencies. However, the psychiatrist, as a physician, is also trained in the science and use of a wide spectrum of medicines used to treat mental illness/emotional problems. This is extremely important because medicines are being employed in the treatment of mental illness/emotional problems on an ever-increasing and more reliable basis.

As the Group for the Advancement of Psychiatry (GAP) states in a report to which I have previously referred,[28]

> there is clear evidence that drugs do more than offer mere symptom relief. For example, lithium appears to alter CNS [central nervous system] functioning in a manner which is crucial to the treatment of manic-depressive illness. Phenothiazines have specific antipsychotic effects. . . . The successful treatment of a psychotic state by drugs may still leave the patient with serious neurotic and social problems, but without resolution of the psychotic state these problems may be untouchable by psychotherapy. . . . For schizophrenia, the literature reveals that (1) the major tranquilizers (e.g., phenothiazines, butyrophenones) are central for producing symptom remission and improving social effectiveness, and that (2) the value of insight or uncovering therapy as a sole treatment or as an adjunct is dubious. . . . In depression, recent and preliminary data suggest that pharmacotherapy and psychotherapy affect different dimensions of the illness and have additive effects.

The GAP goes on to state: "A careful review of the literature shows that there is no systematic evidence whatsoever that appropriate psychotropic agents, at appropriate dosages, interfere with the psychotherapy of schizophrenia, depression or neuroses. Statements to the contrary are editorial and opinionated and are clearly based upon ideological commitments." Most psychiatrists would agree with the GAP tenets I have just quoted. They would hold that specific medicines now play a paramount and proprietary role in the treatment of many syndromes, including lithium for manic-depressive illness, antidepressants for certain major depressions, and major tranquilizers for many psychotic disorders; they would also hold that although the prescription of psychotropic medication is most often vital to the successful treatment of these syndromes, some form of psychotherapy will most often be of additional value in their treatment.

I have previously noted that 29% (or approximately one in three) of all persons being treated by (nonpsychoanalyst) psychiatrists on an outpatient basis receive medication as a part of their treatment.[18] If we count both inpatients and outpatients being treated by psychiatrists, the percentage would be somewhat higher. (This is because the person who is hospitalized for treatment of his mental illness/emotional problems is usually suffering severe symptoms; typically, the psychiatrist will prescribe some medication for him.) In any case, I believe the total number of persons for whom psychotropic medication will be prescribed in the future is bound to grow as new, safer, and more effective medicines become available for the treatment of mental illness/emotional problems.

In contrast to psychiatrists, other mental health professionals are neither trained in the science and use of medication (psychiatric nurses are an exception) nor licensed to prescribe it. Thus, a person treated by a clinical psychologist or social worker (M.S.W.), for example, can receive medication as a part of his treatment only if and when a psychiatrist (or other physician) is consulted. The psychiatrist will then prescribe medication, if it is indicated, and treat the patient conjointly (or supervise the patient's treatment) with the psychologist or social worker, monitoring the specific requirement for medication and adjusting the dosage as necessary. In fact, this does happen for many persons in treatment, and the patient benefits from dual treatment by a psychiatrist and a nonpsychiatrist MHP. However, nonpsychiatrist MHPs too often work alone. Current state and federal laws permit under many circumstances the independent reimbursement of nonpsychiatrist MHPs for their treatment services. Their patients (clients) are not required to obtain even a single consultation with a psychiatrist or other physician. Therefore, the patients (clients) of many nonpsychiatrist MHPs are often not afforded any contact with a physician—psychiatrist or nonpsychiatrist—from the initiation to the conclusion of their treatment. This may result in poor or inadequate (as well as more expensive) treatment for many such patients. This is because many nonpsychiatrist MHPs, due to the nature of their (nonmedical) training, do not recognize that for many of their patients psychotropic medication, either by itself or in conjunction with psychotherapy, is the treatment of choice. Thus, there are many persons being treated by clinical psychologists (Ph.D.s), social workers (M.S.W.s), and so-called lay therapists who are in effect being denied their best opportunity to get better. In a certain sense, some such persons can be considered to be the victims of malfeasance, if not malpractice—if, for example, they suffer from a "major psychiatric syndrome" and are neither diagnosed as such nor treated with psychotropic medication for it. (I must be careful to make the distinction here that not all persons who suffer from a "major psychiatric syndrome" should receive medication as treatment for it.)

As I discuss elsewhere in this paper, many nonpsychiatrist MHPs are biased against the use of psychotropic medication. In fact, they are often biased to an extreme degree. A relatively small number of psychiatrists, including especially some psychoanalysts, are also unfavorably predisposed, in general, toward the use of such medication. Nevertheless, the vast majority of psychiatrists would agree that although the value of psychotropic medication can be disputed for a particular patient, the general value of such medication in the treatment of mental illness/emotional problems cannot be denied—provided it is employed with due respect and caution. Of course, ultimately, it is up to the individual person to decide whether he (or she) wishes to take medicine, but he should at least be in a position *to be advised* as to whether medication might help him and to have it prescribed for him if he so desires.

I believe the ideal mental health care is delivered when a person is screened on an evaluation basis by a psychiatrist at his (or her) entry point into the mental health care delivery system—even if he is to receive all or the bulk of his subsequent care from a nonpsychiatrist MHP or paraprofessional. At such a screening, the psychiatrist can determine if there is a role for the utilization of psychotropic medication in the patient's (client's) treatment; if there is such a role, the psychiatrist can then afford the patient this therapeutic option. In terms of ascertaining those therapeutic options open to him, it would also be of value for a patient to learn from a psychiatrist, in the course of a consultation, that he *does not* specifically require "psychiatric" (i.e., medical) treatment, that psychotropic medication should not be prescribed for his symptoms, and that he will benefit most from a course of "pure psychotherapy." Perhaps, the psychiatrist will tell him, he might benefit from a short course of psychotropic medication at some point in his treatment—if his symptoms worsen or change in character—but this can best be determined at a later date. Indeed, most persons who see a psychiatrist in consultation will receive such advice (see statistics on percentages of patients for whom psychiatrists prescribe medication, Section 5.3). Their best course, if they then decide to enter into "pure psychotherapy," will be to seek such treatment from the best psychotherapist they can find—whether he (or she) be a psychiatrist, a nonpsychiatrist MHP, or a paraprofessional.

There is an additional and more primary reason for a psychiatric screening besides the determination as to whether a patient can benefit from medication. Many persons suffer from mental illness/emotional problems on an organic (physical) basis; they suffer from an illness that is only secondarily producing mental illness/emotional problems. For example, when a person complains of depression, it is very easy to attribute the symptom to a difficult marital situation or to a disappointment in the person's life, whereas actually the person is suffering from kidney disease, a thyroid condition, or a brain tumor. The psychiatrist, as a physician, is in the best position to initially and thoroughly evaluate the patient. This includes his determining the emotional component, if any, of physical symptoms of which the patient complains and his considering the possibility that the patient's emotional complaints reflect an organic (physical) illness. The psychiatrist supplements this approach to the patient with a purely psychological analysis of his emotional distress. At this point, then, the psychiatrist can plan an appropriate, complete treatment approach for the patient—including the ordering of physical examinations and diagnostic tests on an initial basis, as indicated, and at appropriate times during the patient's treatment. It must be stressed that many organic (physical) illnesses can first make their presence known through their effects on the patient's mood or thinking. Thus, in one study,[31] it was found that of 100 persons admitted to a psychiatric ward, 46% were found to have medical illnesses that directly caused or greatly exaccerbated their symptoms and were consequently responsible for their admission, while an additional 34% of patients were found to be suffering from a medical illness requiring treatment."

This study, then, emphasizes the importance of an integrated medical and psychological clinical approach to the patient who suffers mental illness/ emotional problems. Generally speaking, I do not believe that the incidence of organic illness in persons treated on an outpatient basis for mental illness/ emotional problems will be as high as that reported here. (In two separate studies, that incidence was reported at 9.1%[32] and 20%.[33]) Still, it is clear that we cannot neglect the medical approach to this group of patients in favor of a strictly psychological approach. The data would suggest that most persons who are to receive mental health care on either an inpatient or an outpatient basis should undergo a complete medical history and physical examination at the start of their treatment, or should have done so within a reasonable period of time of the start of treatment, so as to help rule out the possibility that an organic illness is causing or contributing to their symptoms.

In connection with the relationship between organic illness and mental illness/emotional problems, I would comment further here on the role of the psychiatrist. Let me present a very abbreviated case history from my own practice: A patient I once treated suffered from depression and hypothyroidism (decreased functioning of his thyroid gland). The connection, if any, between the two was not immediately obvious since he was taking thyroid medication as prescribed by his internist and his blood level of thyroid hormone was within the normal range. Despite psychotherapy sessions on a one-to-two-times-per-week basis, however, the patient's depression continued and at times was severe—to the point where he was completely immobilized. At this point, I recommended to the patient's internist that we increase his thyroid medication. We did so, raising the patient's blood level of thyroid hormone from low normal to midnormal range. The patient's depression now resolved dramatically and the patient and I mutually decided to terminate treatment. Admittedly, this is an anecdotal report (not acceptable for research purposes) and the patient was lost to long-term follow-up. Indeed, his depression may have resolved spontaneously and only coincidentally with the change in his dose of thyroid medication. I report this case here only to point out the medical–psychological floating "attention set" of the psychiatrist and to demonstrate the special expertise he can bring to the treatment setting.

I must also note that although I believe strongly in an approach to mental health care delivery such as I have outlined in this section—i.e., a full role for all mental health professionals and paraprofessionals, but a central and coordinating role for the psychiatrist—such an approach is often logistically difficult (at best) and can involve complications in patient management as well.

From the logistical point of view, there is a shortage of psychiatrists; it is impossible for a psychiatrist to be involved in the care of every person who requires mental health care. In terms of patient management, it is axiomatic in medicine (including psychiatry) that *someone* (i.e., some *one* person) must be *directly in charge* of the patient's care. However, if a "coordinating" psychiatrist and a nonpsychiatrist MHP who is directly treating a client (in the private outpatient sector) disagree over the particular course of treatment a client should have (e.g., whether or not psychotropic medication should be prescribed for the client), who decides which treatment the client should have? In other words, which treating professional should have ultimate clinical responsibility for the client's treatment? (The obvious answer must be "the professional who has independently contracted to directly treat the client." In many cases, this will leave the psychiatrist without much influence; it will diminish the impact and potential of coordinated care.) And to whom should the client (patient) listen? Realistically, a client cannot be expected to be completely informed as to what course of treatment is best for him. In the first place, he is often suffering symptoms such as depression and anxiety which cloud his judgment. Even with a clear mind, however, such a decision (who he should listen to) is difficult for the patient to make. After all, he is a layperson, not a mental health professional. He must rely to a great extent on the best judgment of those professionals he consults. (This is a reality in all medical care, no matter how well informed a patient is.) If those professionals disagree, the patient will often be very confused.

Under our current mental health care delivery system, psychiatric management of mental health care is effectively mandated (although this is changing) through the schedule by which health insurance structures patient reimbursement for charges for such care. As I shall discuss below, I believe that, in the ideal, it is often desirable to place a psychiatrist directly in charge of the treatment of the person who requires mental health care, even when that person is receiving the bulk of his mental health care from a nonpsychiatrist MHP and the psychiatrist is functioning more or less as a consultant. (This presupposes that the individual psychiatrist "in charge" is well versed in, and applies an eclectic approach to, mental health care.) However, I do not think that as a general rule we should absolutely impose any level of psychiatric care, or psychiatric management of mental health care, on any person who seeks such care—at least as regards outpatient treatment. As I have already suggested, we should encourage the person who suffers mental illness/emotional problems to seek, at a minimum, consultation with a psychiatrist of his choice. Perhaps more important, we should encourage the nonpsychiatrist MHP to coordinate the care he delivers to his clients with that of a psychiatrist of his choice (one with whom he feels he can comfortably work). There should be a clear chain of clinical command as regards the client's (patient's) care. Ultimately, however, coordinated mental health care, if it is to be effective, must depend to a great extent on a *voluntary cooperative arrangement* involving a treating MHP, his client, and a psychiatrist—with the treating professionals working together to provide the client with the best mental health care.

Of course, in clinic and institutional settings (private and public), a multidisciplinary staff is in theory available to treat the patient and to plan for him the best course of care. (In reality, psychiatric manpower is minimal to absent in too many clinics and institutions—especially in the public sector.) I would postulate that in the ideal, the psychiatrist should be assigned the primary clinical responsibility for the patient's (client's) care in these settings. For if the psychiatrist does not supervise the total treatment of the patient, his care may be compromised in the direction of a purely psychological approach to his diagnosis and treatment—as opposed to a combined medical-psychological approach. Indeed, it is ideal, in my opinion, for the psychiatrist to be administratively in charge of the total mental health care a (mental health) clinic or institution delivers. This is so because the administrator has the ultimate power to determine the direction of mental health care that will be delivered in the setting he controls. (The administrator's power exceeds that of the director of clinical care because he can, with some restrictions, decide the type and number of MHPs who should be hired by his organization. He can also choose his personnel on the basis of the specific clinical persuasions or orientations they hold. Further, he can assign their clinical duties in the manner he chooses.) If the administrator is a nonpsychiatrist MHP, he may well hold a bias against a medical approach (combined with a psychological approach) to mental illness/emotional problems and mental health care in general—which will result in an unbalanced and inappropriate psychological approach to mental health care by his clinic or institution. A lay administrator may well hold the same bias, given in part the widespread apprehension of the layperson vis-à-vis the chemical and electrical treatment of mental illness/ emotional problems. In any event, the lay administrator is often neither trained nor experienced to any great extent either in the medical diagnosis of mental illness/emotional problems or in the theory and practice of the various specific modalities of mental health care, whether they be medical or psychological. Consequently, he will have difficulty conceptualizing the proper course, including direction and extent, of treatment any given patient should receive. (In a similar vein, the nonsurgeon administrator will have difficulty, to say the least, directing the surgical clinic or operating room theater.) In all fairness, I must note here that certain psychiatrists favor almost exclusively a "drug approach" to the treatment of mental illness/emotional problems; clearly, a psychiatrist who displays such a predisposition is not the best person to administer a mental health care program, for he practices in accordance with a potentially harmful bias that gives undue weight to the medical as opposed to the psychological approach to treatment. Similarly, a psychoanalyst psychiatrist who abjures the use of psychotropic medication in favor of an exclusively psychological approach to treatment is handicapped as an administrator.

In sum, the successful management of a mental health care delivery system, whether on the clinical or administrative level, is dependent upon an eclectic orientation toward mental health care on the part of the managers. This is the case whether the person in charge is a psychiatrist, a nonpsychiatrist MHP, or a lay administrator. What should be clear from this discussion is that clinical directors and administrators of mental health care units—whoever they are—must be chosen with extreme care. They should be thoroughly versed in and familiar with the medical and psychological dimensions of mental illness/emotional problems and its treatment. (In the ideal, this would include extensive experience on the clinical level.) For as much as the clinicians directly engaged in treating the patient (client), the clinical director of a program in mental health care and the administrator above him can make or break mental health care for the patients (clients) who patronize the clinic or institution they manage. To "make" it (responsible as well as responsive), they must promote an integrated rather than a fragmented approach to mental health care. Under this concept, the psychiatrist is actively involved in the treatment by nonpsychiatrist MHPs and paraprofessionals of persons who suffer mental illness/emotional problems; the psychiatrist functions side by side with these other providers so as to make comprehensive care available to the patient (client) and so as to insure that no patient falls into a semisegregated health care system that will not properly serve his complete mental health care needs. The first dictum of all health care must be "to do no harm" to the patient (client). The second dictum must be "to relieve suffering whenever possible." To effect both of these dictums, we must be sure that the patient is afforded proper diagnosis and treatment that incorporates a multidimensional approach to mental health care and bridges the fields of "medicine" and "psychology". With specific reference to the prescription of psychotropic medication, it is probably true that a large segment of those persons who receive mental health care will require either minimal and infrequent psychotropic medication or none at all. However, as I have noted, it is only through the involvement of the psychiatrist in the mental health care process that this therapeutic dimension—i.e., the prescription of psychotropic medication—can be afforded the patient. (Of course, the nonpsychiatrist physician can prescribe psychotropic medication; it is a role that he has had to fill and will have to fill in the future. Nevertheless, this role poses potential problems. See Section 5.4.) I want to be sure to specify here that I do not seek to compromise the role of the nonpsychiatrist MHP and paraprofessional; rather, I seek to establish the importance of a team approach between the psychiatrist and other mental health professionals and paraprofessionals as regards the provision of mental health care services now and in the future.

The nonpsychiatrist mental health professional should hardly feel threatened by the role of the psychiatrist as I have described it here. Indeed, I might hypothesize an ever-expanding, diversified, and central role for the nonpsychiatrist MHP and paraprofessional in the future as regards the provision of "pure psychotherapy." Further, one can anticipate that new lay superspecialists in psychotherapy will come "on line" to provide this much-needed health care service (i.e., "pure psychotherapy") to persons who suffer mental illness/emotional problems. They will be produced by innovative, comprehensive psychotherapy training programs that are even now evolving and in some cases are already producing these advanced superspecialists in psychotherapy. It can be anticipated that before too long, the "new psychotherapist" will be specially trained in principles of psychopharmacology and as such will be qualified to prescribe psychotropic medication under the supervision of a psychiatrist. Thus, he (or she) will be in a position to conceptualize and practice that balanced approach to mental health care (combining the utilization of "pure psychotherapy" and psychotropic medication) that is now only in the domain and within the expertise of the psychiatrist. Further, he will be able to complement the psychiatrist's role (again, with supervision by the psychiatrist) as a "coordinator" of mental health care; specifically, he will consult with clients of MHPs and paraprofessionals who are not qualified to prescribe psychotropic medication and he will recommend the prescription of medication for such clients as appropriate. Thus, in the future, the psychiatrist will have assistance from "within the field" as well as from nonpsychiatrist physicians in meeting the "medical needs" of those persons who require mental health care, and he will be freed to assume additional duties and functions. In this connection, the psychiatrist's role will evolve from what it is now. He will be the primary provider of specialized mental health care for those persons who primarily require a medical approach (e.g., the prescription of psychotropic medication) as treatment for their mental illness/emotional problems. He will become increasingly involved in liaison-consultation with nonpsychiatrist physicians as well as with his fellow mental health professionals—especially as regards meeting the medical needs of those patients (clients) they treat. In addition, the psychiatrist, as a member of the "medical team," will devote much of his therapeutic efforts to "biobehavioral medicine," that new branch of medicine that deals with patients who suffer "pure" organic (physical) symptoms and/or illness, and "psychosomatic" symptoms and/or illness and attempts to effect their complete treatment by a combined psychological and medical approach. Still, the psychiatrist will continue to practice psychotherapy *per se,* in accordance with his personal preference to do so, be that "pure psychotherapy" or psychotherapy that employs psychotropic medication when and as required by the patient.

Indeed, we must expand the base of specialized providers of mental health care under NHI. If we do not, too many persons who suffer mental illness/emotional problems will continue to be forced to get the mental health care they require on a nonspecialized basis from nonpsychiatrist physicians. I have previously discussed the tendency of the nonpsychiatrist physician to overutilize psychotropic medication (see Chapter 4). I would like to supplement that earlier general discussion here with data from the National Ambulatory Medical Care Survey (1973–1974).[34] That survey examined (among other things) the types of treatment/service delivered when the patient's principal diagnosis was mental disorder. The survey found that the nonpsychiatrist physician employed "drug therapy" in 67% of all "patient visits" for mental disorders. By contrast, the psychiatrist employed "drug therapy" in 32.2% of such visits. Also, the psychiatrist utilized psychotherapy or "therapeutic listening" in 91.2% of patient visits, while the nonpsychiatrist physician utilized this therapeutic modality (in which he has little training and most often must confine himself to offering "support") only 21.8% of the time. Thus, the data would indicate that the nonpsychiatrist physician, in addition to relying heavily on drug therapy for his patients who suffer mental disorder, prescribes such therapy much too often without adjunct psychotherapy, a practice that is unwise at best and contraindicated at worst for most patients. In my opinion, a person should be entitled to receive specialized mental health care and access to the appropriate specialists must be made available to him under NHI.

It should be obvious from my remarks in this section that I feel very strongly that many nonpsychiatrist MHPs and paraprofessionals are extremely capable psychotherapists. Indeed, this must be beyond dispute. My only contention here is that they too often practice a singular approach toward treating their clients—unless they work in tandem with the psychiatrist. The psychiatrist, by contrast, approaches the patient variably, employing the most appropriate treatment modality, be that "pure psychotherapy," psychotherapy with adjunct medication, or medication alone. In this connection, the psychiatrist, because of his multiplex, diversified approach to his patient and his ability to apply a wide therapeutic spectrum to his patient's treatment, is less likely to be biased toward or against a particular mode of treatment. The nonpsychiatrist MHP, on the other hand, is more likely to be biased against those treatment forms he cannot provide his client and is more likely to treat him in accordance with the isolated therapeutic modality he is qualified to practice. Some way must be found of overcoming the potential therapeutic gap that may result from the secular approach to mental health care practiced by nonpsychiatrist MHPs and paraprofessionals. This is essential since, realistically speaking, they will function in the future as first-line providers of mental health care, and they will clearly provide the majority of mental health care.

I should emphasize that in drawing certain distinctions between the psychiatrist and the nonpsychiatrist MHP, I do not wish to exclude the latter as providers of mental health care to any major category of patients. Thus, in the total, abstract ideal, the psychiatrist may be the provider of choice for persons who are suffering the emotional sequelae of organic (physical) illness. With proper training, though, the nonpsychiatrist MHP can assist the psychiatrist in treating such persons as a member of a mental health team supervised by the psychiatrist. (Indeed, with the psychiatrist in short supply, the team approach is essential.) It is true that some patients experiencing organic (physical) illness will strictly require treatment by a psychiatrist who will coordinate the patient's total health care, as necessary, with his (the patient's) primary physician. However, many other patients suffering organic illness, carefully selected, will be able to benefit equally well from psychotherapy administered by a qualified nonpsychiatrist MHP operating completely independently of the psychiatrist. Like the psychiatrist, the MHP shall, as indicated, conduct treatment in liaison with the patient's physician.

Let me amplify here my vision of the roles of the various mental health professionals under NHI. As I have noted, arguments that arise between the psychiatrist and the nonpsychiatrist MHP on this score often stem from their respective political-economic self-interests. I must admit that I do not think I can resolve finally and completely in this paper the question of the proper provider roles for the various mental health professionals under NHI. In any event, I am more concerned here with combating unfair and unwise limitations on coverage for mental health care under NHI. For if there is severely limited coverage, it will not matter who specifically does not provide care.

Nevertheless, I do wish most keenly to dispel in this book the myths concerning the superiority or inferiority of one professional group or the other as relates to their treating persons with mental illness/emotional problems. It is true that I envision and have proposed herein a special role for the psychiatrist under National Health Insurance, a role that centers on and utilizes his medical as well as his psychological expertise. It would be an understatement for me to acknowledge that many nonpsychiatrist MHPs would not agree in totality with my views as to this special role for the psychiatrist. Rightly or wrongly, many nonpsychiatrist MHPs wish to achieve total parity with the psychiatrist. The ultimate issue, then, is rather simply expressed: Is the highly trained nonpsychiatrist MHP as capable and qualified a provider of mental health care as the psychiatrist? In my opinion, the answer is most definitely yes in many respects. My only contention is that the psychiatrist, by dint of his medical background and expertise, can complement the (nonmedical) skills and expertise of the nonpsychiatrist MHP and is in the best position to coordinate the functions of all professionals involved in the delivery of mental health care.

Let me then state one more time here that when it comes to the practice of "pure psychotherapy"*—where it has been determined that the patient does not require psychotropic medication of any kind—the nonpsychiatrist MHP who is as highly trained as the psychiatrist qualifies on an equal basis with the psychiatrist as a provider of care—except in some cases where the patient concurrently suffers organic (physical) symptoms or illness. Consequently, nonpsychiatrist MHPs must be included under NHI as providers of psychotherapy—under a financially equitable formula that takes into account, in determining fee for service, degree of training, special qualifications and certification, and experience.

In calling for the inclusion under NHI of nonpsychiatrist MHPs as providers of mental health care, I am hardly being revolutionary. Freud himself

---

*Pure psychotherapy—see Chapter 1.

was certainly in favor of lay analysts treating persons with mental illness/ emotional problems, and he actively promoted the concept of their practicing his new technique of psychoanalysis. Freud might have had a somewhat different view if he had had specific prior knowledge of the advances that would be made in the field of mental health care in terms of the medicines that have become available to treat persons with mental illness/emotional problems. Still, I doubt that his views toward the practice of "pure psychoanalysis"* would have changed.

Ultimately, it seems to me, we need to devise a system wherein we can identify the successful practitioner of pure psychotherapy—whatever his background and training. Perhaps we can develop a system analogous to the medical specialty certification boards whereby we would certify psychotherapists. (The psychiatry specialty boards in fact do not measure or reflect in any way on the psychiatrist's ability to perform psychotherapy *per se*.) Unfortunately, it will be complicated at best to develop such a system because of the varying backgrounds of the various MHPs and the multiple psychological schools to which they adhere, no matter what their particular profession. Also, it will be exceedingly difficult to develop any certification examination for the psychotherapist because the successful practice of psychotherapy involves much more than a knowledge of psychotherapeutic theory and technique *per se* on his part. It involves the psychotherapist's ability, as previously described, to relate to his patient (client) in a warm, compassionate, and empathic manner. In other words, the psychotherapist, in order to be effective, must possess certain desirable human qualities! It is easy to imagine an examiner, himself lacking in these qualities, attempting to judge them in others. Still, I think we must strive to institute some system whereby we can judge the skill and capability of the individual practitioner of psychotherapy. The system must evaluate the practitioner's knowledge of psychotherapeutic theory and technique. It must measure on an equal basis how he relates on the personal level to his patient (client).

Of course, I would agree that if we expand the base of practitioners of psychotherapy under NHI to include clinical psychologists (Ph.D.s), social workers (M.S.W.s), and others, we might be faced with a situation where the nation, financially speaking, will have difficulty in providing full coverage for psychotherapy as a specific form of mental health care. I suggest, though, that we can afford to provide full coverage for psychotherapy under NHI or under existing insurance programs if we only define "psychotherapy" and the proper roles of the various MHPs more exactly. I have already suggested that when the patient requires only "emotional support," the services of a psychiatrist *per se* are not strictly required. I also think that under NHI we

---

*Pure psychoanalysis—psychoanalysis in which the utilization of psychotropic medication is eschewed at all times during the course of the treatment. (*Pure psychoanalysis* is an artificial term. I use it in the same sense that I have used the term *pure psychotherapy* to reflect treatment that does not involve the utilization of psychotropic medication.)

shall probably have to exclude from eligibility for psychotherapy those persons who require only "education." Indeed, psychiatrists and clinical (Ph.D.) psychologists are too highly trained to engage in purely educational functions. When it is a lack of education *per se* about how to deal with the common problems and dilemmas of life that is the primary source of a person's difficulties, we must develop some other resources besides psychotherapy to meet the person's educational needs. I believe that a large percentage of people who are "frustrated" or who are having "difficulties" can be dealt with outside of formal psychotherapy. We should reserve psychotherapy, and its reimbursement under NHI, as a form of mental health care for those persons who suffer from distinct mental illness/emotional problems—where the cause of such goes far beyond a lack of education on their part.

I am not saying here that education does not play a large role in psychotherapy. It most certainly does. A person must learn about himself (or herself) if he is to moderate or resolve his symptoms and enhance his level of functioning. He must develop a cognitive awareness of himself that includes an understanding of who, how, why, what, and where he is. No, I am not demeaning here the importance of the educational experience that psychotherapy and other forms of mental health care entail. Rather, I am only proposing that we must develop and foster educational programs outside of formal psychotherapy that emphasize concepts of mental health and problem solving. This would include, for example, simple counseling. This can be especially useful for persons who do not already suffer from classifiable mental illness/emotional problems, or whose mental illness/emotional problems are minor in degree. It can well forestall, in true preventive medicine fashion, the future need for mental health care.

In connection with the concept of providing a person with "psychological education," as opposed to formal psychotherapy, I would like to comment here on the teaching of so-called coping strategies and coping techniques. In fact, the teaching of such strategies and techniques often constitutes a large part of "behavioral psychotherapy" as it is currently practiced. Although it is undoubtedly useful for many persons to learn and to employ such tools of coping, they can frequently be taught (when they are the modus operandi of the "treatment" process) outside of formal psychotherapy by mental health paraprofessionals, former patients (clients) (e.g., employed in the treatment of phobic persons), skilled persons (e.g., "successful parents" employed to teach distraught parents how to manage their children), and others. Let me emphasize that any brand of psychotherapy, if it is to be worthwhile, must ultimately convey to the patient (client) alternative ways of thinking, feeling, and behaving, ways that will be more effective and successful for him or her. In this sense, all legitimate forms of psychotherapy must impart coping skill to the patient. However, for most persons who suffer mental illness/emotional problems and who are engaged in formal psychotherapy, such skill is most often (though not always) imparted only *as a part of* or as *a result of* a complex, integrated treatment process. (For further discussion of the definition of psychotherapy, see Chapter 7 and the Appendix.)

Essentially, here, I am suggesting that we provide appropriate civilian intervention for persons who do not require formal mental health care. At the same time, we should refine our mental health care delivery system in terms of defining roles for the various mental health professionals. The most appropriate care can be delivered and considerable cost savings can be achieved by selecting the appropriate MHP for any given patient (client). Thus, in the same way that a nurse or physician's assistant can in many cases care for a patient's medical or surgical needs (under supervision) once a physician has determined the exact treatment needs of the patient, I feel strongly that "lower level" MHPs and nonprofessional providers of mental health care can meet many persons' mental health care needs and deliver appropriate treatment (under supervision) once a psychiatrist has evaluated a person and determined his or her mental health care needs. Careful triage of patients, then, will be crucial under NHI to establish exactly who should be treated and who should treat. If we are to have triage, though, the most qualified professional should perform the triage rather than the lesser qualified professional. (The opposite is currently practiced in many triage operations.) The psychiatrist, with his multisystem understanding of and approach to patients, is the logical choice here. Why should the most qualified professional supervise a triage operation? Because the lesser qualified professional is likely to miss cases where there is a serious problem that is not patently manifest in the patient's presenting symptoms. Responsibility for care must therefore be relegated downward rather than upward.

The triage psychiatrist will determine which individual persons suffer from classifiable mental illness/emotional problems and can benefit from treatment. Further, the triage psychiatrist will decide, with the patient's full participation, which particular course of treatment (medication, psychotherapy, etc.) is best for that individual patient and what level MHP or nonprofessional should administer his care.

In discussing who should provide mental health care, it is important that we do not become totally lost in making distinctions among the various mental health professionals. We must upgrade the practice of psychotherapy no matter who the practitioner is. One thing that very much bothers responsible practitioners of psychotherapy is the fact that the consistency and the quality of psychotherapy practiced by MHPs of all types and psychological persuasions is often less than desirable. One can hardly say that this is unique to the practice of psychotherapy, however. It is a phenomenon associated with the practice of medicine in general. There are good physicians and physicians who are, to be polite, less than good, and there is every grade in between. I believe that a large proportion of the poor results obtained in psychotherapy occur in cases where the patient (client) is treated by an MHP who is in one way or another not personally suited or prepared to practice psychotherapy.

These practitioners lack the skill and personal qualities necessary to carry out successful psychotherapy. To further complicate matters, they have a tendency to set treatment goals for their patients (clients) that are neither realistic nor appropriate and thus not achievable.

In appraising the efficacy of psychotherapy, we must focus on the capacities of the psychotherapist as well as on the validity of the particular system of psychotherapy he employs. Unfortunately, most efforts to date, either planned or already implemented, to study and judge the relative merits of psychotherapy have concentrated to a great extent on the latter. As I have pointed out, however, the "person" and skill of the individual psychotherapist plays as large a part in the success or failure of the psychotherapy that he practices as does the system of psychotherapy he employs. To neglect this verity in favor of an analysis of the effectiveness of particular psychotherapy systems or an analysis of the abilities of particular provider "classes" of psychotherapists misses the mark. I suggest that when we are able to more carefully select individual psychotherapist candidates for training (no matter which specific mental health profession they are entering) and when we are able to refine our training of them as regards teaching them both the diagnosis and the treatment of mental illness/emotional problems [e.g., educating nonpsychiatrist MHPs as to when they should refer their clients for psychiatric (medical) consultation and/or treatment], we will see a much higher success rate for psychotherapy. This will stem in part from the fact that patients (clients) will receive the most appropriate treatment or combination of treatments.

Let me recapitulate here: The psychiatrist–physician is in a unique position to evaluate, diagnose, and effectively treat persons who suffer mental illness/emotional problems, and, in addition, to consult with, and to coordinate the care of patients (clients) of other professionals and workers in the mental health field. Clearly, though, we need to make room under NHI (and under our existing mental health care delivery system) for other mental health professionals such as clinical psychologists (Ph.D.s), social workers (M.S.W.s), and psychiatric nurses. We need to develop some formula for a consortium of mental health professionals and paraprofessionals to treat patients who suffer mental illness/emotional problems. We also need to develop an equitable formula for providing payment to the various mental health professionals—based on their level of training and their level of patient responsibility. Unfortunately, the situation now exists where there is often not much difference among the fees of the various categories of mental health professionals and "counselors." Fees for service of private practitioners too often do not reflect differences in their levels of training. We must change this if we wish to afford the private patient (client) real choice of provider and if we desire the mental health care delivery system to work more cost-efficiently. With regard to the psychiatrist's role under NHI, we must remember that there are not enough psychiatrists available to provide all levels of mental health care. We must also remember that it is neither appropriate nor necessary for the psychiatrist to treat all patients. Well-trained mental health professionals and paraprofessionals of all categories will always be needed in private settings as well as in the public sector. However, we must be exceedingly careful in planning and enacting coverage for mental health care under NHI: We must not allow practitioner reimbursement—and in essence give "license to heal"—to everyone who claims to know what mental health and mental health care are.

At the risk of being repetitive, I would like to expand here on the basic concepts I have presented in this section of my paper. Mental health care differs from other forms of medical care, insofar as both outpatient and inpatient care are concerned, in that the cost of care on both the diagnostic and therapeutic level is largely derived from professional services, that is, care delivered directly by the professional (or paraprofessional), rather than from professional services plus ancillary services—such as laboratory tests and X rays. (Of course, there is often a professional component to the cost of such ancillary services.) Mental health care is manpower-intense, rather than technology-intense; therefore, the professional level at which mental health care is delivered will have a relatively greater impact on the total cost of mental health care than will the level at which professional care is delivered for other types of medical care—although the potential for savings, by appropriate assignment of patients to the proper level of care, is, of course, immense as regards *all* medical care.

The first and primary responsibility of all health care professionals, no matter what their specialty, is to insure that every person who suffers any illness is provided state-of-the-art health care. Yet the medical professional, and I include the mental health care professional in this category, must now more than ever be aware of the cost of the diagnostic and treatment services he provides his patients (clients). Thus, although many persons who are ill require highly specialized care, it should be the concern of the medical professional to design the individual patient's care so that he receives the full and complete care that he needs, but at the same time receives it at the appropriate health care level.

The fact is that medical care is becoming increasingly more complex and the role for the physician-specialist, whether he be a psychiatrist (or other high-level mental health professional), orthopedist, neurologist, cardiologist, etc., is ever expanding. Still, we can allocate our professional medical resources much better than we now do. Clearly, physician-specialists (and nonphysician mental health professionals) are often misused. It is possible for less specialized practitioners of health care to carry out—with clinical supervision and oversight by the physician-specialist (or MHP) that most often includes examination of the patient (client) at periodic intervals—many of the clinical duties and responsibilities that specialists in all medical fields have assumed up to now. As medical care becomes increasingly more expensive, we should strive to reorganize the health care delivery system so that we make the most appropriate use of all medical professionals and paraprofessionals. By doing so, we will significantly reduce the cost of medical care at the same time that we preserve quality of care for the individual patient (client).

All physician-specialists, and mental health professionals of all types, should be willing to identify patients (clients) who can be successfully treated by health professionals or paraprofessionals who are less highly trained than themselves. In reverse fashion, health professionals and paraprofessionals should look to refer to more highly trained health professionals patients (clients) who are beyond their level of expertise. Of course, this is the *ideal* and we can expect that the private practitioner, no matter what his specialty, who operates on a fee-for-service basis may be reluctant to refer his patients (clients) to other practitioners. At least, he will not be economically motivated to "give up" his patients. Yet, lest we be too critical in our attitude toward the private practitioner, let us also remember that the physician-specialist, and the various mental health professionals, working in HMOs and other organized private health care plans and in the public sector may too readily and willingly refer patients (clients) to practitioners who are less well trained than themselves due in large part to the pressure their health care organization places on them to control and minimize operating costs.

I have purposely framed the above discussion in the context of medical care in general, as opposed to mental health care *per se,* because I do not wish to convey the false impression that mental health care is a singularly wasteful modality of health care. We must not make mental health care a whipping boy for the inefficiency of our entire health care system. It is true that we often have the situation in mental health care where the psychiatrist, the psychologist, the MSW, and the psychiatric nurse provide virtually the same type and level of care to identical categories of patients—with equal efficiency and success. However, it is also true that we often have the situation in *all of medical care* where the physician-specialist and the generalist provide virtually the same type and level of care to identical categories of patients. It is the entire health care system, not any specific modality of care, that often functions inefficiently. Although we must strive to remedy this, it is unlikely we will be able to find a complete cure. No matter how well we organize our health care delivery system, no matter how ingeniously we match patients (clients) to their proper slot within the system, the physician-specialist (or the MHP) will often wind up treating the same categories of patients the generalist treats—and he will frequently care for his patients in much the same fashion as the generalist cares for his. Why? Simply because much of the time, it is difficult or impossible to cleanly and clearly divide general health care from specialized health care. The nature of medical care is such that the generalist usually provides at least some specialized care and the specialist usually provides at least some general care. To state this another way, the "pure" specialist and the "pure" generalist do not represent the typical health care practitioner. More commonly, the specialist and the generalist deliver care along a continuum that both diverges and intersects. This is especially obvious—although, I must stress, hardly unique—if we examine the functions of the various practitioners of mental health care.

Let me now focus on the mental health care delivery system, itself, and consider in brief how we can streamline it. First, the mental health professionals must make all possible efforts, as I suggest in this paper, to determine exactly who needs to treat whom for what. We have yet to conclusively ascertain this, although it seems clear that the patient (client) is often best served by treatment by a combination of mental health professionals and/or paraprofessionals. In fact, although there is varied opinion on the subject, we do not even yet know whether the specific level of training of the practitioner of mental health care plays a significant role in the eventual outcome of treatment for many, but certainly not all, categories of patients. Most definitely, the practitioner requires a certain minimal and substantial level of training. Yet I have tried to underscore in this paper the point that the persona of the psychotherapist, whatever his profession, plays a major role in his ability to successfully conduct psychotherapy. Thus, it may well be that if we have a particular person well suited on the personal level to provide psychotherapy—that is, he (or she) possesses certain favorable personality characteristics, emotional maturity, and a high level of psychological sophistication—and if we then provide this person with a requisite level of training, this may suffice to allow him to effectively treat patients (clients) who suffer from many types of mental illness/emotional problems. Further, for a great many patients, it seems likely that the most important factor in the success of treatment relates to common, nonspecific "healing elements" of the psychotherapeutic process, itself, no matter who is conducting the treatment. (In an analogous fashion, much of the success we have in treating medical-surgical patients can be attributed to nonspecific healing elements that are common to all medical care.) Within these confines, let me propose, as I intimated earlier in my paper, that in evaluating the mental health care needs of every person who suffers emotional distress, we should first determine whether he (or she) requires formal psychotherapy or counseling. Of course, psychotherapy is really a generic term. Thus, parallel with all medical care, some patients (clients) will require the most highly specialized and sophisticated psychotherapy, as delivered by the most highly trained, sophisticated mental health professional, while many other patients will benefit from a basic, elementary course of psychotherapy that, indeed, approximates, in many respects, counseling—which I will simplistically define here, for purposes of our discussion, as the provision by a counselor to a client of emotional support, advice, and "psychological education." Leaving aside those persons who require only counseling, and this constitutes a large group of those persons who suffer emotional distress, the fact is, and I have repeatedly maintained this, that the psychotherapy, as distinct from counseling, that many patients (clients) require can be provided by fully trained and qualified mental health paraprofessionals, including "aides," "workers," etc. If we can only appropriately triage patients into the therapeutic niche in which they belong, and this is a big "if," we can provide them with the complete mental health care they require, do so at the appropriate level of care, and do so in an affordable fashion. This is not necessarily the case *now*, I should point out, but, one hopes it will be when we develop sufficient numbers of paraprofessionals (again, I must stress) fully qualified and trained to deliver psychotherapy and, furthermore, operating within a mental health care delivery system wherein every patient is guaranteed access to a medical approach to his mental illness/emotional problems. In line with this, the mental health care delivery system we ultimately evolve must be flexible enough that no patient is ever locked into any isolated fraction of it; the patient must be able to flow, in accordance with his mental health care needs, from level to level of care.

Each of us, if we are ill, from no matter what cause or condition, wants to be assured that we will receive the most expert care. Even as we restructure our mental health care delivery system, and our entire health care delivery system, let us make sure that it delivers such care. It is no easy task to determine exactly into which slot we should place the patient (client) who requires mental health care or medical care of any variety. Let us always err on the side of providing the individual patient health care at a higher level than he actually requires, rather than at a lower level. Let us appropriately despecialize medical care—but let us also be anxious to encourage appropriate specialized care for the patient. We can cause great harm to a great many patients if we are too anxious and too eager to despecialize health care, if we absolutely and rigidly confine patients to receiving their care at specified (lower) levels of the health care delivery system. In accordance with the philosophy of triage I outlined earlier in this paper, I do believe that under any health care system we ultimately evolve, every patient should have at least initial access to health care at the highest professional level; he should also have full access to follow-up of his case by a specialist.

Indeed, under many currently operating HMOs and private prepaid health plans and, of course, in the CMHC, despecialized mental health care, and often other medical care, is already the rule. Of course, patients (clients) at the CMHC have little choice in the matter, but many patients in the private prepaid plans accept this—for whatever reason—perhaps only as the price they must pay for lower premiums for their health care. In this connection, I propose that as we evolve our existing health care delivery system, we should organize the system to advise and educate all patients (clients), and every person before he becomes a patient, as to the nature of mental health care, and all medical care, and the proper role and function of the specialist and the generalist. Medical care by its very nature must always remain somewhat magical, and we should not—indeed, we could not, even if we wanted to—reduce it to plain, logical, cold clinical nuts and bolts. At the same time, we must demystify mental health care and all medical care as much as we can. In this way, the patient (client), working with his physician or mental health professional, will gradually come to understand that he does not always require the most specialized health care and he will become more accepting of general care. By educating the patient, as well as by reorienting the physician-specialist (and all mental health professionals), we can foster the development of a health care delivery system that meets both the clinical and the psychological needs (the two are inseparably intertwined) of patients and operates on the most cost-efficient basis.

Of course, if we are to institute a broad-based approach to mental health care that effectively utilizes all the different groups of mental health professionals, we need to defuse the antagonism that too often exists between the various groups of MHPs; we need to encourage cooperative efforts between them if we are to organize and deliver inclusive and appropriate mental health care. Each professional group must recognize the skills and expertise of the other. Thus, the psychiatrist must acknowledge the legitimate right of other types of mental health professionals to practice "pure psychotherapy" on an independent basis—although not under all circumstances. For example, the psychologist, and perhaps other MHPs, can treat on an independent basis some persons who require hospital care, consonant with the hypothesis that not all such persons require psychiatric (medical) care *per se*. However, the majority of such persons will require specialized psychiatric care, and mental health care must be structured so as to insure that they will receive such care.

I would note here that the nonpsychiatrist physician, who is not a specialist in mental health care, is currently entitled to deliver broad-based mental health care on an independent basis—i.e., without clinical oversight by the psychiatrist. I do not see how we can continue such a policy under NHI, or under existing health insurance programs, and at the same time deny the specialist in mental health care, even if he is not a psychiatrist, the right and privilege to provide independent mental health care. In advocating such a "right" (for the nonpsychiatrist MHP), I can only hope that when a person chooses a nonpsychiatrist MHP as his psychotherapist, he (the psychotherapist) will appropriately coordinate the care he delivers to that person with a psychiatrist. This presupposes that the nonpsychiatrist MHP is trained to recognize when his client requires specialized psychiatric intervention and that he is willing to refer his client to the psychiatrist when his client's clinical condition dictates it. The underlying premise must be that the nonpsychiatrist MHP accepts the validity of specialized psychiatric care. Although there are many nonpsychiatrist MHPs who subscribe to this premise, too many, unfortunately, do not. A significant number of nonpsychiatrist MHPs do not view the psychiatrist as possessing any special expertise; they do not believe in the validity of psychiatric (i.e., medical) diagnosis or in psychiatric (medical) treatment—especially when it entails the prescription for the patient of psychotropic medication or electroconvulsive therapy. (See my discussion in Chapter 4 on the purpose of prescribing and the proper utilization of psychotropic medication.) Such an attitude on the part of many (but certainly not all) nonpsychiatrist MHPs immensely complicates the provision of mental health care; it jeopardizes proper mental health care for many persons. It is one major reason many psychiatrists are unwilling to advocate independent provider status for nonpsychiatrist MHPs.

I am fully aware that the policy I have just advocated will create unfortunate gaps in mental health care. Under it, some persons will fall through "holes" in the mental health care delivery system; they will not receive the mental health care they require—because the treating (nonpsychiatrist) MHP will fail to correctly diagnose his client's mental illness/emotional problem and will fail to realize, as well, that his client requires specialized psychiatric treatment for it. (It is equally true that gaps currently exist in the delivery of medical-surgical care. Thus, some patients fall through holes in the health care delivery system at large. Many a patient does not receive the specific health care he requires because his physician does not properly diagnose his condition; the physician does not realize that a particular patient requires specialized care that he himself is not capable of providing.) However, in spite of the shortcomings of the policy I propose, it is also true that, under it, some persons will be able to avail themselves of better treatment than they would have received if they had been confined to seek their treatment from a psychiatrist. Thus, there are many nonpsychiatrist MHPs who practice "pure psychotherapy" better than many psychiatrists (and vice versa, of course). At the same time, it must be realized that we cannot at this date prescribe specific absolute treatments for many types of mental illness/emotional problems—just as we cannot prescribe specific medical treatments on an absolute basis for many illnesses. In view of this, we should allow a wide spectrum of therapeutic choice to any person who seeks mental health care. We can insure the availability of such "therapeutic choice" to the patient (client) by allowing him to seek his care from a wide spectrum of fully trained and fully qualified mental health professionals. Thus, if a person wishes to pursue a course of "pure psychotherapy" (with a nonpsychiatrist MHP) as treatment for a particular mental illness/emotional problem, as opposed to a course of treatment (from a psychiatrist) that combines psychotherapy and psychotropic medication, he should have this option since the same therapeutic results can often be achieved through either of these approaches to treatment—regardless of the cost of treatment. Of course, the situation I have just described is not unique to mental health care. There is a wide variety of equally effective therapeutic options available to the patient for many medical illnesses. Some of these options cost more than others. Yet we afford the patient the right to choose the specific treatment he desires—largely by insuring the costs of different types of treatments. I am not proposing here that we allow a patient (client) who suffers mental illness/emotional problems to embark on an extravagantly costly course of care (by insuring that care) when less costly care will afford him the same clinical results; still, there must be some leeway for the patient to choose among different courses of care even when the relative costs of these different courses of care vary from one to another.

Let me add one word of caution: I do believe very strongly that there are certain mental illnesses for which it is unthinkable at best to withhold psychiatric (medical) treatment—e.g., the utilization of psychotropic medication. For example, it seems to me that it is difficult, if not impossible, to justify withholding lithium (at least on a trial basis) in the treatment of (many) persons who suffer classical "manic–depressive illness." In addition, as I have just suggested, the great majority of patients who require inpatient mental health care will benefit greatly from psychiatric (medical) care—i.e., psychotropic medication and in some cases electroconvulsive therapy. We cannot be so clinically abstruse or even negligent as to deny such persons the opportunity to receive medical as well as psychological care. We have entered an era in the treatment of mental illness/emotional problems in which psychiatric (medical) diagnosis and psychiatric (medical) treatment can afford many persons, especially those who are severely ill, the opportunity to achieve relief of their symptoms. Yes—we must expand the pool of providers (mental health professionals) who are authorized to treat persons who suffer mental illness/ emotional problems; however, we cannot deny the severely mentally ill person—whether he is being treated on an inpatient or an outpatient basis—the possibility and opportunity of receiving psychiatric (medical) care as appropriate to his condition.

I can only hope that as mental health care becomes more refined, and as the various elements of psychiatric treatment (particularly the use of psychotropic medication in the treatment of mental illness/emotional problems) become better understood by and more acceptable to the nonpsychiatrist MHP (and to the layperson as well), the various providers of mental health care will be able to and willing to organize and deliver clinically appropriate mental health care services to all persons who intersect the mental health care delivery system at whatever level.

Of course, no matter how well the mental health care delivery system is structured and organized in terms of provider roles and functions, no matter how well its patients (clients) are appropriately slotted into the system, no matter how well we define mental health care services *per se* as distinct from educational, support, social, and rehabilitation services, and no matter how well the mental health care system is staffed and patients have financial as well as physical access to it, the system will not work if the *care* it offers is marginal or inadequate. Therefore, I must emphasize that the psychiatrist and other MHPs must now redouble their efforts to define what constitutes the best, most appropriate treatment for persons who suffer mental illness/ emotional problems. This is an elementary and vital provider function. As I have previously suggested, however, the politics of psychological treatment, both in the past and at present, have too often precluded the exposition of definite, meaningful guidelines for mental health care. Clearly, though, the psychiatrist (and other MHPs) must now catalog the advantages and disadvantages of such disparate treatment forms as behavior therapy, psychoanalysis (all schools), psychodynamic psychotherapy (all schools), and chemotherapy. He must also carefully scrutinize and examine the "medical model" as it applies and does not apply to the evaluation and treatment of mental illness/emotional problems. The medical model is certainly pertinent and applicable much of the time. However, it cannot be used by the psychiatrist in all cases to exclude nonpsychiatrist mental health professionals from the practice of mental health care.

I have already expressed the thought that I do not think we will ever arrive at a total, unanimous consensus as to what constitutes the best specific treatment for any individual person who suffers mental illness/emotional problems. Further, I believe that the MHP working with his patient (client) can often arrive at the same treatment end through different treatment approaches. (The differences between treatment approaches are often more apparent than real.) Still, as for any medical care, the successful practice of mental health care, specifically psychotherapy, will depend to a great extent upon the method of practice and the theoretical orientation of the practitioner. As the physician (nonpsychiatrist) continuously evaluates his treatment approach to the patient, the psychiatrist must now do the same. As medicine and surgery have advanced, they have replaced obsolete treatment forms with more effective treatment modalities. The nonpsychiatrist physician has defined guidelines for the diagnosis and treatment of various illnesses. It is time for the psychiatrist and other mental health professionals to make this a priority as well.

In a similar context, the physicist, as his science has progressed, has replaced (or supplemented) older, pre-Einstein models of the external, physical world with new models that better explain the dynamics of the universe. The psychiatrist, too, must be willing to update his theories—the psychological cornerstones of his treatment philosophy. He must revise his old model of the inner, psychic world to reflect the new data and evidence as to its dynamics. Unfortunately, there has been a certain reluctance to do so. Many practitioners, blinded by their set visions, refuse to modify and continue to espouse older theories of psychology and human behavior. I am not saying in this respect that psychoanalytic theory,* for example, needs to cede to "learning theory." I am suggesting, rather, that the best *combined* theory as to how the mind works must be hypothesized, committed to experiment, and applied in terms of treatment technique. Only in this way can we insure the efficacy and relevance of mental health care. Only in this way, too, can we develop effective peer review mechanisms that will be necessary if mental health care is to be cost-effective. After all, one cannot review treatment unless one has guidelines as to the best treatment approaches and the mechanism by which treatment works. To do so would be unfair to both the recipient and the provider of care.

---

*The term is vague. There are various schools of psychoanalytic thought, just as there are different schools of psychotherapy that espouse different theories.

In this connection, though, I must caution against any precipitous or premature establishment of firm treatment guidelines for mental health care. For example, within the present political climate, there is substantial, if not inordinate, pressure operating on the psychiatrist (and other MHPs) to find that a short course of treatment, designed and implemented in a specific way, constitutes the best care for those persons who suffer mental illness/emotional problems. Unfortunately, for the patient first and for the financial underwriting of mental health care second, such treatment will be effective and useful for only a certain group of persons. However, as I have constantly maintained, persons who suffer from many categories of mental illness/emotional problems will always require long-term, expensive care (even if it is only sometimes marginally effective), although we can hope to refine our clinical approach to such persons so as to abbreviate their treatment to the maximum extent possible. When the nonpsychiatrist physician testifies to a similar situation with regard to the patients he treats, his point of view is seen as acceptable and even obvious. Although the symptoms of mental illness/emotional problems and the results of treatment are often difficult to see and understand (for the layperson), as compared to the corresponding symptoms and results of treatment for medical-surgical illness, we should translate this concept of health care for medical-surgical illness to health care for mental illness/emotional problems.

6

Mental Health Care and Its Relationship to General Medical-Surgical Care of the Future

Throughout this paper, I stress the interface between organic (physical) illness and mental illness/emotional problems (see Chapters 2 and 3). I believe that in the future, the orientation of medicine will change—as it is already doing—to focus more and more on psychological factors as they affect health and illness. Medical care will pay more specific attention to the patient's unique personality as it makes him (or her) susceptible to disease or exacerbates illness. It will take into account as well the patient's emotional reaction to the stress of his illness and its effect on the course of that illness. This will result in an ever-increasing demand for mental health consultation and care. However, I feel that appropriate intervention by the psychiatrist (or other mental health professional) in the health care process will contribute to the stabilization of the total cost of medical care and may even decrease that cost, as illustrated by the following examples:

A patient reacts with excessive anxiety and depression to a hospitalization for an illness. In the hospital he (she) must ultimately rely for his well-being on his physician and the hospital staff. This patient, however, cannot tolerate not being in total charge of his life and not being able to control his own destiny. His main psychological "flaw" is that he is afraid of being dependent on anybody. He finds it difficult to trust others. With each day in the hospital, where one is never more like a child and more dependent, he becomes more depressed and anxious. He becomes frustrated and angry as well at his physician and the hospital staff, but he wishes to be a "good patient" so he keeps his feelings to himself. In fact, his depression and anxiety are hardly noticeable to others. His body is quite aware of them, however, and his condition worsens as his emotions exert a negative effect on the course of his illness. Fortunately, with the help of a mental health team his physician calls in, this patient is able to partially resolve his fear of dependency that is at the core of his depression, anxiety, and anger. His condition now gradually improves and he is discharged from the hospital.

This extremely common example demonstrates how the patient's emotional reaction to his (her) illness, whether or not he is in the hospital, will

influence the severity of his illness and the rate at which he is able to recover.*
In this case and in many others like it, the physician's attention to the patient's emotional state, rather than his prescription of specific medicine, was
the key that allowed the patient to get better.

Of course, at the present time, medical-surgical patients are for the most
part reluctant to accept evaluation and treatment from a psychiatrist. They
feel this demeans them; they fear that their physician in ordering such care
does not accept their illness as "real" and views them as "hypochondriacal."
Indeed, physicians today do often only resort to calling in a psychiatrist when
they consider the patient just that. Therefore, changing the attitudes and
prejudices of both patients and physicians toward the role of the psychiatrist
in treating illness is a first step in creating a more modern, responsive, and
effective health care system.

> Instead of obligating his patient to thousands and thousands of dollars
> of health care costs for *post hoc* treatment of a heart attack, a physician
> provides his patient, instead, with preventive mental health care before
> he suffers his heart disease. He chooses to treat the patient's "type A
> coronary" (predisposing to a heart attack) personality while the patient
> is still healthy. In so doing, he modifies, if he does not eliminate, the
> psychological factors operant in the patient that predispose him to a
> heart attack and a likely early and untimely death. (This is not to exclude
> the role of genetic factors in the etiology of heart disease for many
> persons, or the role of diet, smoking, and other factors. Compulsive
> smoking, eating, and drinking, of course, are hallmarks of emotional
> distress.) It may cost many dollars to provide preventive mental health
> care to this person and to others like him. In the end, though, a cost
> saving will be achieved—both in terms of medical care *per se* and in
> terms of a "save" of a productive member of society.

This example demonstrates the fact that by treating the patient's personality and by enabling him to recognize and deal appropriately with stress, we
can and shall, I believe, reduce the frequency and severity of illness. It is not
that we shall treat one particular personality type to prevent one particular

---

*A paper published after the completion of my paper, Mumford E, Schlesinger HJ, Glass GV: The
effects of psychological intervention on recovery from surgery and heart attacks: An analysis of
the literature, *American Journal of Public Health* 72:141–151, 1982, reviews "34 controlled studies
[that demonstrate] that, on the average surgical or coronary patients who are provided information or emotional support to help them master the medical crisis do better than patients who
receive only ordinary care . . . on the average psychological intervention reduced hospitalization
approximately two days . . . the evidence is that psychological care can be cost-effective." This
paper reviews multiple studies that demonstrate that patients' rates of survival and/or recovery
from illness and their response to medical care is dependent on their psychological (emotional)
state at the time of their illness and treatment. The paper also clearly documents the potential or
psychological intervention, even on a minimal generic basis, to favorably alter the course of a
patient's hospitalization.

disease; rather, we shall deliver mental health care that makes a person aware of and then helps him to resolve or moderate potentially pathogenic (in the physical and emotional sense) dammed-up feelings of frustration, anger, insecurity, "hurt," anxiety, depression, etc. Such emotions, if unmastered or repressed (held in), have the potential to produce disease in many body tissues and organs.

A patient develops peptic ulcer disease (ulcers) at the age of 25. Over the next 10 years he suffers continual symptoms of ulcers and he is hospitalized three times for severe exacerbations of his condition. Three years later, when his ulcers begin to bleed severely, he is hospitalized again. This time his physician recommends surgery to remove a portion of his stomach as the only definitive cure for his ulcer disease. He has the surgery and is discharged from the hospital. However, he remains well for only 6 months. Now he develops severe headaches. He undergoes an extensive medical work-up for his headaches, which includes skull X rays, an electroencephalogram, and a CAT scan. No definitive cause for his headaches is found and he is treated with medication. His symptoms continue over the next decades. He experiences not only headaches but various other physical symptoms. He misses work and is forced to curtail his social life at times due to the severity of his headaches and other physical complaints. He continuously takes medication to control his headaches, but the medication is only marginally effective.

A second patient, age 25, presents to a different physician with peptic ulcer disease. A diagnostic work-up is performed and treatment is begun. This physician elects to refer the patient to a psychiatrist, however, because he recognizes that the patient's peptic ulcer disease is directly related to his (the patient's) overreaction and misreaction to certain stresses in his life. Over the next 2 years, the patient works with the psychiatrist on a once-a-week basis. During this time, he develops moderate depression accompanied by anxiety. Through working with the psychiatrist, though, he is able to ascertain why he is depressed and anxious and he manages to overcome these symptoms. In the process, he becomes aware that he has been depressed and anxious for at least the preceding 3 years. He realizes that rather than allowing himself to experience these painful symptoms, he "buried" them. He recognizes that these feelings were "eating him up inside" and contributed to the development of his ulcers.

When this second patient's symptoms of depression and anxiety were "uncovered," and as they resolved with specialized mental health care, his ulcer disease went into remission. He is now symptom-free in all senses. Although he experiences the normal discomforts of life and suffers minor symptoms and illnesses, he essentially remains disease-free over the next 30 years.

Table 7. Summary Table for 25 Studies[a,b]

Study[c]	Setting	Time		Study group size	Comparison group				Impact on medical utilization (study group vs. comparison groups)
		Before ADM care	After ADM care		Size	Psychiatric match	Utilization match	Demographic match	
Mental Health									
1. West German (Duehrssen) (1962)	Clinic	Unstated	5 years	845	None	—	—	—	85% reduction in days of hospitalization
2. Kaiser Permanente (Follette) (1967)	HMO	1 year	5 years	152	152	Yes	Yes	Yes	62% decline for all medical visits vs. +13%; and 68% decline for all inpatient days vs. −6%
3. HIP (Fink) (1969)	HMO	1 year	2 years	112	106 116 97	Yes No Yes	No No No	No No No	8% decline for physician services vs. +5%, +3%, and −6%; and 15% decline for lab and X-ray services vs. −25%, −3%, and +1%
4. GHA (Goldberg) (1970)	HMO	1 year	1 year	256	None	—	—	—	31% decline for physician services and 30% decline for lab and X-ray visits
5. Kaiser Oregon (Uris) (1974)	HMO	1 year	1 year	45	45 45	Yes No	Yes Yes	Yes Yes	11% decline for medical visits vs. −16% and −28%
6. Puget Sound (Kogan) (1975)	HMO	5 years	2¼ years	148 171	148 165	No No	No No	Yes Yes	17% and 20% declines in total outpatients visits (including psychotherapy) from year before psychotherapy to 2nd year after vs. +5% and −3%

Study	Setting			N					Findings
7. Blue Cross W. Pennsylvania (Jameson) (1976)	CMHC	About 2 years	About 2 years	136; 26	1,500; 521	No; No	No; Yes	No; No	57% decline in inpatient and outpatient medical expenditures; 87% decline for high utilizers vs. −61% for comparison high utilizers
8. HIP Medicaid (Fink) (1977)	HMO	1 year	1 year	169	141	Yes	No	No	12% decline for all physician services vs. +7%; and 25% decline for lab and X-ray services vs. +28%
9. Mexican-American (McHugh) (1977)	Health center	About 6 months	About 6 months	119	None	—	—	—	72% increase in medical encounters
10. 4 Settings (Regier) (1977)	HMOs; health center	Mental Health care received at some time during the 1-year period studied		987; 541; 258; 957	172; 379; 555; 491	Yes; Yes; Yes; Yes	No; No; No; No	No; No; No; No	6%, 30%, 28%, and 21% fewer medical visits, respectively, by the four study groups
11. GHA (Patterson) (1978)	HMO	3 months; 12 months	3 months; 12 months	952; 426	None; None	—; —	—; —	—; —	Declines of 19% (medical services), 14% (lab), and 30% (X-ray) for 3 months after; declines of 5%, 16%, and 33% for 12 months after
12. Minority Children (Graves) (1978)	Health center	1 year	1 year	21; 21	21; 21	Yes; No	Yes; No	Yes; Yes	36% decline in medical visits vs. +30% and −9%
13. Columbia Medical Plan (Kessler) (1978)	HMO	1 year	1 year	1,155	None	—	—	—	8% decline in medical visits

(continued)

Table 7. (*Continued*)

Study[c]	Setting	Time		Study group size	Comparison group					Impact on medical utilization (study group vs. comparison groups)
		Before ADM care	After ADM care		Size	Psychiatric match	Utilization match	Demographic match		

Study[c]	Setting	Before ADM care	After ADM care	Study group size	Size	Psychiatric match	Utilization match	Demographic match	Impact on medical utilization (study group vs. comparison groups)
Alcohol									
14. Illinois Bell (Hilker) (1974)	Employee-based	5 years	5 years	402	None	—	—	—	Cases of sickness disability down 46%
15. Philadelphia Police Dept. (1975)	Employee-based	Unclear	1–2 years	170	None	—	—	—	Sick days down 38%; injured days down 62%
16. Philadelphia Fire Dept. (1975)	Employee-based	Unclear	6–12 months	77(51)	None	—	—	—	Sick days down 47%; injured days down 2%
17. Oldsmobile (Alander) (1975)	Employee-based	1 year	Up to 1 year	117	24	Yes	No	No	33% decline in S & A benefits vs. +66%; and 52% decline in lost manhours vs. +10%
18. Kennecott (1976)	Employee-based	1 year	Apparently 1 year	12	18	Yes	No	No	48% decline in hospital, medical and surgical costs vs. +87%
19. ATC (IWK Int.) (1976)	ATCs	1 month	6th month	4,777	None	—	—	—	Reduction in hospitalization pointed to total health care savings of more than $1,000 per client
20. G.M. Canada (Lunn) (1976)	Employee-based	About 1 year	About 1 year	104	48	Yes	No	No	48% decline in S & A benefits vs. + 127%; and 64% decline in WC benefits vs. +79%

Study	Setting	Before ADM care	After ADM care	Study group size				Results
21. California Pilot (Holder) (1976)	Employee-based	1 year	3–20 months	240+	None	—	—	—	26% reduction in medical utilization; 5.41 savings in medical expenditures for every $1.00 spent on alcoholism treatment
22. U.S. Navy (Edwards) (1977)	Rehabilitation program	2 years	2 years	148	None	—	—	—	Hospital days down 69%; all illness diagnoses down 79%
23. AHP (Hunter) (1978)	HMO	6 months	1 year	90	90	No	No	Yes	38% reduction in inpatient and outpatient medical expenditures vs. −9%
24. GHAA (Brock) (1978)	HMO	0–24 months	6–31 months	704	None	—	—	—	40% reduction in outpatient medical care utilization
25. Kaiser S. California (Sherman) (1979)	HMO	2 years	2 years	64	85	No	Yes	No	27% reduction in inpatient and outpatient medical care expenditures vs. +53%

[a] Taken from *Medical Care* 17 (December suppl., 1982): 1–82. The table is in the public domain.

[b] This table summarizes the 25 studies reported on in the ADAMHA report.[35] It is divided into columns as follows: (1) *Study*—Lists each study by name. (I have also provided a "reference" list from the ADAMHA report that specifies the identification of each study in greater detail than can be found in the table itself and provides specific references that allow a more detailed examination of each study.) (2) *Setting*—Describes the setting in which the health care was delivered. (HMO = Health Maintenance Organization. CMHC = Community Mental Health Center. "Employee-based" means that a program was set up for the employees. ATC = Alcohol Treatment Center.) (3) and (4) *Before ADM care* and *After ADM Care*—These two columns refer to the time at which data were collected. Thus, for study number 2, the Kaiser Permanente Study, the baseline for medical benefits utilized was taken 1 year before ADM (alcohol drug abuse and/or mental health) care, and the effects of ADM care on utilization of medical benefits were measured 5 years after ADM care. (5) *Study group size*—Delineates the number of persons who were investigated in

(continued)

Table 7. (*Continued*)

each particular study. (6), (7), (8), and (9). *Comparison group*—Delineates the nature of the group, if any, that was studied in comparison to the actual group under study. *Psychiatric match* indicates whether the groups were matched for presence of psychiatric disorders. *Utilization match* indicates whether the groups were matched for prior level of medical utilization. *Demographic match* refers to whether the groups were matched on critical demographic variables. (10) *Impact on medical utilization (study group vs. comparison groups)*—This is the critical column that reports the impact on medical benefits utilization (study group v. comparison group). If there was no comparison group, the results are reported strictly for the study group, and if there was a comparison group, the results for each group are reported and compared.

References: **Mental Health Studies.** 1. *West German Study.* Duehrssen, A.: Katamnestische ergebnisse bei 1004 patienten nach analytischer psychotherapie (Catamnestic results on 1,004 patients after analytic psychotherapy). Translated by the Congressional Budget Office. *Zschr. Psychosom. Med.* **8**:No. 2, 1962. 2. *Kaiser-Permanente Study.* a. Follette, W. T., and Cummings, N. A.: Psychiatric services and medical utilization in a prepaid health plan setting. *Med. Care* **5**:25, 1967. b. Cummings, N. A., and Follette, W. T.: Brief psychotherapy and medical utilization. *In:* The Professional Psychologist Today: New Developments in Law, Health Insurance, and Health Practice. H. Dorken, Ed. San Francisco, Jossey-Bass, 1976, pp. 165–174. c. Cummings, N. A.: Prolonged (ideal) versus short-term (realistic) psychotherapy. *Prof. Psychology* **8**:491, 1977. 3. *HIP Study.* Fink, R., Shapiro, S., and Goldensohn, S. S.: Psychiatric treatment and patterns of medical care. Unpublished report to the National Institute of Mental Health, Project MH 02321, July, 1969. 4. *GHA Study.* Goldberg, I. D., Krantz, G., and Locke, B. Z.: Effect of a short-term outpatient psychiatric therapy benefit on the utilization of medical services in a prepaid group practice medical program. *Med. Care* **8**:419, 1970. 5. *Kaiser of Oregon Study.* Uris, J.: Effects of Mental Health Utilization and Diagnosis on General Medical Care Utilization in a Prepaid Clinic Setting. Boulder, Colorado, Western Interstate Commission for Higher Education, 1974. 6. *Puget Sound Study.* Kogan, W. S., Thompson, D. J., Brown, J. R., and Newman, H. F.: Impact of integration of mental health service and comprehensive medical care. *Med. Care* **13**:934, 1975. 7. *Blue Cross of Western Pennsylvania Study.* Jameson, J., Shuman, L. J., and Young, W. W.: The effects of outpatient psychiatric utilization on the costs of providing third-party coverage. Blue Cross of Western Pennsylvania, Research Series 18, December, 1976 and *Med. Care* **16**:383, 1978. 8. *HIP Medicaid Study.* Fink, R., and Goldensohn, S.: Use of mental health services by Medicaid enrollees in a prepaid medical group practice. Unpublished report to the National Institute of Mental Health, Contract number HSM-42-71-70, February, 1977. 9. *Mexican-American Study.* McHugh, J. P., Kahn, M.

W., and Heiman, E.: Relationships between mental health treatment and medical utilization among low-income Mexican-American patients: Some preliminary findings. *Med. Care* **15**:439, 1977. 10. *Four Settings Study.* Regier, D. A., Goldberg, I. D., Burns, B. J., Hankin, J., and Hoeper, E. W.: Epidemiological and health services research findings in four organized health/mental health service settings. Unpublished paper presented at the ADAMHA Health Maintenance Organization Conference, Chicago, Illinois, November, 1977. 11. *GHA Study.* Patterson, D. Y., and Bise, B.: Report pursuant to contract #282-77-0219-MS. Unpublished report to the National Institute of Mental Health, January, 1978. 12. *Minority Children Study.* Graves, R. L., and Hastrup, J.: Effects of psychological treatment on medical utilization in a multidisciplinary health clinic for low income minority children. Unpublished paper presented at the Southwestern Psychological Association Meeting, New Orleans, Louisiana, April. 1978. 13. *Columbia Medical Plan Study.* Kessler, L.: Episodes of psychiatric care and medical utilization in a prepaid group practice. Unpublished Doctor of Science thesis submitted to the School of Hygiene and Public Health of the Johns Hopkins University. May 1978. **Alcohol Studies.** 14. *Illinois Bell Telephone Study.* Hilker, R. J.: Untitled and unpublished paper presented to the North American Congress on Alcohol and Drug Problems, San Francisco, California, December, 1974. 15. *Philadelphia Police Department Study.* Anonymous: Two tales of one city: Police program. Labor-Management Alcoholism J. **4**:1, 1975. 16. *Philadelphia Fire Department Study.* Anonymous: Two tales of one city: Fire program. Labor-Management Alcoholism J. **4**:17, 1975. 17. *Oldsmobile Study.* Alander, R., and Campbell, T.: An evaluative study of an alcohol and drug recovery program, a case study of the Oldsmobile experience. *Hum. Res. Manage.* **14**:14, 1975. 18. *Kennecott Study.* Anonymous: Insight. Unpublished papers, Utah Copper Division of the Kennecott Copper Corporation, 1969–1976. 19. *ATC Study.* JWK International Corporation: Benefit-cost analysis of alcoholism treatment centers. Unpublished report to the National Institute on Alcohol Abuse and Alcoholism, Contract number ADM-281-75-0027, December, 1976. 20. *General Motors of Canada Study.* Lunn, C. R.: Remarks. Unpublished paper presented at the Ontario Blue Cross Symposium on Alcoholism in Industry, Toronto, Ontario, May, 1976. 21. *California Pilot Program Study.* Holder, H. D., and Hallan, J. B.: A study of health insurance coverage for alcoholism for California state employees. Unpublished report to the National Institute on Alcohol Abuse and Alcoholism. Contract number ADM-281-75-0027, December, 1976. 22. *U. S. Navy Study.* Edwards, D., Bucky, S. F., Coben, P., Fichman, S., and Berry, N. H.: Primary and secondary benefits from treatment for alcoholism. *Am. J. Psychiatry* **134**:682, 1977. 23. *Arizona Health Plan Study.* Hunter, H.: Arizona health plan cost-benefit study. Unpublished report to the National Institute on Alcohol Abuse and Alcoholism, Grant number 5H84AA01745. November, 1978. 24. *Group Health Association of America (GHAA) Study.* Brock, C. P., and Boyajy, T. G.: Alcoholism within prepaid group practice HMOs. Report prepared for the National Institute on Alcohol Abuse and Alcoholism, Grant number 5H84-AA01745, December, 1978. 25. *Kaiser-Permanente of Southern California Study.* Sherman, R. M., Reiff, S., and Forsythe, A. B.: Utilization of medical services by alcoholics participating in an outpatient treatment program. *Alcoholism Clin. Exp. Res.* 3:115, 1979.

The point of this example, and the preceding examples as well, is that when mental health care services are made available to a patient population, great potential exists for a subsequent decline in the overall utilization of medical care—including hospitalization—by those patients receiving mental health care. For some time now, investigators have been attempting to correlate the relationship between the utilization of mental health care by a patient and his subsequent utilization of other types of medical (i.e., medical-surgical) care. The hard-core data are not conclusive at present—although a psychological analysis of the reasons why many persons seek medical care, combined with data, previously presented, indicating that a significant percentage of patient visits to physicians of all kinds stem from psychological or emotional distress and/or disorder, would clearly indicate that mental health care, if it is effective, should reduce a patient's tendency to seek and his need for medical-surgical care. Let us examine, in this connection, a key review of 25 health care studies by the Alcohol, Drug Abuse, and Mental Health Administration (ADAMHA).[35] ADAMHA reports that in 12 of 13 studies dealing with a general population, there were reductions of 5 to 85% in medical care utilization subsequent to mental health intervention for the patients involved. The median reduction was 20%. The other 12 studies reported specifically on medical care utilization after treatment for alcohol abuse. It was found that there were reductions of 26 to 69% in either medical care utilization or "surrogate measures of such utilization" (sick days and sickness and accident benefits). The median reduction was 40%. It should be noted that the studies reported on had some methodological difficulties that make it impossible to completely validate their findings. (I am including herein a summary table from the ADAMHA review "Impact of Alcohol, Drug Abuse, and Mental Health Treatment on Medical Care Utilization." See Table 7.)

To critically balance the ADAMHA review, I shall review and critically analyze in depth here one additional study[36] that brings into question whether or not total health care savings can in fact be achieved by providing patients with mental health care services. This study was a report on the approximately 2.3 million people insured under Michigan Blue Cross and Blue Shield during the year 1975. It was shown that persons who utilized mental health benefits under this program incurred higher mean hospital and physician charges for all diagnostic categories except infectious diseases and injuries. The authors suggest that this may be because "people with mental disorders are older than the population as a whole and therefore more likely to be high users of medical care." The authors pose other hypotheses as well to account for the higher charges: (1) the "detection" hypothesis, namely, that "individuals who encounter the health care system for one reason are more likely to be screened for other conditions, which would then be detected and treated"; (2) the "labeling" hypothesis, namely, that "people who are high users of services for any condition are likely to be thought of as 'hypochondriacal and referred for psychiatric care" (this then constitutes mental health care *after the fact* of medical or surgical care); (3) the "association" hypothesis, namely, that "anxiety and depression are commonly associated with and may be diagnosed along with physical disorders." (Naturally, medical or surgical illness is very distressing to the sufferer.)

The data in this report hardly invalidate the concept that appropriate mental health care can decrease the overall cost of medical and surgical care. In the first place, appropriate mental health care, including psychotherapy or psychotropic medication or both, may reduce the total cost of an episode of illness through controlling the patient's emotional reaction to illness—e.g., anxiety and depression. Thus, although hospital and physician charges may be higher for the medically ill patient who utilizes mental health care services than for the patient who does not, the patient's illness might have been even more expensive had he not sought or been referred for mental health care. (His mental illness/emotional problems might have prolonged and/or complicated his illness.) Further, it should be pointed out that in the insurance program under consideration, outpatient mental health benefits were limited to $400 per year—in fact, a totally inadequate benefit. If the benefits had been more generous or unlimited, we would have been able to get a better gauge on the effect of full and complete mental health care on the incidence, severity, and, ultimately, cost of medical-surgical illness. The patient whose mental health benefits are limited may be unconsciously "forced" to express his emotional symptoms in medical-surgical illness once his benefits run out.

I would also point out that this study reports on charges incurred by the patients in a single year. Thus, mental health care in one year may decrease utilization of medical services in succeeding years. The patients reported on in this study who utilized mental health benefits should be restudied in 5 or 10 years to determine if their total charges for health care over the period are less than those for a comparable group who had not initially utilized mental health benefits. Long-term follow-up in these kinds of studies is essential. No firm or final conclusions can be drawn without it.

Finally, the data in the study indicate that patients who utilized mental health benefits had lower utilization rates of medical services for infectious diseases and accidental injuries. This is highly significant as it has been demonstrated that injuries, which are often extremely costly, may result from mental illness/emotional problems and that they are often not truly "accidental." In addition, a person's emotional health may influence whether or not he contracts an infectious disease. A person's resistance to infectious disease, from the common cold to more serious infectious illnesses, is often partially dependent upon his reaction to stress.*

*Let us not confuse the issue. The point is not whether a person who suffers mental illness/ emotional problems requires more medical care than the person who does not suffer mental illness/emotional problems. Indeed, this may be the case—just as it is likely that the judicious use of mental health care will reduce the overall utilization of medical care by the person who suffers mental illness/emotional problems. A recent in-depth study, published after the completion of my paper (D. A. Regier, I. D. Goldberg, B. J. Burns, *et al*, "Specialist/Generalist Division of Responsibility for Patients with Mental Disorders," *Archives of General Psychiatry* 39(1982): 219–224), seems to confirm both hypotheses for the short clinical run, at least. (The study does not include long-term follow-up of patients.) Ultimately, however, the point is that any person who

In fact, we need many more studies to correlate the relationships between mental illness/emotional problems and medical-surgical illness and the effect of treatment of the former on the latter. Ultimately, I firmly believe, we shall consolidate the view that there is a strong continuum between mental illness/emotional problems and medical-surgical illness. We shall demonstrate that physical symptoms and organic (physical) illness are often an expression of emotional distress. Applying this principle, we shall call upon the psychiatrist and the mental health team he leads to reduce expensive outpatient medical-surgical diagnosis and treatment for the huge numbers of persons who in reaction to psychological stress seek but do not really require medical-surgical evaluation and care—or require it only in a secondary and limited way. We will provide such persons instead with *appropriate* mental health evaluation and care. The psychiatrist will evaluate the patient's emotional and physical state and judge how they are interconnected. Quite often, then, he (the psychiatrist) and his team will be able to alleviate the patient's symptoms or cure the patient without needing to call in other physician specialists or minimizing such intervention.

Of course, the psychiatrist, if he is to be successful in the capacity I have just described, will need to have full treatment resources at his command. When health planners and legislators consider limits on mental health care coverage under NHI, they should realize the implications of such limits for patients such as I have just described. Inadequate limits pose the threat of locking these patients into high-frequency utilization of unnecessary and costly medical-surgical care for their entire lives. Indeed, many "perennial patients" will often require extensive mental health care to allow them to break their old care-seeking patterns. This is because their reluctance to recognize their "real" mental illness/emotional problems is often severe.

Besides the formal studies reported above, there is a plethora of anecdotal reports by physicians to the effect that the recognition and resolution of emotional problems by patients leads to a decrease in the physical symptoms and illness they experience, with a consequent reduction in their need for medical-surgical diagnosis and treatment. The author himself has treated many patients who demonstrate this phenomenon. When the patient, as a result of psychiatric treatment, is able to accept the reality of an underlying depression or anxiety state, he (she) is able to deflect his symptoms from the somatic sphere and, instead, to experience symptomatically his primary emotional discomfiture—which he can then begin to resolve.

It should be noted that simply providing increased coverage for mental health care is not the total answer to reducing medical-surgical health expenditures (via the intervention of a psychiatrist). Unnecessary outpatient treatment and hospitalizations such as I have described are often a result of preju-

---

suffers mental illness/emotional problems deserves full and complete mental health care based on his medical need for such care—as opposed to any other criteria, e.g., the cost-effectiveness of such care.

dices and attitudes of both the patient and the physician toward mental illness/emotional problems. I must emphasize that both the patient and the physician are often unwilling to acknowledge the patient's real problem: emotional distress. The physician actively "conspires" with the patient to treat his medical problems as though they are purely organic (physical) problems; expensive medical evaluations are performed for symptoms such as fatigue, dizziness, headaches, stomachaches, or backaches. Medication is prescribed and needless operations are performed that do not alleviate the patient's symptoms—or if they do, others spring up to take their place and the patient requires further diagnosis and treatment on either an outpatient or an inpatient basis or both. This endless cycle of misplaced, misdirected medical care is perpetuated because both the patient and the physician are unwilling to face the patient's real problem—underlying emotional distress. We must remove the stigma that surrounds mental illness/emotional problems and encourage the patient to acknowledge and accept his emotional upset instead of hiding it in physical upset.

Of course, we can never completely eliminate the necessity for medical-surgical diagnostic studies. When a patient complains of physical symptoms to his physician, these symptoms must be investigated as appropriate—no matter what the status of the patient's emotional health.

Essentially, I am suggesting in this section that the physician in the future will approach the patient from a combined biological, psychological, and social perspective in terms of both preventing illness in the first place and then treating it once it has occurred. (Indeed, this multiple perspective is being currently applied in the new field of "biobehavioral" or "behavior" medicine.) The biological approach to the patient is nothing new. It is a feature of the "biomedical model" we currently follow. I have discussed the psychological approach to the patient above. This leaves the social approach to the patient. It takes into account the fact that no man or woman is a physiological island, that every person lives within a social network, and that that network not only contributes to illness but also reacts to it. The specific way in which those persons who make up the patient's social network react to his illness will influence the course and outcome of that illness. In addition, the patient's illness can cause serious consequences for the physical and emotional health of those persons who make up the patient's social network. Thus, the patient's physician, working in tandem with the psychiatrist and other MHPs, must evaluate and treat as necessary not only any given patient but persons within that patient's social network as well. Often this will entail mental health care and/or separate emotional support services.

Mental health care will always play a primary role for persons who are not "physically ill" and who suffer mental illness/emotional problems. As can be seen, however, it can also evolve into a major medical resource *per se*. The psychiatrist will play a special role in coordinating comprehensive care for the patient, although nonpsychiatrist MHPs can be expected to play a major role as well in the treatment of the patient and persons who make up his social network.

NHI must make provisions for these basic changes that are going to, or at least should, occur in the nature of medical-surgical care. They are another reason why we must expand mental health care services and coverage under NHI, rather than limit them. Poor coverage for mental health care will retard the process of evolution of general medical-surgical care. It will encourage the partially antiquated exclusively biological approach to the patient we now often practice, an approach that for the most part divorces medical-surgical care from psychological care and social intervention, yields less effective health care, and in the process increases the total cost of health care.

7

The Poor Image of Psychotherapy as a Roadblock to Coverage: A Corrected View and Some Thoughts on Validation

Psychotherapy* has a severe image problem. This is still another major factor that militates against full coverage for mental health care under NHI. True enough, laypersons, including health planners and legislators, can see a value in the treatment of serious mental illness such as the psychiatric syndromes. When a person is psychotic, they recognize the necessity for mental health care. However, when symptoms are not that apparent, as in the person who suffers chronic symptomatic maladjustment (see Chapter 3), the public too often does not understand what is to be gained by treatment—or how. The layperson is frequently of the opinion that mental health care, especially psychotherapy, consists of little more than a conversation between a patient and a psychiatrist. He does not conceptualize psychotherapy as any special process. Nor does he believe that any special skills are required to practice it. As a result, the layperson is reluctant to spend his money—or his constituents' tax dollars if he is a legislator—on what he perceives to be a vague, interminable, and meaningless treatment.

If the psychiatrist is to be successful in securing full coverage for mental health care under NHI, it is therefore incumbent upon him to explain the process of psychotherapy in some detail and in a manner that the layperson can understand. The plethora of misconceptions attached to psychotherapy must be dispelled. The psychotherapist (psychiatrist and nonpsychiatrist) must be seen in his proper light—not just as listener, teacher, advisor, friend, advocate, and model, although he is that, but as a highly skilled technician who employs a unique method that frequently transcends to a large extent the various psychological "schools." The layperson must come to realize that psychotherapy does not seek to fit a person into some strange, wild (mad?) theory; nor, practically (clinically) speaking, does it concern itself with the sexual derivation of mental illness/emotional problems—as classical psychoanalysis has done in the past.

---

*Many of my comments in this section about psychotherapy apply to psychoanalysis as well.

Volumes have been written about psychotherapy; it is as impossible to define it within a short space as it is to define "medical care." Within these confines, let me proceed: The psychiatrist and other MHPs must make clear to the layperson that psychotherapy, in the most simple terms, is a therapeutic method that aims to enable a person to achieve partial or whole relief from specifically defined clinical symptoms (as opposed to general upset, confusion, boredom, unhappiness, etc.) from which he (or she) suffers. The psychiatrist must relate that to effect such ends, psychotherapy focuses on enabling a person to *perceive* and *understand* himself. Equally important, a person learns, as a part of the process of psychotherapy, how he *mis*perceives and *mis*understands how others think and feel about him and behave toward him as well as how he relates and reacts to them. Ultimately, psychotherapy strives to allow a person to see himself—his thoughts, feelings, and behavior—and others objectively. Through psychotherapy, a person learns autonomy; he also learns to function in a more adaptive way in terms of relationships with others, work, and play. He becomes conscious and aware, in the fullest possible sense, of the decisions and choices he makes in his life, and he recognizes his ability and option to make different, more appropriate, and ultimately more gratifying decisions and choices. Psychotherapy unshackles a person from his past, allowing him the freedom to think, feel, and behave in a positive, personally rewarding way instead of in the unsatisfying way of his past. [Of course, the psychotherapist's patients (clients) achieve the objectives of psychotherapy to a greater or lesser extent, or in some cases not at all, just as medical-surgical patients respond to their treatment to varying degrees and sometimes fail to receive any benefit from it.] Psychotherapy, it must be stressed, involves much more than the patient's acquiring "information" about himself in an "intellectual" fashion. The patient also reexperiences past emotional "hurts" and traumas as an integral part of his psychotherapy. It is the understanding and assimilation of both the intellectual and the emotional experience of psychotherapy that allows the acquisition of "insight" ("knowledge") that incorporates both cognitive and affective elements) by the patient. It is this insight that to a large extent (although hardly exclusively) allows psychotherapy to work—i.e., to reduce the patient's level of symptoms. I should stress here that psychotherapy does not work in a magical therapeutic vacuum wherein it extracts isolated symptoms with keen surgical precision. It can effect symptom relief for a person only through the process I have just described, a process that seeks to explore a person's view of his inner personal world and the external world around him and seeks to adjust his interaction with both of those worlds.

I must emphasize that psychotherapy, when employed as a treatment for either acute or chronic symptoms, does not make a totally "new person" from an "old" one. It does allow for increased adaptation and enhanced functioning. However, although a person may change significantly, and in some cases extremely, through the process of psychotherapy, he (or she) retains many, if not most, aspects or components of his personality (or "character"). He learns, though, to recognize and manage his personality "flaws" so as to be able to react with more choice and control to those situations that are difficult for him. His symptoms are most often not completely abolished as a result of psychotherapy, but they should be less painful for him. (In the same sense, many, if not most, medical-surgical patients get partial relief from their symptoms and enhancement of functioning as a result of their treatment, but they are not cured of their disease process, and they experience symptoms of varying intensity from time to time to which they will ideally be able to adapt.) I believe that we can attribute a certain portion of the generally prevailing negative opinion of psychotherapy to the unrealistic expectations of many persons as to what it should be able to achieve. If we are to be able to correctly judge the value of psychotherapy (or of any form of health care for that matter), we must evolve a realistic attitude as to exactly what constitutes the beneficial results we should expect of it. We must view psychotherapy as a treatment process in the same context that we view medical-surgical care. We should evaluate the efficacy of psychotherapy neither less stringently nor more strictly than we evaluate the efficacy of medical-surgical care.

Relatively simple, though comprehensible, definitions of the process and goals of psychotherapy such as I have set forth here are not often communicated to the layperson—with the result that the meaning and value of psychotherapy are obscured. To reemphasize: The mental health professional must concentrate his efforts to explain psychotherapy if he is to achieve full coverage for mental health care under NHI.

The above description of psychotherapy does not detract from my earlier contention that mental health care—including psychotherapy—must aim primarily at the triad of (1) symptom cure, amelioration, or control; (2) remission maintenance, prevention of symptoms from recurring; and (3) symptom prophylaxis—prevention of symptoms. It recognizes, though, that management of symptoms often can only be arrived at through gradual personality change or modification, as opposed to a surgically swift removal of symptoms on an isolated basis. It acknowledges that, for many persons, symptoms are not discrete, encapsulated entities that can be erased by medicines or persuasion, but rather that they result from intrapsychic conflicts that a person must resolve if he is to achieve short-term and, more important, long-term relief. I should also point out that such a model of psychotherapy does not disparage the use of psychotropic medication (e.g., antidepressants) in the psychotherapeutic process. As I have emphasized, such medicines are often an extremely important adjunct to psychotherapy. As I have further pointed out, the psychiatrist—or other mental health professionals working in conjunction with the psychiatrist—must appropriately integrate a medical and a nonmedical approach to the patient (client) in order to effect his emotional health. For some patients, the resultant psychotherapeutic approach will be mainly medical and, as such, will primarily entail the use of medication (e.g., antidepressants) with minimal psychotherapy. For many other patients, however, the approach will be exclusively nonmedical, employing only psychotherapy.

I would be the first to acknowledge that the above model of psycho-therapy is somewhat incomplete and limited. For example, psychotherapy also works through simple catharsis, through the process of "desensitizing" the patient to the psychological traumas he has experienced in his life, through a process of promoting the patient's self-esteem ("strengthening the ego"), and through a process that aims at allowing the patient to accept and "forgive" himself and to treat himself less harshly (decreasing the strength of the superego.)* As far as it goes, though, it is a model, I think, with which the majority of my colleagues would generally agree—with the exception of some psychoanalysts and "learning theorists" (behavior therapists).

To assuage my colleagues of these persuasions, I acknowledge that any model of psychotherapy must be based to a certain extent on the underlying assumption that human behavior is predicated on sexual and aggressive in-stincts (drives) since man is in the first instance an "animal." I would also admit that human behavior is *learned* and follows a particular pattern based on selective reinforcement (both positive and negative) and nonreinforcement of thinking, feeling, and behaving. Nevertheless, a person is not a crocodile who reacts purely on an animalistic level any more than he is a robot who reacts in a mechanistic, programmed manner. Many psychotherapists too often neglect the "human quality" in their approach to treatment. Here I am referring to the human need, desire, and spiritual inclination—if not in-stinct—to form permanent bonds and relationships with other persons, to achieve, to realize oneself as an individual person, and so forth. De-emphasis of such "human qualities" in theoretical models of psychotherapy often leads to the assumption by the layperson that psychotherapy is of little practical use. Worse, it reinforces the pervading public apprehension about psycho-therapy. Indeed, I believe that many persons unconsciously view psycho-therapy almost as an alien force that invades one's mind, stripping one of one's individuality. Of course, it does not. It promotes one's sense of indi-viduality ("ownness")—which is not only important in itself but is a prerequi-site precursor to the ability to relate in a complete, mature fashion to others.

I should add here that the psychiatrist (or other MHP), in communicating an understanding of psychotherapy to the layperson, must also explain that the positive results of psychotherapy depend to a great extent on the special and exclusive nature of the "therapeutic relationship"—the total relationship between the psychotherapist and his patient. The psychiatrist must differenti-ate this relationship from other "helpful" pairings and delineate how it is a key factor in the curative or restorative process of psychotherapy (see Appen-dix). Finally, the psychiatrist must explain why psychotherapy in practice is often a time-consuming method, why it is difficult to achieve results with it in a short time span. In this connection, the psychiatrist must emphasize the fact that when he first begins to treat his patient (client), he is often dealing with a

---

*For some patients—in particular those who suffer from certain personality disorders, e.g., the antisocial personality disorder—the superego needs to be strengthened.

person whose symptoms have been formed, shaped, and reinforced over years, if not decades. For such a person, significant and lasting symptom relief cannot often be accomplished in the course of 20 psychotherapy sessions, the current upper limit of outpatient treatment (in the private sector) for which coverage would be available under current NHI legislation. This should be obvious, but it is neither acknowledged, accepted, nor understood. This underlines once again the imperative to educate the layperson about psychotherapy in terms of not only its methods and mechanics but its potential and its limitations as well. Only in this way can psychotherapy overcome the myth that surrounds it. Only then can it overcome the prejudice and discrimination associated with mental illness/emotional problems and mental health care in general. Psychotherapy must defeat a further obstacle: its youth and its "radical" notions. Psychotherapy is really a 20th-century phenomenon. It is the new kid on the health care block and it is a revolutionary child at that—challenging the way people see themselves, their personal worlds, and the world at large around them. This can lead to a benign defensiveness on the part of the layperson toward it, but it can also lead to a hostile, nonrational rejection of it by him.

In the final analysis, the psychiatrist, no matter how well he explains psychotherapy, cannot really expect the layperson to believe *prima facie* that psychotherapy "works," although unless and until he does, he will be unwilling to accept it or endorse or sponsor it (if he is a legislator) as a legitimate form of health care. The layperson, as stated, generally questions the value of psychotherapy. He is often of the opinion that psychotherapy, no matter what is claimed for it, simply "doesn't work."

In fact, many, if not most, surveys and studies on psychotherapy, whether critical or positive, demonstrate limited to little validity. Too often, for example, they do not take into account the quality, duration, or importance of therapeutic changes the patient (client) experiences. (Admittedly, these entities can be difficult to measure.)

It is beyond the scope of this paper to review the wide body of research on "psychotherapy outcome" or to arrive at any final determination regarding the ultimate accountability of mental health care—in particular, psychotherapy. In this connection, however, I will quote briefly from a report prepared by the Congress of the United States, Office of Technology Assessment.[37] The report states, "If one considers only the trend of findings reported by scholarly reviews and analyses of the psychotherapy outcome literature, it would appear that psychotherapy treatments, under some conditions, have been shown to be efficacious. . . . Although the evidence is not entirely convincing, the currently available literature contains a number of good-quality research studies which find positive outcomes for psychotherapy. There are also a large number of studies which report positive effects, but whose methods or generalizability are difficult to assess." (The report also comments on the cost-effectiveness of psychotherapy, concluding that "for some treatment system characteristics and for some problems, psychotherapy appears to be cost beneficial.") I will also quote here from a report to the National Academy of Sciences by Parloff[38] summarizing his work and that of others at the NIMH on the effectiveness of psychotherapy. Parloff's conclusion is that "patients treated by psychosocial therapies show significantly more improvement in thought, mood, personality, and behavior than do comparable samples of untreated patients." Parloff also refers in his paper in this volume to "A recent review [that] summarized nearly 700 published and unpublished studies, each of which included an untreated group. This design permitted the estimate of relevant rates of spontaneous recovery in each study. It was found that in over 90% of the experiments, the psychotherapy group improved more than the control group. The median person receiving psychotherapy was better off than 80% of the untreated controls. The authors conclude that their survey of research findings overwhelmingly validates the benefit of psychotherapy."

The above studies not withstanding, if we are to correctly assess the validity of psychotherapy, future studies must be conducted over sufficient lengths of time (5, 10, or 20 years and even longer) to allow a thorough evaluation of the long-term effects of psychotherapy. This would include measurements not only of short-term and long-term symptom relief but also of social adjustment, work productivity, and success at interpersonal relationships achieved by those persons undergoing psychotherapy, tabulated in terms of their own goals as well as accepted norms.* The effects of psychotherapy should also be measured in terms of reductions in medical care utilization experienced by persons undergoing psychotherapy. All studies, when possible, should include well-matched control groups. (It is often very difficult to include such groups in psychotherapy studies.) In addition, studies of psychotherapy in the future, if they are to be valid, must attempt to control for the quality of the provider's clinical work. This is important because if in any given study the providers of psychotherapy—i.e., the psychotherapists—possess inferior skill or if they are not suited in personality to practice psychotherapy, the particular study can only yield a negative outcome that in turn only reflects on the persona and clinical practice of the psychotherapists involved in the study, as opposed to the particular method of psychotherapy under investigation.

There are at present several comprehensive reviews and studies of psychotherapy either proposed or under way. The Commission on Psychiatric Therapies of the American Psychiatric Association is engaged in the compilation of a Psychiatric Treatment Manual (PTM-I) that will seek to set forth the best type and course of psychotherapy for any given person suffering any given condition. Within the governmental sector, the National Institute of Mental Health (NIMH) has embarked on a long-term research project designed to measure the relative efficacies of different forms of psychotherapy.

---

*We must be exceedingly careful in defining "accepted norms."

In addition, a bill (S647) was introduced in the United States Senate (on March 6, 1981) that, if passed, would create a federal commission (the National Professional Mental Health Services Commission) that would theoretically study the safety and efficacy of various forms of psychotherapy. Finally, ADAMHA is considering initiating its own study on the safety and efficacy of psychotherapy. It is worthwhile to note that it is certainly appropriate for governmental agencies concerned with health planning and health care delivery to become involved in the evaluation of psychotherapy and other forms of mental health care as treatment methods. However, as I have related, this should not occur on an exclusive basis. All forms of health care, including mental health care, should be subjected to fair and vigorous evaluation as regards their safety and efficacy. It is also to be hoped that when such evaluation is conducted within the government or under governmental auspices, political and cost considerations will not preclude the planning and carrying out of comprehensive studies spanning adequate time periods. Such studies, as I pointed out above, should measure as completely as possible the long-term effects of health care. I should emphasize here that symptom relief, especially in the short term, is only one measurement of the validity of any treatment method. This obviously includes psychotherapy.

I must add that the federal commission (the National Professional Mental Health Services Commission) proposed in S647 would not appear to foster a genuine and thorough scientific inquiry into the value of psychotherapy and other mental health care services. It seems designed to effect strict control of the cost of mental health care rather than to examine the legitimacy of such care. S647 seeks to narrowly evaluate mental health care—by January 1984—in terms of whether it is "reasonable and necessary to prevent the patient's institutionalization, [prevent the patient's] inability to carry out activities in society which are generally accepted as being essential, or [prevent the patient's] becoming a danger to himself or others." This, it seems clear to me, does not constitute a proper definition of the purpose of mental health care. Rather, it views such care strictly as a mechanism to insure skeletal maintenance of a person within society. S647 in essence discriminates against mental health care. The same criteria of validity imposed by S647 for mental health care applied to other forms of health care would rule out all but emergency care and stopgap chronic care for the patient whose functioning has been severely compromised. (Even if S647 falls by the legislative wayside, it is possible that other similarly styled bills will find their way to the congressional docket.)

In addition to calling for new, more thorough, and more complete psychotherapy studies, the psychiatrist and other mental health professionals must forthrightly acknowledge that many of those already conducted raise serious questions as to the manner and mode in which treatment—psychotherapy and psychoanalysis—is and should be conducted. The psychiatrist, now and in the future, must use legitimate data from psychotherapy studies to modify his treatment approach to his patients: e.g., to develop more specific criteria for determining which persons can benefit from psychotherapy (including from which form(s) of psychotherapy), to better match particular practitioners to particular patients (clients), to modify old methods, theories, and techniques, and to revise training for the practitioner and the student.

Although I do not believe that any studies on psychotherapy or psychoanalysis conducted to date conclusively demonstrate the ultimate and absolute superiority of one form or length of psychotherapy (or psychoanalysis) versus another, the majority of psychiatrists, I think, will already be willing to conclude, on the basis of the general trend of well-conceived studies on psychotherapy and on theoretical models of psychotherapy (and psychoanalysis) and practical clinical experience as well, that certain forms and concepts of treatment should be replaced or extensively modified, that long-term intensive psychotherapy and psychoanalysis, although they have a definite role, have been overutilized in the past, and that treatment can be shortened or decreased in frequency for many patients (clients) without sacrificing quality of care. I must be quick to point out that short-term psychotherapy, although it is clinically valid and useful for many patients, clearly has its limits. And no wonder! Any physician (or mental health professional) working in any specialty field empirically knows the most simple of clinical verities: namely, that different patients (clients) require different levels of care. This has been, is, and always will be the case, and all the research studies in the world, no matter how carefully and flawlessly they are designed, will never demonstrate otherwise. (In this connection, there is a great question as to whether it will ever be possible to design the perfect research study into mental health care. The nature of such care and the nature of the results of such care make it extremely difficult to structure studies and to evaluate them on a purely "scientific" basis.) It is not that long-term care or short-term care is valid or invalid; rather, the clinician must ascertain for which particular patient (client) a particular level as well as type of care is clinically appropriate. Unfortunately, when it comes to mental health care, and only mental health care, there is the tendency to look at long-term care as black (and somehow "clinically dirty") and short-term care as white (and "clinically clean"). Let us not be therapeutically color-blind when it comes to mental health care. Let us be willing to acknowledge that a particular patient (client), whether he suffers medical-surgical illness or mental illness/emotional problems, will require a unique shade and hue of treatment carefully selected and applied out of the broad therapeutic spectrum. Let us study all medical care, including mental health care, on such a theoretical and real basis. We must be willing to examine and evaluate the applicability of particular forms of treatment to classes and subclasses and subclasses of subclasses of patients (clients). It seems to me that studies of mental health care, especially psychotherapy, will be valid and applicable only so long as we apply this method—which follows a basic and fundamental principle of medical research, a principle that is essential to the evaluation of all medical therapeutics.

To state the general case, as well as the case of the individual patient (client), health planners and legislators will have to accept at some point the fact that short-term psychotherapy can never completely replace long-term psychotherapy. Yes, the psychiatrist will become more efficient in his treatment methods and he will be able to successfully treat more patients (clients) on a short-term basis. However, many patients, especially those who are severely ill and those who suffer chronic symptomatic maladjustment (CSM; see Chapter 3) will require intermediate to long-term psychotherapy. By this I mean, on average, 50 to 400 treatment visits over roughly 1 to 4 years. (By some standards for long-term psychotherapy or psychoanalysis, this constitutes short-term treatment!) In my opinion, this will be the case no matter what extraordinary medicines the psychiatrist may develop and no matter how well he may refine his methods.

The good physician knows that it is a cardinal sin to overtreat his patient; he also knows it is a cardinal sin to undertreat him. In this connection, since I have just spoken out against the overutilization of long-term, intensive psychotherapy (and psychoanalysis), I emphasize here that we must be exceedingly cautious in evaluating the results and merits of short-term (or brief) psychotherapy. Yes, short-term psychotherapy is indicated for many patients (clients); it can constitute a full and complete course of care. However, we must ask whether we can attribute the positive results of short-term psychotherapy, in many cases, to anything more than the nonspecific generic therapeutic *contact* of the patient with the medical healer—i.e., to the healing process attached to the physician (MHP)–patient (client) relationship. We must question whether short-term psychotherapy results in real (partial or whole) resolution of a patient's mental illness/emotional problems or whether, too often, it only dulls, masks, or covers the patient's symptoms. To draw a somewhat hyperbolic analogy, the physician can successfully treat, in the short run, pain from almost any cause or condition by prescribing high doses of narcotics for his patient. By doing so, however, he may harm the patient and even cause his death. At the least, the physician will most often not affect the patient's disease process itself by simply treating his pain. Therefore, it is a general rule in medicine that the physician should not attempt to relieve the patient's pain until he knows what is causing it. And then, although the physician may have to prescribe an anodyne for his patient to afford him symptomatic relief in the short run, the physician attempts to therapeutically attack the patient's pain by treating his disease *process*. In other words, the physician is not so much concerned with treating pain *per se* as he is concerned with treating the cause of the patient's pain. To draw the analogy back to short-term psychotherapy, it is possible that such treatment is too often directed at treating the patient's overt emotional pain, that this type of care too often pays insufficient attention to the patient's underlying cause of pain, that is his basic mental illness/emotional problem. If this is true, although he may receive immediate relief of his symptoms from short-term (or brief) psychotherapy, the patient (client) may eventually experience se-

vere and sometimes catastrophic illness due to the fact that his illness/prob-
lem was not properly and thoroughly addressed and treated when it came to
the attention of the clinician. To return to the medical metaphor, the physician who treats an infectious disease process in his patient is not so much
concerned with reducing his patient's fever as he is with eradicating the
source of infection. Thus, even after the patient's fever has subsided, (and
although the patient often wants to stop his treatment at this time), the
physician will continue the patient's course of antibiotics. Now, although the
mental illness/emotional problems from which most patients suffer is not the
result of an infectious process (although who knows what the future will
reveal about the etiology of certain psychiatric syndromes), I hope the point I
have developed here is well taken: namely, all medical care, including mental
health care, should be directed at treating the patient's (client's) underlying
illness or disease process, not just the symptoms of illness as they are variously manifested in any particular patient. Even after the patient's pain has
subsided, the treating professional must be sure that he has contained, if not
cured, the illness from which the patient suffers to the maximum extent
possible—in spite of the fact that the patient is no longer complaining of pain.
[Every mental health professional knows that patients (clients) too often terminate their treatment prematurely; their emotional distress or symptoms,
which prompted them to seek treatment, are often quickly relieved to a substantial extent by even the briefest treatment; yet their illness/problem has
hardly been diagnosed, addressed, or appropriately treated.] If the physician,
or MHP, cannot treat the patient's illness or problem itself, then and only
then should he treat the patient's symptoms alone. To apply these principles
to the treatment of mental illness/emotional problems means, in the first
instance, that we are ready and willing to conceptualize mental illness/emo-
tional problems as *processes* rather than as *isolated symptoms* or *constellations of
symptoms*. Yes, let us appropriately prescribe short-term (or brief) psychotherapy for those patients (clients) who require this modality of care; however, let us not wish or attempt to dispense with—or, more politely, discharge
from care—as quickly as possible the patient who suffers mental illness/emo-
tional problems. Rather, let us accept him into the mainstream of health care
and treat him accordingly.

It would be ideal, in terms of both minimizing human suffering and
containing the cost of mental health care, if the psychiatrist could routinely
practice a therapeutic magic and dispense with his patients' symptoms in
rapid order. The reality is, though, that for most patients (clients) there is
simply no shortcut—no fast way—to symptom relief and emotional well-
being. If in fact there were, it would be a relatively easy task to solve all the
suffering of mankind—individually and collectively. It is true, as I have pointed out, that some persons with specific kinds of mental illness/emotional
problems do respond to short-term psychotherapy employed with or without
psychotropic medication. Thus, the majority of persons who suffer acute
"adjustment reactions" (transient situational disturbances) and some persons

who suffer emotional "crises" are likely to require only short courses of psychotherapy. This is especially the case if the person is relatively mentally healthy to begin with. Nevertheless, for the larger number of persons who suffer mental illness/emotional problems, improvement through change can only be a slow and gradual process—a process that begins with psychotherapy and continues long after psychotherapy is completed. This is the basic reality that planners of mental health care delivery systems for National Health Insurance must grasp. Logically, this should not be a difficult truth to recognize and accept, although its implications are profound and costly.

Although it is unfashionable today in some circles to quote Freud, his comments on the necessary length of treatment are quite concise and relevant here. In 1913 Freud[39] wrote,

> An unwelcome question which the patient asks the physician at the outset is: How long will the treatment last? What length of time will you require to relieve me of my trouble? . . . The answer is like that of Aesop in the fable of the Wanderer; on being asked the length of the journey, he answered 'Go,' and gave the explanation that he must know the pilgrim's pace before he could tell the time his journey would take him. . . . As a result of the lack of insight on the part of patients combined with the lack of straightforwardness on the part of physicians, analysis* is expected to realize the most boundless claims in the shortest time. . . . [However,] no one would expect a man to lift a heavy table with two fingers as if it were a little stool, or to build a large house in the time it would take to put up a wooden hut, but as soon as it becomes a question of neurosis† (which mankind seems not yet to have fitted into the general scheme of his ideas) even intelligent people forget the necessity for proportion between work, time, and success—a comprehensible result, too, of the deep ignorance which prevails concerning the aetiology of neurosis. Thanks to this ignorance a neurosis is generally regarded as a "maiden from a forest"; the world knows not whence it comes, and therefore expects it to vanish away some day. . . . The shortening of the analytic treatment‡ remains a reasonable wish. . . . Unfortunately, it is opposed by a very important element in the situation—namely, the slowness with which profound changes in the mind bring themselves about. . . .

*All psychotherapies as well as psychoanalysis—ED.
†Or a question of chronic symptoms of any kind—ED.
‡And treatment that entails psychotherapy—ED.

8

Attitudes That Affect Mental Health Care Coverage; The Psychiatrist in Perspective

There is probably no form of health care that is as controversial as mental health care in terms of its theories, aims, methods, and potential impact on individual persons and society as a whole. Mental health care is an extremely emotionally laden area of health care. Our thoughts and feelings, our attitudes and our prejudices toward mental health care are bound to affect individual and societal acceptance of it—and thus influence our health policy toward it. This obviously includes the manner and extent to which we shall provide coverage for mental health care under our health programs—including, in the future, NHI. Therefore, let us briefly examine in this section common attitudes that color our perception of mental illness/emotional problems and mental health care. Let us also consider here the psychiatrist (and other mental health professionals) in perspective, detailing what he can and cannot achieve.

I believe that the proposed limits on mental health care under NHI reflect to a certain extent our anxiety as individual persons about our inner selves. I believe in part we have relegated mental health care to second-class or even third-class status because of a negative "emotional" attitude that we possess toward our mind and its workings. We would often prefer not to think in great psychological depth about ourselves. We know we are emotionally complicated and that we experience powerful conflicting thoughts and feelings. We sense that they are best left alone, that exploring them can only open a psychological Pandora's box that will lead to obfuscation rather clarification, complication rather than resolution, emotional disturbance rather than emotional calm. We are, in sum, often afraid of our emotions, no matter how "normal" we are. Because we are afraid, we tend to shy away from people who experience emotional problems—or even worse, "mental illness." And ultimately, we shy away from treating them.

Our fear of our emotions stems in part from our view of the mind as some dark, unfathomable recess where our thoughts and feelings "happen" mysteriously and beyond our control. We should see this now for the myth it is. The mind, whether in a state of health or illness, does not operate in a random, haphazard manner any more than the heart, kidneys, or liver operate on the basis of spontaneity and chance. There is reason, rhyme, and method to the way we think, feel, and behave. If we can accept this, we can begin to recognize the pervasive impact of our thoughts, feelings, and actions on our total lives—past, present, and future. We can acknowledge that it is only in our best interest to know and understand ourselves so that we do not repeat the mistakes of our past, so that we can learn and grow, and so that we may be productive and fulfilled as individual persons.

However, it is one thing to urge such a view as I have expressed here, another to effect it. Our irrational anxiety about our inner selves and our fear of our thoughts and emotions constitute a universal psychological dynamic. We must first deal with it if we are to propose the validity of mental health care and seek its acceptance in theory and practice. Until we overcome our fear of our emotions, all the facts, data, statistics, and arguments that speak to the importance and affordability of mental health care will be wasted.

A further factor that results in a negative view of mental health care concerns an attitude we often possess toward the general role of the psychiatrist and other mental health professionals. Some opponents of comprehensive mental health care are quick to point out that even the best professional mental health care will not solve all of a person's problems. They urge severe restrictions on mental health care under NHI on the pretext that the psychiatrist (or other MHP) is mainly engaged in treating the untreatable—the common dilemmas and problems of life that all people must face and deal with as best they can. This is a misconception that must be dispelled if we are to gain proper coverage for mental health care under NHI. To do so, I would first refer the reader to Chapter 3 for a listing of specific mental illnesses/emotional problems for which mental health care is indicated. I would then fully agree with the concept that emotional discomfiture is part and parcel of the privilege of life. We are all bound to experience major disappointments and losses in our lives and with them will come our share of hurt, grief, and other emotional pain. However, emotional well-being and mental health for a person partially depend upon how well he or she is able to cope with life's "common" dilemmas and problems. We can complicate them for ourselves very easily. We can magnify and distort them; we can make them much more difficult and painful than they should be. We can create "common" problems and dilemmas; we can bring tragedies upon ourselves by the way we behave toward and relate to others as well as by the way in which we view ourselves.

The role of the psychiatrist (or other MHP) is first to treat specific symptoms such as depression and anxiety and to help a person to lead his life in such a way that his symptoms are either stabilized or do not recur (remission maintenance and symptom prophylaxis). However, the psychiatrist has a further goal in treating the patient who comes to him unable to cope with life's "common" dilemmas and problems. For such a person they are not "common" at all; rather, because of the person's intrapsychic makeup, they are extremely painful, unsolvable obstacles to his conduct of everyday life. (This is the key concept critics of mental health care must grasp.) The psychiatrist seeks to control and minimize the impact of life's dilemmas and problems for such a person and to help him to deal with them with the least amount of pain, suffering, and distress possible. For example, it is much easier for a person to cope with the death of someone close to him if he does not experience pathological guilt about the way he behaved toward that person while he was alive. Similarly, a person can cope with and recover from a divorce less traumatically if he (or she) does not hold himself exclusively or mainly responsible for that separation. The psychiatrist (or other MHP) cannot *change* reality, but he can help a person to *see* reality, to dispel the myths he holds about himself and his relationships with others, fictions with which people often punish themselves and others.

To reemphasize: The psychiatrist and other MHPs are not concerned with eliminating the problems of life. They couldn't even if they wanted to. Mental health care is not designed for this purpose. What the psychiatrist strives to do is to moderate a person's pathological emotional reactions to the negative events and circumstances of his life. We must promote a realistic view of the psychiatrist (and other MHPs); we must view his function in proper perspective if we are to understand the purpose of mental health care and insure it properly under NHI.

There is a further common attitude that affects our outlook toward mental illness/emotional problems and mental health care. It is that mankind has a standard burden imposed upon him to shoulder the woes of the world and for the most part to live quietly and in desperation. In my opinion, this is a pathological attitude, an attitude symptomatic of depression. It is true that the events and circumstances of life often conspire to make life exceedingly difficult, stressful, and painful for many. However, psychologically speaking, the average person has the emotional potential to achieve a certain level of satisfaction in his life and to be fulfilled to a greater or lesser degree as a person. It is not events and circumstances that deny a person pleasure, but he himself who does so. Unless we accept this postulate, we will have difficulty granting the value of mental health care to help the person who suffers discrete mental illness/emotional problems that result in painful symptoms and a negative personal and world view.

A final word with regard to life's "common" problems: We can never just dismiss them, even if many of them are unavoidable. They are not simply minor emotional aches and pains that result from our exercise of life. Out of balance, they can exact a heavy toll upon us, if not in psychic pain, then in physical pain and distress. As I have pointed out, many if not the majority of visits to physicians of all kinds are caused as much by the patient's "poor" emotional response to life stresses as by anything else. To refer to the previous examples I have given, such visits are made for the diagnosis and treatment of both "simple" headaches, stomachaches, backaches, "other aches," and major debilitating illnesses. Those so-called normal problems of everyday life can severely disable us or literally kill us.

9

Epilogue
A Final Perspective

I have tried in this paper to demonstrate the importance of and the necessity for full and complete coverage for mental health care under National Health Insurance—controlled and limited by careful professional monitoring rather than by public law. I hope it is not too late for us to effect such a policy. The wheels are in motion to severely limit mental health care under NHI. We must put on the brakes and reverse the trend.

It may be that we as a society shall have to decide that we cannot afford to fund completely certain modalities of health care that are extremely expensive. For example, we may not be able to afford to insure heart transplants on an unlimited basis under NHI. Of course, much of the most expensive medical-surgical care is consumed by the very few. This would include many burn victims, shock and trauma victims, and sufferers of certain chronic illnesses (e.g., renal disease). In principle, I am against the limitation of legitimate medical care for any condition. My bias is not grounded solely in humanitarian concerns. Rather, I feel that the development of widely applicable and cost-effective advanced treatment techniques for common and rare illness and injury depends upon the liberal funding of experimental and first-phase treatment modalities. In terms of heart transplantation, for example, current experimentation and treatment may lead to the development of cost-effective mechanical heart devices and/or the development of relatively inexpensive techniques to resolve the autoimmune reactions that complicate human organ transplantations.

If, indeed, we decide to limit medical care under NHI, I think we must be very careful to limit only those treatments that benefit the very few. (How many constitutes a "very few" is a question that is exceedingly difficult to answer. If we are ever unfortunate enough to become a member of that group, it becomes an emotional majority for us.) In this connection, it seems to me that mental health care has the potential to reach and improve the lives of countless numbers of persons. Perhaps some limitations on certain forms of "optional" mental health care will be necessary in the future. Here I am referring to long-term intensive psychotherapy and psychoanalysis for the patient who has achieved a satisfactory level of adaptation and functioning but who wishes to proceed further with his treatment in order to resolve certain emotional issues and conflicts. (The borderline between "necessary" and "optional" treatment may be very difficult to draw.) Perhaps, also, it will be necessary for us to expect some patients to partially defray the cost of their medical treatment (all kinds, including mental health care) in accordance with their personal income and financial state. I am basically against initial deductibles for health care wherein the first portion of the patient's medical expenses are not covered by insurance. Such deductibles do theoretically save money, but they encourage the patient to put off his health care until the last moment. We should encourage him instead to seek early medical intervention to insure his well-being as well as to minimize health care costs that result from undiagnosed and untreated "first-phase" illness. Nevertheless, we might have to formulate a plan for National Health Insurance wherein reimbursement to the patient for his medical expenses begins at a certain level that is dependent upon his financial status. This would allow the cost of all medical care to be spread across the population more equitably.

In the first analysis, the future of mental health care is out of the hands of the psychiatrist and other mental health professionals. It is ultimately the responsibility of state, county, municipal, and federal health planners and legislators. Members of that group who have either personally experienced mental illness/emotional problems, or who have had a family member or good friend experience them, should realize full well that the proposed limits on mental health care lack medical purpose, usefulness, and compassion. In the latter instance, I refer to "feelings." In this connection, we must acknowledge the role emotion plays in the establishment of national priorities and policy. It is an integral part of legislative decision-making processes. Certainly emotional response should not override the rational consideration of a problem and its solution. Still, after reason has prevailed, there must be room in designing and implementing policy on important issues for concern and compassion toward those who will be affected by the policy being deliberated. This is no earth-shaking revelation. Most significant social policy evolves in large part from what is judged to be "right" and "necessary." This includes health care policy directed at the treatment of chronic medical and surgical illness. However, we seem to have forgotten what is right and necessary when it comes to mental health care. All this is not to detract from the logical arguments presented herein for complete coverage of mental health care under NHI. It is to suggest that we cannot lose track of the *human plight* of the individual person who suffers mental illness/emotional problems, as well as his true need for mental health care, as we implement national health insurance and plan complete health care for our society.

In concluding this paper, I would be remiss if I did not state that responsible psychiatrists (and other mental health professionals) worry extensively over the general validity of psychotherapy with particular reference to the manner in which it is often practiced. We are obviously extremely concerned, for the patient's (client's) sake, that our services should be efficacious. In this connection, I do not think it would be unfair to hypothesize that a significant percentage of the practitioners of psychotherapy achieve a limited to modest success with a fair percentage of their patients but do not do so in any way that we can attribute directly and specifically to the application of their stated theories and methods. However, this does not constitute as severe an indictment of psychotherapy as it sounds. A significant percentage of all patients will improve no matter what specific diagnostic and therapeutic methods any physician employs. As a corollary to this, many medical-surgical patients get better in spite of their treatment—or they get worse no matter what treatment is employed. The point is that there are a great many nonspecific factors operative in the health care process that are palliative or curative for the patient (client). This is the case with regard to both medical-surgical care and mental health care (although we should not conceptualize these two varieties of care as separate entities). Thus, we cannot blindly criticize psychotherapy for a certain vagueness and imprecision of theory and method that it sometimes appears to display. We must instead view psychotherapy in terms of a vagueness and imprecision of theory and method that characterizes all health care. Generally positive results are often obtained in psychotherapy through the play of phenomena nonspecific to the psychotherapeutic process but rather attached to the health care process in general—including the physician–patient relationship—no matter what the symptoms or illness being treated and no matter what the form of treatment. Such phenomena may include the actual experience by the patient (client) of being *cared for and about* in the emotional sense by "the healer" (as manifested by the latter's patient listening and general empathy and sympathy). The physician may also effect the patient's improvement or cure by acting as a general authority figure for the patient and "commanding" him (directly or indirectly, consciously or unconsciously) to get well (see footnote on p. 155). In addition, the actual suffering of symptoms by the patient may ultimately be curative to a small or large degree in terms of the gratification it affords of the patient's psychological need to suffer as a form of expiation for (most often) imagined "misdeeds" or "bad" thoughts and feelings. In this sense, the physician ultimately acts to "forgive" the patient or to allow the patient to forgive himself.

In evaluating the efficacy of various modalities and specific methods of health care, we should also consider the following: Many illnesses and individual symptoms run a distinct course of their own. They possess an intrinsic natural history that plays itself out independent of or parallel to medical intervention for many, but not all, patients. In the same sense, external stress may precipitate or exacerbate pathological internal physiological response— i.e., external stress can provoke isolated symptoms or illness of an organic (physical) or emotional nature, or both. As the external stress diminishes, the symptoms or illness tend to moderate or resolve of their own accord. However, because some patients (clients) improve without treatment, on a tangent with treatment, or even with the wrong treatment, this does not invalidate the specific methods and forms of health care that allow patients who suffer from the same symptoms or illness to improve or recover. (Because some patients' ulcers heal naturally or spontaneously, this does not invalidate the medical treatment of ulcers. Because some patients' anxiety and depression quiesce or resolve naturally or spontaneously, this does not invalidate the treatment of such symptoms via various modalities of mental health care.)

I do not think, in sum, that we will ever be able to separate from the total health care process those therapeutic and coincidental factors that are in the purest sense "nonmedical." The health care experience must always remain to a large extent a "soft," spontaneous, and nonspecific process directed at meeting the patient's emotional needs as well as a physical and clinical method that employs specific "hard" therapeutic modalities. We should have reasonable expectations as to what we think any modality of health care should be able to achieve, and we should fund such health care on the basis of whether it reasonably achieves such expectations. We should not disallow funding for a specific form of health care because we do not recognize or understand exactly how and why it works.

I believe that on careful examination, it becomes apparent that much, if not most, health care, from mental health care to surgical care, is derived from, embodies, and applies (whether consciously or unconsciously) psychological methods in order to effect the physical and emotional welfare of the patient (client). This should reinforce the concept of the importance of mental health care, distinct from or congruent with medical-surgical care, as a basic and integral part of the total health care process.

Let us leave aside in this paper the question of the absolute right of persons to absolute quantities of health care. Though I personally believe we have an obligation to make complete health care available to those persons who require care, the question itself is beyond the scope of this paper. My only contention here is that in terms of delivering health care, mental health care should be provided on a quantitative and qualitative par with other health care services. Another way to state this is that once we make a decision to supply health care to any person, no matter through what system, sector, or agency, we should do so in a fashion that meets the complete health care needs of that person. (This does not mean we have an obligation to provide any variety of health care *ad absurdum*.) At the same time, we must strive to provide health care that is efficient and attentive to fiscal constraints. On both accounts this makes for a strong role for mental health care in the total health care delivery process. I hope my remarks in this paper with regard to the "rights" of persons to mental health care and our responsibility to provide it will be viewed in this context.

Let me also caution here that if we are to accurately evaluate the efficacy of mental health care, we must not idealize what we think it should be able to achieve for any person (any more than we should idealize the potential of other forms of health care). Yet we have a tendency to do so at the same time that we are prone to denigrate the need for such care or the process itself. I have previously addressed the nature, derivation, and meaning of the negative viewpoint toward mental health care, so I shall only comment on the idealistic viewpoint here. Too often, we expect the end product of mental health to be "happiness," when this concept has very little to do with such care. As often, we look for miracles from mental health care. We expect dramatic emotional rebirths of persons who receive such care. Because this does not happen for most persons, because mental health care does not meet our unrealistic, idealistic expectations for it, we can then further disparage it. However, the fault is not with mental health care; rather, it is with our conception of it. In evaluating the viability of mental health care, we must keep firmly in mind the reality that although some persons receiving such care will improve dramatically, a large group will receive modest benefits and a large group will receive minimal benefits. (This distribution of the efficacy of mental health care is, as I have pointed out, what we would expect to find for most forms of health care.) We should also remember that the benefits to be derived from mental health care are often not fully realized at the end of such care. For as I have previously noted, it is in the nature of mental health care to provide a way and a method of "coping" that must be refined, extended, and applied by the recipient of such care over a lifetime.

Finally, I must add that I anticipate and look forward to the controversy that is likely to surface surrounding this white paper and this book. Such controversy could be forthcoming on multiple accounts: First, many psychoanalysts may feel that I have unduly spoken out for restrictions on psychoanalysis under NHI; on the other hand, those who strictly favor short-term mental health care may feel that I have been too lenient in my calls for "full and complete" coverage for mental health care under NHI. Second, those who are strong proponents of a pharmacological approach to the treatment of mental illness/emotional problems may feel I have not been a strong enough advocate of this approach; others more wedded to "pure psychotherapy" may feel I have been too strong an advocate. Third, those who are generally pessimistic about the value of psychotherapy may feel I have been extremely optimistic in my assessment of its value and potential; those who are convinced of the merits of such treatment may feel I have been overly restrictive in my definition of what it does and does not constitute. (Other disagreements over my conception of the definition, purpose, function, application, and technique of mental health care are bound to follow.)

Fourth, those who are in favor of an NHI health care delivery system based for the most part on the CMHC or HMO will feel that I place too much emphasis in this paper on the role of the private sector—especially the private practitioner—as a provider of mental health care services under NHI. The private sector (notably the private practitioner), on the other hand, may be critical of my remarks regarding the need to control to the maximum extent possible the length and cost of mental health care under NHI, a position that will necessitate standards and guidelines and ultimately limitations on the manner and mode in which mental health care should be prescribed and administered—thus abridging the freedom of the mental health professional to practice exactly as he or she wishes and discouraging by excessive regulation or the threat thereof the mental health professional from practicing in the private sector. Fifth, those who are especially concerned with controlling the cost of mental health care under NHI may feel that I am too "care-oriented" without regard to the cost of such care; those who are indeed largely or exclusively care-oriented may feel that I am too "cost-oriented." Sixth, health planners and policy-makers (including mental health professionals themselves who work in such capacities) may feel that my paper is biased on the side of the practitioner of mental health care, whereas the practitioner may feel that I am biased on the side of the planner and policy-maker. Seventh, the various mental health professionals may feel that I have not fairly or completely represented the specific role and function of their particular professions. Last, patients and clients of mental health professionals, including various patient-consumer groups, may also disagree over certain positions I have taken in this paper. However, of one thing I am sure: They will not want their rights or access to legitimate mental health care curtailed in any manner.

In sum, the issue of coverage for mental health care under NHI is an extremely emotional one that involves not only theoretical, logistical, and economic considerations, but also basic attitudes and philosophy toward mental illness/emotional problems and mental health care. Discussion and argument regarding this white paper and this book should be considered in this context.

The reader should also consider the discussion of mental health care herein in the following light: Though mental health care, as I have shown, has much in common with medical-surgical care, it is in many respects a unique form of health care that requires a separate planning and review process. Keeping in mind the admonition that we must first and always remain totally aware of the best interests of the patient (client), we must seek during such a process to establish the best working theoretical models for mental health care, to develop the best health care systems to deliver such care, and to institute a high degree of quality control as regards the training, licensing, and actual clinical work of the various providers of mental health care. Though most health care can only be as effective as the person who provides it is competent, this holds especially true for mental health care where the provider and the process of care are often inseparable—more so than for other forms of health care. (In literary terms, the MHP's psychotherapeutic "style" creates to a large extent the "content" of psychotherapy.)

In the end, I hope this white paper and this book will engender useful debate on its subject and begin a process that will lead to the delivery of responsible mental health care responsibility monitored and controlled in terms of both quality and cost. This should be a national health policy goal both before and after the institution of National Health Insurance.

Appendix

Understanding Psychotherapy
The Psychotherapist and His Client

As I have repeatedly maintained, every person involved in theorizing or formulating health policy or in planning or administering mental health programs should strive to develop a basic understanding of mental health care—including, especially, psychotherapy. It seems to me that such an understanding is necessary if we are to organize and deliver appropriate mental health care services under NHI or under existing health insurance.

In this Appendix, I shall recapitulate and expand upon certain aspects of the form and function of psychotherapy as presented in other sections of my paper. I shall discuss the "therapeutic relationship," the *total* relationship between the psychotherapist—whether psychiatrist, (clinical) psychologist, social worker (M.S.W.), psychiatric nurse, or other—and his or her client (patient)* that develops over the course of psychotherapy and that is an integral part and an exclusive feature of the process of psychotherapy (as opposed to other "helping methods"). I shall also comment on the special role of the psychotherapist within that relationship, a role that makes him unique and separates him from others who help people to "feel better." The views I present here are fairly basic in scope, and I would hope that most mental health professionals would agree with them in the broad sense—especially as they apply to intermediate to long-term psychotherapy.†

Let me begin this Appendix by attempting to promote a proper perspective of psychotherapy (and mental health care). I might first remind the reader what psychotherapy is and what it is not. Psychotherapy cannot function as a psychological salve or an emotional balm for all troubled persons at all

---

*I use the generic *psychotherapist* in this appendix. For this reason it seems appropriate to use the general term *client* to refer to the recipient of care (see footnote on p. 13).

†This appendix deals with the "therapeutic relationship" between psychotherapist and client and other aspects of psychotherapy with specific reference to *individual psychotherapy*. Conjoint (marital) therapy, family therapy, and group therapy call for specific psychotherapeutic techniques and client management, which I do not discuss herein. Nevertheless, these therapies do share many common elements of psychotherapeutic technique with individual psychotherapy. In addition, many components of the therapeutic relationship itself are maintained across all formats of psychotherapy.

troubled times. However, for many persons who suffer emotional pain, it constitutes a treatment that, in the most simple terms, promotes relief from such pain to the maximum extent possible. Psychotherapy works in part by allowing a person to first recognize his ways and modes of thinking, feeling, and behaving, and then to gradually alter his thinking, feeling, and behavior in an adaptive manner. For many persons, psychotherapy is most—or even only—effective when combined with the prescription and utilization of psychotropic medication; for many other persons, however, the use of such medication is inappropriate, if not contraindicated, and "pure psychotherapy" (see Chapter 1) offers the best approach to treatment.

It is important to remember here that although a person may (rarely) enter into a course of psychotherapy or (more likely) continue it beyond a certain point strictly or primarily to enhance "the quality of his life," such "treatment," although I endorse its purpose, cannot in any sense be construed to be "health care." In order to qualify as (insured) health care, psychotherapy, consistent with the function of other medical care, must be (1) designed and implemented to relieve or stabilize the *clinically defined* symptoms of *medically recognized* mental illness/emotional problems a person suffers (see reference 9) or (2) utilized to prevent the onset of mental illness/emotional problems that may develop on a secondary basis as a complication of an immediate mental illness/emotional problem from which a person suffers or that may develop on a primary basis as a result of a traumatic life stress to which a person has been exposed—e.g., illness, loss of job, divorce. (Typically, in the latter case, the person will be experiencing some symptoms, i.e., some degree of emotional distress, at the time psychotherapy is contemplated or initiated.)

I will be the first to acknowledge that utilization control over the practice of psychotherapy—as psychotherapy is carried out by independently licensed psychiatrists, psychologists, and social workers working in the private fee-for-service sector—is not what it should be. (By contrast, control of psychotherapists' clinical practice in organized health care settings such as CMHCs and HMOs is often excessive and contrary to the best interests of their clients.) Yet we cannot simply rely on third parties who finance health care to monitor and regulate health care of any modality. Their agenda is often in juxtaposition to that of those persons who require a particular health care service; they are primarily motivated to control the cost of health care, too often at any expense. In this connection, I have commented in my paper on the value of peer review as a means of insuring medical and fiscal oversight of all varieties of health care. If this system has flaws, including the tendency of a profession or a segment of it to maintain its role "at all costs," it is also more likely to insure that clients will receive the proper quantity and quality of care.

Notwithstanding the need to regulate the delivery of psychotherapy, as well as other care, one should not get the idea, as I have repeatedly emphasized, that psychotherapy (or other mental health care) is overutilized or misused any more than other modalities of health care. It should not be assumed, as many critics of mental health care do assume, that psychotherapists are out to provide their clients "free," extraneous "health care." (Such a theorem stems largely from emotional bias against persons who suffer mental illness/emotional problems and those who care for them.) The fact is that beyond any obligation to a health care organization or an insurance company, a psychotherapist has a clinical responsibility to his client to make sure that when that client reaches a point (and that point is often difficult to exactly determine) in his treatment when further psychotherapy is primarily designed to improve the client's "quality of life," he (the client) must assume responsibility for payment for his psychotherapy. This is in accordance with a basic goal of psychotherapy, which is to teach a person to "take care of himself"—to take responsibility for himself. (This includes monetary responsibility.) Clearly, if a person is to do this, he cannot depend inappropriately (that is, when he is not suffering symptoms) on someone or something (a health care system) to take financial care of him. This is inconsistent with a model of "mental health." Not only can it not be encouraged, it cannot be tolerated by the psychotherapist.

Indeed, for a long time now, there has been much theoretical debate among psychiatrists as to whether it is therapeutically beneficial for a person to pay for his psychotherapy—even if he is suffering acute symptoms—on one basis, among others, that if a person pays for his treatment, it will encourage him to take responsibility for his (mental) health. There is some validity to this argument. However, it could also be said, but this is not often discussed, that we could encourage persons who suffer organic (physical) illness to take more responsibility for their health if we forced them to pay for their health care. If we did so, they would be more likely, for example, to maintain a proper weight, exercise, not smoke, and curtail alcoholic intake if for no other reason than to control their health care expenses; further, people who suffer psychosomatic symptoms or illness (and who account for a great percentage of the cost of health care) would be more likely to live with their physical distress or "cure it" themselves. Nevertheless, although a particular practitioner—psychotherapist or physician of any specialty—may find it therapeutically beneficial for a particular client or patient to work out an arrangement with him wherein that client or patient would pay for his care, I think it would be a grave misjudgment for us to deny any person who suffers medically recognized symptoms of any type insurance coverage for health care. (Of course, insurance deductibles and required copayments, in addition to supposedly encouraging a person not to abuse health care, can function in theory to encourage a person to take more responsibility for his health. In my opinion, though, they too often have the effect of scaring the average person away from health care when he needs it.)

In pronouncing judgment on psychotherapy (and other mental health care), we should also consider that the average person, for psychological and emotional reasons, is more likely not to use the mental health care benefits to which his insurance entitles him, in comparison with any other benefit. Fur-

ther, even when a person does seek psychotherapy, the mental health professional, as often as any other professional, will not allow him to indulge in
"cheap" (i.e., useless) care. Because he is attuned to the psychology of his
clients' "need" for care, the psychotherapist makes his clients squarely confront their health problems in their full dimensions. This includes making
them face any improper utilization of medical-surgical care—as well as mental
health care. By contrast, other health care practitioners, no matter what their
specialties, are more likely to reject "difficult patients" out of hand—and, in
effect, shuttle them down the therapeutic road to other sources of care. (The
process repeats itself *ad infinitum*.) Alternatively, practitioners will counte-
nance and oblige their patients' demands for health care—whether or not
they are appropriate—often damaging their patients in the process. In sum,
the average physician is too often unwilling to confront his patient with his
clinical judgment that he (the patient) is using health care inappropriately and
excessively (usually due to recognized or unrecognized emotional distress).
The irony of viewing psychotherapy (and other mental health care) as useless, wasteful, or exorbitant is that the only way it is possible for many
patients to reduce their dependency on and use of health care in general is
through the utilization of psychotherapy (or other mental health care).

We face an obvious imperative: We need to control and contain the cost
of all health care while at the same time we promote the best health care for
any given person. However, in our efforts to manage health care from the
economic point of view, we cannot scapegoat psychotherapy, or other forms
of mental health care. My efforts to define and explain psychotherapy in this
appendix and elsewhere in my paper are designed to allow us to view and
treat psychotherapy, and other mental health care, fairly, and in the context
of other types of health care.

Before moving on to consider the question of *how* psychotherapy works,
let us briefly reconsider the question of *if* it works. In other words, what is the
efficacy of psychotherapy and how do we judge it? The studies on psychotherapy outcome I previously summarized in my paper hardly completely
establish the efficacy of psychotherapy, including any specific form of psychotherapy. I have acknowledged as much in my paper. Though there is
among experts a general consensus that psychotherapy "works," to be hon-
est, there is to date no clear-cut, overwhelming consensus as to the total
merits of psychotherapy—i.e., the dimensions and extent of its applicability
and usefulness. In this connection, I never did intend that my paper or this
book should focus exclusively on a complete debate or discussion as to the
efficacy, cost-effectiveness, etc., of psychotherapy or mental health care in
general. This is a subject for a complete volume in itself.

For a thorough review of the difficult theoretical, methodological, and
practical problems inherent in evaluating the efficacy of psychotherapy, I
refer the reader to papers published by London and Klerman[40] and Parloff.[41]
Perhaps the reader, after studying these papers, will agree with Toksoz B.
Karasu, chairman of the American Psychiatric Association's Commission on

Psychotherapies, who has stated,[42] "Regardless of whether evaluation [of psychotherapy] is in the hands of an advisory body, a panel of experts, a panel of clinicians, or a panel of researchers, it is apparent that unequivocal conclusions about the effectiveness of psychotherapy may never be possible. At best, we may be able to create a framework that can provide only partial answers."

I hope the reader will consider Dr. Karasu's remarks within the general context I have repeatedly stressed in my paper—namely, it is difficult to validate the efficacy of much of medical care. It is often impossible to separate the effects of particular medical interventions from the milieu in which health care takes place and the complex total process health care involves. In this connection, "medicine" (medical care) is an art as well as a science. One does not measure art by statistics. The further implication is that some physicians (or psychotherapists), independent of their scientific (medical) knowledge or technical skill, are better able to heal their patients (clients) than others because they are better at practicing the *art* of healing. In addition, the success of medical care often depends on the patient (client) himself; some patients, independent of the medical science or art being employed on their behalf, are better able to get well than others because of their willingness and ability (skill) to work toward getting well. Another way of stating this is that different physicians of all specialties (or psychotherapists) employing the same care (on a technical level) achieve different results with the same types of patients (clients), and different patients receiving the same care (on a technical level) get different treatment results.

If we do not exactly know, and can never precisely and absolutely know, why the patient (client) who avails himself of psychotherapy "gets better," we also often do not know exactly why the medical-surgical patient gets better. A patient may improve after a visit to the doctor for many reasons— including a sympathetic smile from a secretary while he registers for his care, a chat with an empathic nurse while he waits for his care, or the aura of simply entering and staying for a while in a physician's office. You will notice that in these examples I have left out the physician himself as an instrument of healing.

In sum, if we are to determine the reasons for the success or failure of "treatment" for many, if not most, patients (clients), no matter from what illness they suffer, we need to conduct a multifactorial analysis of that treatment that extends far beyond an evaluation of the specific medical technology being employed. Health care is not just "biological intervention," whether we are talking about a psychiatrist treating schizophrenia with psychotropic medication or a surgeon taking out an appendix. Let us view psychotherapy, and all medical-surgical care, as a complex psychological, emotional, social, and cultural interaction between a "healer" (psychotherapist or physician of any specialty) and a patient (client) that includes and extends beyond the application of specific health care technology. Only by adopting such a perspective can we properly understand and fully appreciate the value of therapeutic approaches to both mental illness/emotional problems and medi-cal-surgical illness.

Let me be clear here. I strongly believe that psychotherapy, properly prescribed, practiced, and conducted at the appropriate professional (or para-professional) level, is a most powerful and cost-effective "weapon" in our health care armamentarium. In focusing on hard data as to the efficacy of psychotherapy (or the lack thereof), I do not mean to disparage psycho-therapy, but only to place it on a scale with all health care. This, I hope, will lead to a philosophy of mental health care that is fused to a philosophy of health care in general. From that should follow a pragmatic approach to psychotherapy (and all mental health care) that will not differ from our ap-proach to other modalities of health care.

Psychotherapy works in large measure through the complex "therapeu-tic relationship." This is a very special relationship between psychotherapist and client marked by a genuine caring, concern, and affection on the part of the psychotherapist toward his client. In this respect, the relationship is not especially unparalleled. A person may have relationships with other people who care about him just as much and who are just as concerned about his welfare. However, the relationship between the psychotherapist and his cli-ent differs in a profound way from all other relationships the client may have. In many respects, it is a one-way relationship. The psychotherapist receives his fee, which allows him to practice his profession. He enjoys his craft, even if he finds it difficult, and he learns and grows from all of his relationships with his clients. He is gratified by the opportunity and privilege to help his client to resolve or stabilize his symptoms. Aside from this, however, the relationship between the psychotherapist and the client *exists for the client;* ultimately, it does not exist for the well-being, pleasure, gratification, or hap-piness of the therapist. The psychotherapist, although his work often fulfills him on a certain professional and personal level, must satisfy his own emo-tional needs elsewhere. The client is "there" (in psychotherapy) for himself; he is not there for the psychotherapist. What is the effect of this? It enables the client to work toward his health within a special relationship in which nothing is expected of him (or her) except that he try to reach the therapeutic goals he sets for himself in terms of his emotional well-being. (The client does not set vague and abstract goals for himself; rather, he sets his goals in conjunction with his psychotherapist, who has evaluated his clinical condi-tion, judged the type and severity of his mental illness/emotional problem, and considered the therapeutic adjustment it is possible for the particular client to make in terms of resolving, ameliorating, or stabilizing his symp-toms.) Thus, there is no pressure on the client to be "a certain way," to conform, to please, to amuse, or to do right by the therapist. The client's only business with the psychotherapist is to work toward getting well—or as well as possible. In this connection, the psychotherapist must always offer his client, stated or unstated, the *hope* that he will get well or better. (Indeed, such

a message must be considered to be a crucial component of the psychotherapeutic process.) Nevertheless, the psychotherapist must be exceedingly
careful not to push his client too hard or too fast. This can put too much
pressure on the client to control his emotions, to progress, and to change,
when perhaps he is not at a given time capable or ready to do so. In fact, the
relationship between the psychotherapist and his client is structured the way
it is so that the client will not feel any pressure to be *any* way. To the extent
the client does perceive pressure, the therapist gets a good clue as to the
client's emotional needs—e.g., his need to please others, to conform, or to be
"accepted." (Sometimes, when the psychotherapist prematurely and force-
fully pressures his client "to be healthy," a false cure or a pseudocure results.
The client *acts well* to avoid rejection by or to please his psychotherapist; he is
then discharged from treatment but soon regresses to his "sick state." He has
only temporarily covered or masked his symptoms; he has not really dealt
with his mental illness/emotional problem. Nevertheless, it is sometimes appropriate for the psychotherapist to encourage the client to "cover" his symptoms rather than to work them through or resolve them. Such a technique is
often utilized in crisis and short-term (or brief) psychotherapy, where the
psychotherapist often attempts only to restore the status quo. It may also be
utilized for some clients who are extremely ill on a chronic basis.)

The psychotherapist does not want or expect anything from his client
other than that he commit himself to work toward his health.* The client's

---

*It may sometimes appear to the layperson that the psychotherapist is not concerned with either
the length and expense of treatment or even the ultimate treatment outcome itself. This is not or
should not be the case. However, as I have noted in the text, the layperson must realize that the
psychotherapeutic process in its full dimensions cannot be forced on the client. If psychotherapy
is to work, the client must gradually develop during the course of psychotherapy, with the
psychotherapist's assistance, a readiness and a willingness "to change." Psychotherapy, it must
be realized, is a complex, integrated process, rather than a single, discrete therapeutic intervention or even a series of such interventions. Thus, the psychotherapist cannot demand in an
authoritarian fashion that the client change. In fact, the essence of psychotherapy can be construed to be the process of gradually getting the client to overcome his resistance to change. For
the most part, this occurs sequentially, in small steps, not in quantum leaps. The layperson must
understand that the psychotherapist does not take a *laissez faire* approach to psychotherapy—
even if he sometimes appears to be passive and inactive. It is just that the psychotherapist must
often be exceedingly patient. Often he must wait for his client "to come to him"—with his, the
psychotherapist's, assistance, even if this assistance be quiet and gentle. It is difficult to observe
much of what takes place during the process of psychotherapy. The healing process it involves
takes time, much as all medical-surgical healing processes take time.

I should note here that if the psychotherapist truly feels that his client is unwilling and
uncommitted to work toward his emotional health, he will, or should, discharge that client from
treatment. Here, though, we must remember that all clients are at times during psychotherapy
highly resistant to working toward their health, some for longer periods than others.

Finally, let me comment that *any* physician does not want or expect anything from his
patient other than that he commit himself to work towards his health. Thus, the sentence that
prompted this footnote should be viewed in the general as well as the specific context. If we are
to understand psychotherapy we must strive to see the similarities between mental health care
and medical/surgical care at the same time as we note the distinctions between the two.

relationship with others will not be so undemanding. Most people have their own needs, which they rightly expect to be met in their relationships with others. They want something back for themselves—or for the interest or institution they represent—when they interact with another person. It is the essence of human relationships; it is also what complicates them all. Thus, in almost all the relationships a person has with others, he has to be generally agreeable to be with, considerate, thoughtful, conforming to expectations, etc. However, in the relationship a person has with his psychotherapist, he can be angry to the extreme, depressed, ungiving, dissatisfied, demanding, rejecting, etc. The good psychotherapist will expect this and will not become upset. He will not become frustrated, and he will neither retaliate against nor reject his client. In fact, he looks at the expression of such feelings by the client (within the framework of the client's overall commitment to work toward his health) as crucial and necessary to the success of psychotherapy and he welcomes it! No, the psychotherapist is not looking for the client to be "nice" to him. He is only looking to clarify the conflicts and contradictions in his client's life and to help his client to resolve them.

I must add that although a great deal of intimacy may develop between a client and his psychotherapist, there are no grounds for the psychotherapist to involve his client in his (the therapist's) own personal, emotional life. I have suggested this before, but I must emphasize it now: The psychotherapist's problems are his own, and his client is not engaged in psychotherapy to help him (the psychotherapist) solve any of his problems or to make life better for him. The sum of all this is that the client can feel safe in his relationship with his psychotherapist. The client doesn't have to concern himself that his life will be "wrecked" any more than he perceives it to be already by personal demands placed upon him by another. I should add that the psychotherapist does not espouse any causes, other than that of mental health, and he does not attempt to impose his personal or world view on his client. He conducts treatment in a manner that resonates to his client's personal and world view (which may change during the course of psychotherapy as the client sheds pathological psychological constructs).

In the psychotherapist–patient relationship, the client also enjoys the opportunity to learn trust and intimacy, difficulties over which are at the core of many persons' problems. A major goal of psychotherapy is to allow a person to succeed in establishing or improving other relationships of an intimate nature. It aims to help him to realize and to stop doing the things by which he defeats himself time and time again in relationships. (It also aims to help him choose persons with whom to have relationships who will interact with him in an emotionally mature, "healthy" manner.) The client learns how to do this in part by overcoming in psychotherapy the difficulties, concerns, and fears he encounters in his relationship with his psychotherapist. Therefore, the client's relationship with the psychotherapist is in part a practice relationship—or a preparatory relationship—although it is a very real relationship and a meaningful one in itself.

We have seen that psychotherapy does not involve just another, if extremely special, "nice, warm, and beautiful" relationship between two people. It does partly consist of a very intense person-to-person relationship that is mutually rewarding for both the client and the psychotherapist (although in different senses). However, the psychotherapist, in his work relationship with his client, is very much interested in experiencing and allowing his client to experience that "part" of himself (i.e., the client's self) that he consciously or unconsciously tries to hide from other people and often hides from himself as well. The psychotherapist is completely open to the expression of this other "part" of his client. The psychotherapist wants to see and interact with the person who is difficult to live with, not only the person who is "a joy forever." This is crucial if the psychotherapist and his client are to come to recognize and understand when, why, and how the client misperceives and misreacts to people and circumstances. (Such a recognition and understanding constitutes an extremely important step in the process of change that the client undergoes during psychotherapy.) Therefore, psychotherapy, in addition to encompassing a very special relationship, involves a complex, intricate, and objective study of the client's entire "personality"—his ways of thinking, feeling, and behaving. The client can't just get this analysis and assessment anywhere. There is a skill as well as an art to conducting psychotherapy. There is a structure, process, and technique to psychotherapy.

Without getting too abstruse, I should mention in this connection a phenomenon that displays itself in the way the client relates to the psychotherapist in ongoing psychotherapy. It plays a very important role in the therapeutic relationship. The phenomenon is known as *transference*, and it is to promote its development—as well as to remain objective—that the psychotherapist maintains a certain "distance" from his client. By distance I mean that the psychotherapist does not reveal a full, complete picture of his own life and personality and that he may remain silent at times. (If the therapist feels he has something worthwhile to say, he says it, contrary to popular opinion.)

Simply put, the essence of the transference is that the client transfers thoughts and feelings that he (or she) has about others onto the psychotherapist. Some of the time the client actually thinks, feels, and behaves unconsciously toward the psychotherapist as though he were not the psychotherapist but rather an important other person in the client's life. This is not surprising. Once our personalities are formed, we tend to be fairly consistent in the way we relate toward people with whom we are intimate. As an example of the transference phenomenon, we can site the situation where the client becomes severely angry at the psychotherapist for no ostensible reason and the anger persists even though the client perceives that there are no valid "real" reasons for the anger. Similarly, the transference phenomenon is operative when the client consistently feels that the psychotherapist is displeased with him (or her) despite the fact that the psychotherapist does not indicate any displeasure and does not in fact feel any. The transference then, is the client's distortion of his relationship with the therapist. (It may be a positive as well as a negative distortion.)

The transference is a valuable tool in psychotherapy because it reveals to both the psychotherapist and his client, once the client realizes that his feelings have been misplaced and are not appropriate to the situation, how he distorts, misperceives, and misunderstands how others think and feel about him and behave toward him. At the same time, understanding the transference enables the client to see how he misperceives and misunderstands others. By working with his client toward an understanding of the transference, the psychotherapist enables his client to see himself (his thoughts, feelings, and behavior) and others objectively. (This may not bring about therapeutic change in itself, but it is a prelude to such change.) Of course, the analysis of the transference is only one of many technical elements of the psychotherapeutic process. I should also mention a few other basic elements of that process. These would include the analysis by the psychotherapist of the client's history (the "story" of his past and present life as and how he relates it), the client's patterns of thinking and feeling, his nonverbal expression ("body language"), and the nature of his "resistance" to therapeutic change. Such analyses are really made possible by the structure of psychotherapy. They would be difficult to achieve under any other method. Of course, different psychotherapeutic approaches utilize the different techniques of the psychotherapeutic process to different extents. Thus, psychoanalysis uses the transference to a great extent, while at the other extreme, behavior therapy at least purports not to use it at all.

I must reiterate here that the person-to-person relationship between the psychotherapist and his client plays a crucial role in the psychotherapeutic process. In many ways this is a nurturing relationship for the client. To some extent, it must be because psychotherapy itself is often a frustrating, demanding, and painful experience for the client. In fact, the intensity and manner of a client's reactions to the vicissitudes of psychotherapy gives the psychotherapist insight into the client's personality and mental illness/emotional problems. The client, too, must be asked to examine his emotional reaction to the process of psychotherapy; this is an integral part of his treatment. Indeed, the very design of psychotherapy makes it unique as a helping and healing method. For example, psychotherapy by its basic structure forces a client to confront his dependency needs; it allows him to "work through" (resolve by repeated examination from multiple perspectives) pathological dependency. ("Dependency" is not intrinsically pathological; it is a state that is part of life, but we must learn to be dependent in a healthy and mature fashion.) The design of psychotherapy also allows a client to work through the psychological conflicts that have prevented him from functioning as an autonomous (independent and self-serving in a healthy way) person. (Problems with dependency and autonomy, which are related, frequently constitute a major component of the psychodynamics of mental illness/emotional problems.) In these respects, the "termination" of psychotherapy is a very important component of the total process of psychotherapy, as opposed to merely an end-point. Much of the work of psychotherapy is accomplished in the termination phase, a phase that can be quite painful for the client. Contrary to popular opinion, psychotherapy, especially intermediate to long-term psychotherapy, is very much trial and ordeal as much as or more than it is sustenance for the client. This raises an important point. Too often, we indict persons who seek out psychotherapy as "weak." Instead, we should view them as possessing a certain strength and determination beyond their suffering. Indeed, it takes courage for a person to enter into and sustain a full course of psychotherapy, properly designed and carried out.

I would add here that even the most "standard" psychotherapeutic technique will vary widely depending upon whether short-term, intermediate-term, or long-term psychotherapy is being conducted. The psychotherapist will also direct the therapeutic relationship along different lines, depending upon the anticipated length of the psychotherapy. In short-term psychotherapy, for example, the psychotherapist may encourage the clients' positive "idealized" view of him (i.e., the psychotherapist) in order to facilitate treatment. In addition, the psychotherapist may offer the client more emotional support and he may offer him as well more direct, immediate, and sustained guidance than he would if psychotherapy were to continue for a longer period of time.

It should be obvious that the psychotherapist's "job description" is a difficult, demanding, and sometimes even impossible one! It is no easy requirement for the psychotherapist to possess and practice at all times the qualities and characteristics that I have implied here are fundamental and essential to the successful practice of psychotherapy. The psychotherapist after all is only human. Still, he (or she) must strive to embody and employ these qualities and characteristics on behalf of his client. He must seek to be caring yet objective, tolerant and neutral, and emotionally independent of the client's emotional needs and demands. The success or failure of psychotherapy often hinges on the psychotherapist's ability to conduct himself along these lines. As if this task were not great enough, the psychotherapist must also constantly and consistently demonstrate a "mentally healthy" way of being and relating to his client, for the client will often "identify with" the psychotherapist and incorporate aspects of his (i.e., the psychotherapist's) personality into his own psyche. (Indeed, this is one element by which the treatment process works.) As I have maintained in this paper, the persona of the psychotherapist is as important to the success of psychotherapy as is the technique he practices.

I do not wish to imply by the above discussion that all good psychotherapists are clones of one another. Psychotherapists differ from practitioner to practitioner. Even though different psychotherapists will utilize the same psychotherapeutic techniques to much the same extent, their "manner" of implementing them will depend largely on their individual personalities. By this I mean that every psychotherapist possesses a certain "style" that is derivative of his personality, and he practices psychotherapy in accordance with that style. In a certain sense, every psychotherapist practices a unique approach to psychotherapy. (In a similar vein, no two physicians—of any specialty—practice in an identical fashion. Even though they may order or perform the same tests and prescribe the same treatment, their exact styles of practice reflect their personalities.) And though there are certain absolute qualities the psychotherapist must possess (patience, compassion, empathy, etc.), I cannot categorically state that the psychotherapist must possess certain absolute quantities of these qualities.

The "personality" of the psychotherapist is relevant to my discussion here because whether we are talking about the treatment of mental illness/emotional problems or medical-surgical illness, the individual client (patient), depending upon his own personality, will respond better in the therapeutic sense to a psychotherapist (or physician of any specialty) who employs a particular "style." Let me demonstrate this in terms of the patient who is receiving medical-surgical care. Some such patients do best when they are treated by a physician who assumes an authoritarian role; others do better with a physician who deals with them on an "equal basis." In other words, some patients feel more comfortable when the physician firmly takes control of their "case" and independently manages their care, while other patients wish to come to joint treatment decisions, to the maximum extent possible, with their physician. It is true that this model is especially valid for medical-surgical care and often is not applicable as regards the treatment of mental illness/emotional problems—especially in terms of the practice of "pure psychotherapy." For example, for the average client, the psychotherapist simply cannot practice psychotherapy in a classical authoritarian manner. Most often the psychotherapist must allow his client to control the pace of psychotherapy. By this I mean that although the psychotherapist is always actively managing and directing his client's care, he cannot force treatment down the throat of his client. The psychotherapist can only meet his client at the psychological and emotional point where he (the client) is operating. Yes, the psychotherapist attempts at all times to facilitate his client's rate of progress; he seeks as rapid a resolution as possible of his client's symptoms. Nevertheless, the psychotherapist can only accelerate the treatment process within certain technical limits. Within these limits, however, some clients do better with psychotherapists who are more aggressive in their therapeutic styles and more overtly demanding of their clients than are other psychotherapists. On the other hand, many clients will not respond well at all to treatment by a psychotherapist whom they perceive as pressuring them.

Of course, the skilled psychotherapist knows that there is a time to "push" and a time not to push any particular client. The psychotherapist will typically be "demanding" of his client at certain points during treatment, while at other points he will be "nondemanding." The client must expect the internal structure of his psychotherapy to vary, no matter what the basic "style" of the particular psychotherapist from whom he is receiving his care.

(Of course, this situation is hardly special to psychotherapy. Different patients of all medical specialists require different therapeutic approaches at various points in their treatment. Thus, the physician will sometimes treat his patient aggressively, while at other times he will take a "sit back and wait and see" attitude toward how the patient's symptoms evolve.) It is the psychotherapist's ability to determine his client's exact treatment needs at various points during his treatment and the psychotherapist's ability to match a therapeutic plan to those needs at any given point that make for a good treatment result for the client in psychotherapy. (The same paradigm holds true for any physician treating any patient.)

Yet, despite the most expert treatment planning by the psychotherapist, the successful treatment of the client is largely dependent on the success of the relationship that develops between the client and his psychotherapist over the course of the client's treatment. (I am really not talking here about the total "therapeutic relationship" as I have defined it in terms of psychotherapy in this appendix, but only about that part of the therapeutic relationship that has to do with the ability of the client and his psychotherapist to relate and to work together positively on a person-to-person level.) The success of the client–psychotherapist relationship hinges on the client–psychotherapist *match*. The personality of the psychotherapist, which will determine the style by which he practices, must suit the personality of the client. Indeed, assuming the client is capable of forming and working within an intimate person-to-person relationship with a psychotherapist, the client–psychotherapist match often plays the determinant role in therapeutic outcome for the client—whether the client requires crisis (emergency), short-term, intermediate, or long-term care. (The patient–physician match also often plays a major role in therapeutic outcome for the patient who requires long-term care for chronic medical-surgical illness. For the patient who requires emergency or acute care for major medical-surgical illnesses, the patient–physician match plays a relatively smaller role in therapeutic outcome than the actual treatment the patient receives—although we cannot even always be sure of this.)

Unfortunately, treatment outcome studies too often neglect the effect on treatment outcome of the client–psychotherapist match. In my opinion, it is a variable that has major implications not only for the individual client (patient) who seeks the best health care possible, but also for the planning and structuring of health care delivery systems. Such systems must recognize that if psychotherapy is to be effective for any given client, that client must be free to receive his care from the qualified psychotherapist of his choice. Not only should the client be free to select the psychotherapist who he feels is "right for him," but he should be able to change his psychotherapist if he feels his treatment is not going well. We absolutely cannot lose sight of the fact that there is a continuous psychological and emotional interplay between the client and his psychotherapist (or between any patient and his physician). Mental health care (and health care of all kinds) is not a series of isolated events that "happen" to a client (patient); rather, it is a multifaceted, integrated process that takes place along a therapeutic continuum. The personality fit of the client (patient) and his psychotherapist (physician) is at the heart of that process. I cannot stress enough how important it is for any person who requires psychotherapy (or health care of any kind) to choose his psychotherapist (or physician) wisely. And unless we build appropriate "patient options" (e.g., choice of practitioners) into the health care delivery systems we evolve in the future, not only will a great many patients not improve symptomatically, but health care delivery systems will reap the expense of treatment failures.

I hope the reader will excuse my sometimes awkward rhetorical juxtaposition above of mental health care, specifically psychotherapy, with medical-surgical care, including my discussion of the common links between the various practitioners of health care in terms of the ways they relate to their patients (clients) and their patients relate to them. Yes, mental health care differs in certain respects from other modalities of health care, and I have pointed out how in this paper. However, even as we note the unique aspects of mental health care and the special problems mental health care delivery poses, we should acknowledge the overriding similarities between mental health care and medical-surgical care. Indeed, only when we are willing to recognize the connection between mental health care and health care *in toto* will we see fit to conceptualize mental health care and treat it as an essential component of health care. My aim throughout this paper has been to show that mental health care in theory and purpose, and in terms of the actual way in which such care is practiced, fits into a unified model of health care.

As often as not, medicine is psychology, and psychology is medicine.

References

1. Psychiatry newsletter. *J Continuing Ed Psychiatry*, December 1978, p 13.
2. President's Commission on Mental Health: Report to the President, vol 1. Washington DC, US Government Printing Office, 1978.
3. The Alcohol, Drug Abuse, and Mental Health National Data Book. US Department of Health, Education and Welfare, Public Health Service, January 1980.
4. Office of Program Development and Analysis: The Financing, Utilization and Quality of Mental Health Care in the United States, Draft Report. National Institute of Mental Health, US Department of Health, Education and Welfare, 1976.
5. Regier DA, Goldberg ID, Taube CA: The de facto US mental health services system: A public health perspective. *Arch Gen Psychiatry* 35:685–693, 1978.
6. Hon. Richard Roudebush: Communication to the US Congress. Veterans Administration, January 1977.
7. Luce BR, Schweitzer SO: Smoking and alcohol abuse: A comparison of their economic consequences. *N Engl J Med* 298:569–571, 1978.
8. Brodie HK: The Treatment of Mental Illness: A Study of Provider Locus. Strecker Monograph Series 17. Philadelphia, Institute of Pennsylvania Hospital, 1980.
9. American Psychiatric Association: Diagnostic and Statistical Manual of Mental Disorders, ed 3. Washington DC, APA, 1980.
10. Holmes TH, Rahe RH: The social readjustment rating scale. *J Psychosom Res* 11:213–218, 1967.
11. Greer S, Morris T, Pettingale KW: Psychological response to breast cancer: Effect on outcome. *Lancet* 2:785–787, 1979.
12. Krizay J: Measuring psychiatric utilization: The rubber yardstick. *Am J Psychiatry* 137:1589–1591, 1980.
13. Office of Technology Assessment, US Congress: Assessing the Efficacy and Safety of Medical Technologies. Washington DC, US Government Printing Office, 1978.
14. Assembly of Life Sciences, National Research Council: Health Care for American Veterans. Report of the Committee on Health Care Resources in the Veterans Administration. National Academy of Sciences, 1977.
15. Cooper T: Cost-containment and self-control: Where the twain meet. *Modern Medicine*, November 15–30, 1979, pp 9–10.
16. Sharfstein SS: Third-party payers: To pay or not to pay. *Am J Psychiatry* 135:1185–1188, 1978.
17. Sharfstein S, Taube CA, Goldberg ID: Problems in analyzing the comparative costs of private versus public psychiatric care. *Am J Psychiatry* 134:29–32, 1977.
18. Marmor J, Scheidemandel PL, Kanno CK: Psychiatrists and Their Patients: A National Study of Private Office Practice. Washington DC, Joint Information Service of the American Psychiatric Association and the National Association for Mental Health, 1975.
19. Goldensohn SS: Cost, utilization, and utilization review of mental health services in a prepaid group practice plan. *Am J Psychiatry* 134:1222–1226, 1977.
20. Craig TJ, Patterson DY: Productivity of mental health professionals in a prepaid health plan. *Am J Psychiatry* 138:498–501, 1981.

21. Sharfstein SS: Will community mental health survive in the 1980s? *Am J Psychiatry* 135:1363–1365, 1978.
22. Health maintenance organizations: Requirements for a HMO. Final regulations. *Fed Regist* 45:72524–72536 (Oct 31), 1980.
23. George Washington University Health Plan Member Handbook, 1979.
24. Towery OB, Sharfstein SS, Goldberg ID: The Mental and Nervous Disorder Utilization and Cost Survey: An analysis of insurance for mental disorders. *Am J Psychiatry* 137:1065–1070, 1980.
25. Krizay J: Mental Illness and the Community Responsibility. Washington, DC, American Psychiatric Association, in process.
26. American Psychiatric Association: Operations Manual of the Board of Trustees and Assembly Procedural Code. Washington DC, APA, 1980.
27. Freud S: An Outline of Psychoanalysis. London, Hogarth Press and the Institute of Psycho-Analysis, 1949.
28. Group for the Advancement of Psychotherapy: Pharmacotherapy and Psychotherapy: Paradoxes, Problems, and Progress. New York, GAP, 1975, pp 427–431.
29. Alcohol, Drug Abuse, and Mental Health Administration: Personnel Needs for Mental Health Services. Report to the Senate. Department of Health and Human Services, Public Health Service, June 1980.
30. Graduate Medical Education National Advisory Committee: Report to the Secretary of the Department of Health and Human Services. Hyattsville Md, Health Resources Administration, Office of Graduate Medical Education, DHHS, 1980.
31. Hall RC, Gardner ER, Stickney SK, et al: Physical illness manifesting as psychiatric disease: II. Analysis of a state hospital inpatient population. *Arch Gen Psychiatry* 37:989–995, 1980.
32. Hall RCW, Popkin MK, Devaul RA, et al: Physical illness presenting as psychiatric disease. *Arch Gen Psychiatry* 35:1315–1320, 1978.
33. Koranyi EK: Physical health and illness in a psychiatric outpatient department population. *Can Psychiatr Assoc J* 17(suppl 2):109–116, 1972.
34. Regier DA, Goldberg ID: National Health Insurance and the Mental Health Services Equilibrium. Bethesda Md, National Institute of Mental Health, Division of Biometry and Epidemiology, 1976.
35. *Med Care* 17 (December suppl):1–82, 1979.
36. Liptzin B, Regier DA, Goldberg ID: Utilization of health and mental health services in a large insured population. *Am J Psychiatry* 137:553–558, 1980.
37. Office of Technology Assessment, US Congress: The Implications of Cost-Effectiveness Analysis of Medical Technology: The Efficacy and Cost Effectiveness of Psychotherapy. Washington DC, US Government Printing Office, October 1980.
38. Parloff MB, et al: Assessment of Psychosocial Treatment of Mental Health Disorders: Current Status and Prospects. Report to the National Academy of Sciences. Washington DC, Institute of Medicine, 1978.
39. Freud S: Collected Papers, vol 2. Authorized translation under the supervision of Joan Riviere. London, Hogarth Press, 1953, pp 347–351.
40. London P, Klerman GL: Evaluating psychotherapy. *Am J Psychiatry* 139:709–717, 1982.
41. Parloff MB: Psychotherapy research evidence and reimbursement decisions: Bambi meets Godzilla. *Am J Psychiatry* 139:718–727, 1982.
42. Karasu TB: Proving the efficacy of psychotherapy to government: A bureaucratic solution? *Am J Psychiatry* 139:789–790, 1982.

Points of View

Richard H. Beinecke
and Bertram S. Brown

Introduction

Proposals for National Health Insurance have been introduced yearly in every session of Congress since 1939. During the 95th and 96th Congress (1979–1980), at least 16 unique bills were submitted by members of the House and Senate. During 1978–1980, four congressional committees (House Ways and Means and Interstate and Foreign Commerce, Senate Finance and Subcommittee on Health and Scientific Research) held at least 15 days of hearings on the subject. Despite this great amount of effort, the United States is probably no nearer to having a comprehensive and coherent national health insurance system now than when the idea was first presented. Two major steps have been the passage of Medicare and Medicaid. However, developing an adequate relationship between these two programs has blocked more progress. Although the Republican party now controls the Senate and the White House and although some persons hope that a form of national health insurance may now be enacted, the history of NHI under both Democratic and Republican administrations suggests that the chances of agreement on a comprehensive NHI proposal are minimal.

The issue of whether a comprehensive national health insurance bill is passed is only the "cover" under which the health care issues churn. However, the NHI debate is useful in and of itself, first, because it is a mirror in which the critical issues in health care can be seen. Second, NHI provides a forum in which health questions can be analyzed and highlighted. In fact, in the early 1980s the NHI issues are being processed through the debate as to the final fate of the future of health planning, PSROs, and the federal support of health manpower, to mention just a few. These ideas are then enacted in

Richard H. Beinecke • Horizon Health Group, Inc., Washington, D.C. 20036. **Bertram S. Brown** • Hahnemann University, Philadelphia, Pennsylvania 19102.

other forms of legislation such as bills for cost-containment, revisions of Medicare and Medicaid, the president's budget, and growing in importance in the 1980s, state legislation.

Seen in this perspective, the national health insurance discussions are particularly illuminating as a lens through which to view mental health issues in the United States. NHI proposals demonstrate how mental health services are discriminated against in health care planning, and how mentally ill persons are still stigmatized by our nation's people. Dr. Joseph English,[1] testifying before the Subcommittee on Health of the House Ways and Means Committee, stated the problem well:

> We have but one request to make to you, Mr. Chairman. All of the bills that are currently under consideration by this committee in the area of health insurance at the moment continue to discriminate against the mentally ill, and our purpose in appearing here is to request nondiscriminatory treatment for the millions of people in this country that suffer from nervous and emotional and mental disorders.
>
> The widespread belief that their benefits have to be limited in ways that the benefits of patients with other illnesses are not limited—for example, in the number of visits they can have with their doctors or the number of dollars that can be committed to their care—I suppose, simply reflects the fact that the stigma which has been associated with mental illness for centuries still exists in this country.

Mental health issues in NHI parallel those of health care but constantly reflect the above bias. This dual system is particularly apparent in the gaps in service and coverage in the nation, in the lack of adequate remedies for these in NHI proposals, and in two critical issues in health care—whether health and mental health coverage should be extended by (a) expanding benefits and services and (b) expanding the providers who may be reimbursed by third-party payers.

Gaps in Funding of Health Care

Gaps

In 1979 public and private health insurance was extensive for 220 million Americans. Major gaps in coverage nevertheless existed. These included the following:

1. Twenty-two million Americans had no health insurance coverage; 7.5 million of these persons had incomes below the federal poverty level. An additional 10 million had family incomes under $14,000. These persons were not eligible for Medicaid, Medicare, or free care through federal delivery systems such as the VA hospital system.

2. Only 35% of the nation's poor were eligible for Medicaid. This was due, first, to federal law, which bars single individuals, childless couples, and most two-parent families from participating in Medicaid no matter how low their income or high their medical expenses, and second, to state restrictions on Medicaid eligibility.

3. Twenty million Americans had inadequate insurance that failed to

cover basic hospital bills, doctor's services, or medical tests; 3.6 million of
these persons had incomes below the poverty level.

    4. An additional 41 million Americans did not have insurance against
very large medical expenses, and 83 million persons were vulnerable to catastrophic expenses.[2]

    5. In 1979, due to these gaps, 50,000 persons declared bankruptcy due to
high medical expenses, and 7 million families incurred medical expenses over
15% of their income.[3]

    In addition, health care services are unevenly distributed throughout the
nation. An estimated 51 million Americans, particularly in rural and inner-
city communities, live in medically underserved areas.[2] Levels of care for the
poor and minority populations, while better than in the past, are still substantially below those for wealthier and white persons.[4] The elderly also receive
less than their fair share of care. Auxiliary and preventive services such as
dental care and early childhood screening for disease tend to be utilized
primarily by affluent populations. Only a small percentage of the population
has access to alternative treatment facilities, such as HMOs (Health Maintenance Organizations), which may have lower costs.

    Thus, despite improvements in coverage during the past decades, there
are still substantial gaps and many Americans do not have access to care that
they need.

Funding

    In the meantime, the costs of health care have risen sharply. In 1950,
$12.7 billion or 4.5% of GNP was spent on health care in the United States. By
1978 the nation was spending $192.4 billion (9.1% of GNP).[5] It is projected
that unless costs are contained, expenditures will rise to $438.2 billion (10.5%
of GNP) by 1985 and $757.9 billion (11.5% of GNP) by 1990.[6] Federal expendi-
tures will rise to $110 billion by 1984 or $.15 of every tax dollar. Average
medical costs for a family of four will rise from $2373 in 1979 to $4064 in 1984;
for a single aged person, from $2259 to $3868.[2]

    Furthermore, there has been a striking shift in who pays for health care.
In 1966, 51.5% of health care costs were financed through direct payments
from insurance. By 1977 this percentage was down to 30.3%. During the same
period, the percentage paid by private health insurance remained relatively
stable (24.7%–27.6%) and those from philanthropy and direct industry contributions were both stable and small (2% in both years). By contrast, third-
party payments from government increased from 21.8% to 40.1%, an increase
caused at least in part by a dramatic rise in the percentage paid of the costs of
care to persons 65 and older (29.8% to 67.0%).[7]

Scope, Gaps, and Funding of Mental Health Care

    1. Thirty-two million Americans or 15% of the population were conser-
vatively estimated to have had mental disorders during 1975. Ten percent of

the population is estimated to have a mental disorder at any given time. Mental disorders are defined as "organic and functional psychoses, neuroses, personality disorders, alcoholism, drug dependence, behavioral disorders, mental retardation and other ICDA Section V disorders. Excluded are the more common 'problems of living' and emotional symptoms affecting the majority of the population."[8]

2. In 1975, 6.7 million persons were seen in the specialty mental health sector, a fourfold increase since 1955. Two points are particularly striking when the settings in which these persons were treated are analyzed. First, the ratio of inpatient to outpatient episodes reversed itself during this 20-year period—from 77 inpatient/23% outpatient in 1955 to 28 inpatient/72% outpatient in 1975. During this period, the actual number of inpatient episodes did grow modestly in most types of facilities. But it fell by 27% in state and county mental hospitals.[8]

Second, most persons who received mental health treatment received it from office-based physicians and general hospital outpatient and emergency rooms. In fact, 73% received that care solely in the general health care sector, only 19% solely in the specialty mental health sector, and 8% in both sectors.[8] Further, it is estimated that at least 60% of patients going to family doctors' offices for physical symptoms have a psychological problem that either is a primary problem or aggravates the physical conditions or interferes with effective treatment regimens.[9] Thus, it is clear that mental health and physical health are closely linked and have a great impact upon each other.

Gaps and Funding

Even though great strides have been made in mental health care during the past 30 years, major service gaps still exist that have been created or exacerbated by the ways in which mental health services are financed. Those gaps are more widespread than for health care as a whole, and they are indicative of the intentional or unintentional discrimination.

1. The costs to society of mental health problems have been estimated for 1975 at $43 billion from alcohol abuse, $10 billion from drug abuse, and $31 billion from mental illness.[8]

2. Of the 8.6% of GNP devoted to total national health expenditures in 1975, 0.9% was spent on ADM (alcohol, drug, mental health) treatment programs. The portion of GNP for mental health treatment was over 9.8%.[8]

3. Total expenditures for alcohol and drug abuse treatment have been growing at a slower rate than and mental health treatment at the same rate as general health care expenditures. Unlike those for health, however, the average costs for mental health expenditures have remained stable. This is due to patient care episodes and total expenditures increasing at the same rate and reflects a shift from inpatient to outpatient care, which is less expensive.[8]

4. In 1975 revenues for mental health expenditures came from the following sources: 21% from federal sources, 30% from states and localities, 15%

from private insurance, and 34% from private, noninsurance sources (mostly patient fees).[8] This is very different from overall health revenues. The federal government and private insurance contribute far less and states and localities and other private sources contribute far more to revenues than in the general health sector. Further, these ratios have remained relatively stable in recent years in contrast to overall health care, where federal expenditures have risen sharply and private payments are far less now than in the past.

Gaps from the Perspective of the Individual

According to the President's Commission on Mental Health,[10]

> these include low-income individuals, and particularly the elderly, children, minorities, the unemployed, and those not expected to work. These individuals are most likely to be unable to finance their own mental health services or to be able to maintain private insurance which includes mental health coverage; they must rely on public categorical programs or public health financing programs. The panel recognized that problems exist for workers as well, especially those who have minimal insurance coverage or difficulty getting time away from their jobs.

The Panel on Cost and Financing of Mental Health of the President's Commission[10] outlined in detail how Medicare and Medicaid prevent adequate mental health services for those populations. These discriminatory provisions include the following:

1. There is a limitation of inpatient psychiatric hospital services under Medicare Part A to 190 days.

2. Under Medicare Part B, reimbursement is provided for medical care of a patient with mental illness on an outpatient basis for no more than 50% of charges or $250 in each calendar year (as compared to 80% and only a $60 deductible for other covered services). This limitation does not apply to physician provided care on an inpatient basis, thus fostering institutionalization.

3. There is a 100-visit limit on home health care, and no home care support services are allowed.

4. Severe restrictions exist on care for partial hospitalization.

5. No reimbursement is given to community mental health centers (CMHCs).

6. There are no coverage increases in mental health provision of Medicare to keep up with inflation, even though monthly premiums for Part B were increased threefold by 1978.

7. Many limitations are placed on mental health services covered under Medicaid, including many outreach and support services. There is an emphasis on inpatient services, with nearly 70% of payments going for these services in 1977.

8. There are often narrow eligibility standards for Medicaid; at least one out of three persons under the poverty line is ineligible for services.

Thus, mental health is treated far differently from health care, leading to inadequate care for many persons.

Gaps from the Perspective of the Region[11]

Mental health care is more available in urban and suburban than in rural communities. Rural areas have fewer hospitals and community mental health centers and fewer mental health practitioners per 100,000 population than do urban and suburban regions. Many underserved minorities live in these areas. Rural persons have many unique service needs—in transportation, education, service linkage, and clinical areas. Structured government programs designed for urban locations are thus often inadequate in providing care to these areas.

Gaps from the Perspective of Services Needed

"Existing means of financing mental health services focus upon the provision of care in institutions. This focus is true for charity support, support through public programs, and support through private insurance plans."[10] While institutional care for severe mental health problems will always be needed, a balance of funding is critical if costs are to be kept down and unnecessary hospitalization is to be avoided. At the present time, outpatient mental health care is discouraged by existing financing mechanisms.

> About 92% of employee benefit plans have *some* coverage of physician outpatient care for mental conditions. All the state Medicaid plans are *supposed* to include such outpatient care. However, support for outpatient mental health services tends to involve large co-payments, limits on the numbers of services supported, and limits on the dollars available for insurance support of these services. These limitations on outpatient services discourage their use, particularly by the poor and near poor, who have very little disposable income.[10]

In addition, day hospitals, halfway hospitals, home health care, transportation, and time spent arranging social services such as housing, financing, provider linkages, shopping, and adult education often do not qualify as reimbursement services.

> Most insurance programs, including Medicare, provide funding only for a diagnosed illness. Preventative services, services to identify high risks, health educational services to advise about warning signs and treatment programs, outreach programs, and other support services are frequently not reimburseable under existing financing mechanisms. The absence of such funding discourages their use, particularly by the low-income population.[10]

As a result of this financing bias, many persons who would benefit from treatment in less restrictive and costly settings are not receiving it. Long-term care in community residences is discouraged, while hospitalization for acute illness is promoted. Ideally, a continuum of care needs to be available and supported by financing mechanisms. This does not exist at present.

Gaps from the Perspective of the Provider

Finally, gaps exist in reimbursement to two types of providers of mental health services—(a) nonphysician providers whose fees are not reimbursable except when they work under the direct supervision of a physician, and (b) settings that are currently excluded from reimbursement.[10]

The last section demonstrated how noninpatient settings are discriminated against by third-party payers. Community mental health centers have particularly been hurt by this provision and, as a result, receive far less monies from insurance programs and rely far more on categorical federal grants than do inpatient mental health providers. Thus, in 1976 CMHCs received 65.7% of their funds from the following sources: federal staffing grants, 19.7%; other federal funds, 7.3%; state funds, 29.5%; local funds, 9.2%. Insurance payments provided only 8.0% of funds; Medicare, 2.4%; Medicaid, 10.4%; patient fees, 4.0%; and other receipts, 5.3%.[8] Severe limitations are also present in Medicaid and private insurance payments to other facilities such as HMOs, ambulatory care centers, and group homes when mental health services are provided. This financing structure sharply limits the development of a wide continuum of caregivers.

Another group that is discriminated against is nonphysician providers such as clinical psychologists, clinical social workers, psychiatric nurses, and especially members of other counseling professions. Psychologists, social workers, and psychiatric nurses usually can be reimbursed only if they work under the direct supervision of a physician, although in some states this requirement is no longer true for Ph.D. psychologists. The other professions seldom are eligible at all.

In sum, while major gaps remain in health care coverage for Americans, persons needing mental health care are particularly hurt by the financing and service delivery system in the nation. While much progress has been made, far more needs to be done if an equitable system is to be designed.

Why There Are Differences

Why do these differences exist? Five factors form the basis of the discrimination between the mentally ill and other persons.

The Devil and Deep Illness Dimension

The basic taproot was expressed well by English[1] earlier in this chapter. Mentally ill persons have experienced long-standing stigmatization by society. Myths that crazy people were the devil come to earth and that these persons had illnesses that were deeper than other medical problems resulted in poor care and often persecution. "Normal" persons' intolerance of differences and our frustration with a problem that has not lent itself to easily defined solutions have contributed to differential treatment of mentally ill persons.

The Total Life Issue

Mental health issues are at the heart of life's problems and the most critical human dilemmas. It is difficult, if not impossible, to set boundaries on these questions. There is a legitimate fear of being drowned unless strict limits are set on these all encompassing sets of concerns.

The Multiprovider Issue

Mental health care, more than strict medical care, is provided in many settings and by many types of professionals. It is often easier to restrict coverage than to govern providers.

State Dominance

Historically, states managed most of mental health care. Only recently have private and multifunded organizations moved in a major way into the field. Health care funding has usually been designed for these groups. Thus, they have not traditionally had an interest in supporting mental health care.

The Deserving Patient Issue

Many mental health problems are seen as self-inflicted and deserving of punishment. We have seen no hesitation in treating emphysema and lung cancer caused by cigarette smoking. Yet drug abusers are treated differently, and only minimal progress has been made in alcoholism being seen as a disease.

Recent NHI Proposals

Overview

The Appendix summarizes the major national health insurance bills before Congress in 1979 and 1980. It outlines the general concept and approach of each bill, its coverage, benefits, administration, and financing, and its mental health components.

One can classify these bills as being in three broad groups, organized from the most to the least amount of government control over insurance programs.

Comprehensive Public Service. The first group of bills is the most comprehensive in coverage and utilizes primarily a public service approach to service delivery. The Dellums bill merges many current federal and private health programs and forms a new system in which all care is provided by the federal government. The Corman bill is the Health Security Act, which has been introduced every year since 1970. It provides for total federal financing of health care, but services are provided by both public and private facilities.

The bill in this category that generated the most interest during 1979 and 1980 was the Health Care for all Americans Act. It is a compromise bill, an attempt to take the planning and coverage aspects of the Health Security Act and combine them with more private sector involvement. The bill provides for universal coverage of the American population with uniform and standard benefits, complete federal control of the health care budget, and top-down planning. The program would be operated by a National Health Board and the Department of Health and Human Services. Private health insurance groups could underwrite policies within budgets negotiated with the board. Hospitals and private practitioners would continue to provide services, but there would be more federal controls upon them. The federal government would allocate budgets for health services to states that would negotiate with four consortia of insurers to set rates. These consortia would cover four types of plans: (1) prepaid group HMOs, (2) independent practice HMOs, (3) Blue Cross/Blue Shield plans, and (4) commercial carriers and self-insurers. In addition, an expanded Medicare program and state and federal purchases would provide for care for poor and other underserved populations.

Catastrophic-Regulated Utility. The second group of bills are those characterized by some form of catastrophic protection. They may be viewed as following a regulated utility approach to health care in that while they rely on the free market to provide services, they recognize that there are gaps in coverage that the federal government needs to help fill, and expanding costs that regulation needs to help control.

There have been many variations of this approach. Closest to the Kennedy bills was the Carter administration's National Health Plan (S 1812-HR 5400). This would set up a dual system of health care financing as the first step toward a more comprehensive program. Private insurance plans would be supported but would be required to meet certain federal standards, including minimum service provisions and a maximum deductible of $2500 for catastrophic illness. In addition, a new program would be set up for all federal health beneficiaries (including Medicare and Medicaid clients) and all persons who would voluntarily want to join it. This program would subsidize premiums for low-income persons and have a sliding fee scale for other individuals and families. Special provisions would be made for elderly persons, and costs would be contained through provisions similar to the administration's cost-containment bill, which was defeated in 1979.

Another set of variations on the catastrophic approach, and for years the prime alternative to the Kennedy-sponsored bills, were those introduced by Russell Long. The three bills are fine tunings of one basic program.

S 350 was the original Long/Ribicoff Bill, which was introduced throughout the 1970s. It has two main sections: (1) a federally administered plan for the unemployed, welfare recipients, the aged, and persons who do not choose private insurance coverage; (2) federally approved catastrophic insurance plans allowed as options for employer groups and the self-employed. S 351 is the same bill, but without the low-income provision. S 760, the most recent version, is the same as S 350, but with some changes in the provisions of the catastrophic program.

Many other variants of the catastrophic approach have been proposed. The Dingell bill has not attracted much attention, probably because it is vague in many of its provisions. It is interesting primarily because of the large role that it gives the state in determining needed services and in administering the program.

Of more importance, particularly since the November 1980 election, are the Republican bills. S 748, the 3-D bill (Dole, Danforth, Domenici) provides catastrophic coverage through, first, required inclusion of such coverage in employer-based plans and, second, expansion of services and coverage under Medicare and Medicaid. By relying on existing administrative mechanisms and focusing on improving primarily catastrophic benefits, this bill, its proponents believe, can fill insurance gaps at minimum cost.

Former Senator Schweiker took a different approach. S 1590 only slightly expands Medicare coverage while, as in the 3-D bill, requiring greater employer coverage. To fill the remaining coverage gap, state-administered private insurance pools would be set up to lower insurance costs, expand covered services, and serve persons ineligible for the private or federal programs.

Another Republican view was former President Ford's NHI proposal, reintroduced as HR 6405. Medicare and private insurance coverage would be slightly expanded to cover catastrophic illness. For those persons not covered under these programs, and to fill the gaps between state Medicaid payments and the new benefits, a new federal program (CAPP) would pay for catastrophic medical expenses when they reached a certain percentage of income.

Finally, Congressmen Martin and Jones introduced HR 3974. This relies on tax credits rather than direct payment to provide protection against the costs of catastrophic illness.

Each of these bills is designed to provide protection against the costs of catastrophic illness. Each defines unacceptable costs in differing ways, setting up varying trigger points for reimbursement. The bills utilize differing mechanisms to administer and finance these proposals, with greater or lesser reliance on federal and state governments and the private sector. Each attempts to limit service coverage while insuring at least minimal benefits for most persons.

Restructuring Private Financing/Free Market. The proponents of the free market approach to national health insurance believe that persons need to have the freedom to choose a health plan that is most suitable for them.

They believe that to facilitate this and to improve care quality, competitive market forces need to be supported. The present system, it is argued, blocks these forces by excessive regulation and excessive federal financing of health care services. The government's role is to intervene only to stimulate competition, which will in turn lead to improved and less costly care.

The main model for this approach is Alain Enthoven's "consumer choice health plan." Although it has never been put in bill form, its outlines are well known.[12] Consumers would be provided with equal subsidies with which they could purchase insurance. These would be in the form of tax credits for employed persons and vouchers for Medicare and Medicaid recipients. Private insurance plans would be required to have annual open enrollment, use community ratings, offer basic health services, and have limits protecting persons against catastrophic costs. In this manner, it is hoped that competition would be stimulated, care improved, and costs held down.

Thus far, four bills have been introduced that incorporate elements of this model. Jones and Martin's HR 3943 would prevent employers from claiming as business expenses contributions toward employee's health insurance covering inpatient care unless certain provisions were met. These would require the employee to pay 25% of these expenses and the insurance plan to limit the costs of catastrophic illness. Ullman's HR 5740 also requires coverage of catastrophic expenses while limiting the employer contributions to health care plans. S 1968, introduced by Senator Durenberger, sets similar standards for plans and, likewise, uses the tax mechanism to limit employer expenses.

HR 7527 is Congressman Gephardt and former Congressman Stockman's proposal. This plan, whose chances of passage are now substantially higher than when it was first proposed, would lead to the greatest change in the health care system. It would modify the tax structure to support purchase of insurance and set up a voucher system to allow poor, elderly, and disabled persons to buy insurance from private carriers with open enrollment. HHS would publicize these plans. In addition, the bill would repeal many health planning regulations to encourage competition.

One final approach has been considered as a method of moving toward national health insurance. As Medicare and Medicaid were viewed by some persons as the first steps toward expanded coverage, some persons believed that extending coverage to children in need could be another step in filling coverage gaps. Marmor in an article in 1977[13] suggested that a bill combining comprehensive services to children and catastrophic coverage could meet critical service gaps while paving the way for a more expanded NHI program at a later date. This proposal was introduced by Senator Hart as S 1014.

The idea of providing expanded child health services also became a leading goal of the Carter administration. CHAP, the Child Health Assurance Program (HR 4962, S 1204), was an administration legislative priority since its introduction in early 1977. CHAP would extend Medicaid eligibility to between 2 and 3 million additional low-income children and pregnant women. The costs of a wide variety of medical, mental health, dental, and prenatal/

postnatal services would be reimbursed. The bill passed the House in December but was killed in the Senate.

Mental Health Provisions

The Appendix lists mental health provisions of national health insurance bills as of December 1, 1980. The benefits in these bills may be summarized as follows:

Only HR 2969 (Dellums) provides for unlimited benefits. Only this bill and HR 21 fund "supporting services" such as health education and social service provision.

On the opposite end, only HR 7527 (Gephardt/Stockman) excludes "items and services related to mental or emotional illnesses or conditions" and "treatment for chronic chemical dependency," although HR 5740 (Ullman) would allow but not require mental health benefits to be included.

In S 1014 and HR 3974, language is unclear as to mental health coverage.

Two bills, HR 3993 and S 1968, continue Medicare and Medicaid as at present with no other reference to mental health. S 1590 modified Medicare only slightly (no reimbursement for long-term nursing home care), as does HR 6405 (190 days/lifetime replaced by 45 days/year). S 1590, S 1968, HR 3943, and S 1014, it should be noted, do have provisions for catastrophic care that could cover inpatient physician-provided care after certain cost limits had been reached.

For inpatient care, all other bills set limits in varying ways. These include 190 days lifetime (S 748), 30 days/year (S 1812 and HR 16), 150 days/spell with 60 days between spells (S 1720), and several variations for different categories in the Long bills.

Outpatient care is limited in two ways. All of these bills pay 80% (20% copayment) up to a specified limit ranging from $400 to $1,000 or 20 visits (S 1720). In addition, S 1812, one part of S 760, and S 748 have a $60 deductible.

Of these bills, only the Medicaid provision of Long's bills specifically reimburses for partial hospitalization (unlimited), while the Kennedy bill allows day care to be substituted up to inpatient limits at the rate of 2 days of day care to one of inpatient.

Home health care is covered by the Long bills and S 760, S 1720, and HR 5740 (100 visits/year) and S 1812 (100 visits/year).

Skilled nursing homes are provided for specifically in S 1720 (100 days/spell), S 1812 (100 days/year), the Long bills, and the other bills that would continue Medicare and Medicaid as at present.

All bills cover medications but in some these drugs must be chosen from an approved list.

Only Kennedy's and Dole's bills extend provider status to CMHCs for all persons, while Long limits this extension to Medicaid services.

Only Kennedy's bill extends provider status to nonpsychiatrists (when practicing in a CMHC or "other provider").

In sum, with the exception of the Dellums bill, which is not currently being seriously considered by Congress, even the most liberal NHI bills such as S 1720 set up far greater restrictions for mental health care than for medical care. Outpatient and inpatient care are limited, the former more than the latter. Inadequate provisions are present for partial hospitalization, day hospital programs, home health care, and various forms of nonhospital institutions such as boarding homes and skilled nursing facilities. Care by psychiatrists is promoted over that of other professions. CMHCs and other organized community settings are discriminated against in favor of inpatient facilities.

Changing Benefits and Services

Two issues can illustrate how most NHI proposals expand financing for health care and yet continue to restrict programs in mental health. The first is how benefits and services are changed.

Health Coverage

Nearly all of the bills expand medical care coverage, using one or more of three mechanisms. First, with the exception of HR 3943, HR 5740, S 1968, and S 350/5760, all of the bills extend services to low-income, elderly, and self-employed persons who in the past have not been able to afford even minimal care. This is done in differing ways. For instance, Gephardt/Stockman provides vouchers to these persons, allowing them to purchase private insurance. The Carter bill sets up a special program to cover these populations. Schweiker's S 1590 organizes state-administered private insurance pools and expands Medicare to cover previously unserved populations. The four bills that are exceptions to this pattern focus on improving services to employed persons only. They leave intact current Medicare and Medicaid provisions and so do not increase numbers of persons served.

Second, there seems to be increasing agreement that some form of catastrophic insurance is needed. Primary differences among bills involve the level of caps; whether these are set by percentage of income, absolute dollars, or some combination of the two; and whether copayments are required.

Other ways of reducing individuals' costs have also been proposed. In the Dellums bill, all care is free, financed by a progressive "health service tax." Kennedy's more realistic proposal insures that all persons are covered by insurance but finances this through individual, corporate, and public payments.

Third, benefit structures provide for reimbursement inpatient and outpatient medical care, usually limited by impacts of copayment provisions. Medical equipment and supplies, labor, and X ray services are also part of most basic benefit packages. There is some dispute over whether costs of medications should be limited by less open-ended coverage, patient cost-sharing, and administrative controls, but generally they are also covered.

Many more limitations are placed on long-term care and preventive programs. In general, these vary according to the continuum of federal to private involvement in a plan. As one moves from the comprehensive bills such as those of Kennedy and Corman to the catastrophic variations and the free market approaches, limits on care in nonhospital settings such as skilled nursing homes appear and home health benefits are curtailed or eliminated. More rapidly (in this order), payments for health promotion and education, preventive care, eyeglasses and hearing aids, and dental care are restricted or dropped. Services to children are the one exception to this rule. Despite the difficulty in getting CHAP passed, even some of the more "conservative" bills include provisions for outpatient and preventive services to children.

If NHI proposals are a guide, the health system of the future will emphasize acute over long-term or preventive care, institution-based rather than community-based treatment, and care that involves high technologies rather than social service provision. From a public health perspective, this is not a sound way to move. From a mental health perspective, it aggravates an already discriminatory situation.

The mental health provisions of NHI bills support the emphasis upon acute care. However, restrictions upon services are far more severe for mental health. This can be illustrated in two areas—outpatient treatment and long-term care.

Outpatient Treatment

The NHI benefit packages reimburse physicians for outpatient care and many services that accompany this care. By contrast, nearly all of the present bills as well as Medicare/Medicaid and most private insurance policies cap outpatient benefits after a certain amount of money is reimbursed. Most plans also require either a deductible or copayments for outpatient mental health care.

These limitations are opposed by most mental health professionals and organizations but are still largely supported by the medical (other than psychiatric) and financing communities. Upton, for instance, has argued in this book for few limitations on outpatient psychotherapy. The Mental Health Association, stressing the importance of Mental Health Service Organizations (MHSOs) such as CMHCs and HMOs, has testified that there should be no outpatient limits in these settings and 30 days' benefits with the first seven sessions fully covered where therapy is provided by a private practitioner.[14]

The issues here are twofold—equity and cost. The Task Panel on Cost and Financing of the President's Commission argued that financing proposals discriminate against the poor. Its report pointed out that limitations and exclusions of benefits, limitations on eligibility of beneficiaries, and deductibles and copayments had served to reduce the availability and utilization of financing for those with low incomes and for those with small health insurance packages. It is these groups, particularly, whose ability to self-finance their mental health benefits is most constrained and who have the smallest propensity to use needed mental health services. Cost-sharing measures deter obtaining services where there is high income elasticity or price elasticity. Both conditions are particularly true for low-income populations with regard to outpatient mental health services. Such methods of cost control of mental health services, when applied to the low-income populations, may be counterproductive and may exacerbate the problems already identified as gaps in mental health financing.[10] Thus, these forms of cost-control discriminate against the poor.

Researchers disagree on whether low-income persons would use more mental health services if such services were better covered by insurance programs. McSweeney has summarized a number of studies showing that poor persons do not use psychotherapy, even if it is free.[15] Crowell[16] has pointed out the distributive problem if this were true:

> If universal insurance plans reduce the costs to those currently using these services, with no substantial increase in demand by persons with lower incomes (i.e., if under federal financing the marginal propensity to consume these services still is greater for the rich than for the poor) then the inclusion of psychotherapy within a national health plan does represent a subsidy to the rich from the poor, resulting in a redistributive effect partially negating the program's overall redistributive goals.

McGuire,[17] however, has taken an opposite view: "I have found that poor people, middle-income people are much more responsive when they have insurance coverage than are upper income people. So that when you include everybody within some financing plan, the poor tend to catch up with the rich in overall utilization."

The primary reason for limiting mental health benefits is not equity but rather that many persons fear that if mental health is more adequately covered in an insurance program, costs will skyrocket. There are two elements to this. First is the fear that if mental health benefits are liberalized, many more persons will take advantage of them. This assumption has not been demonstrated to be true. For instance, Dr. Upton in this book has described a variety of studies that showed both low utilization and low costs of even unlimited coverage. In the Blue Cross/Blue Shield high-option plan for federal employees, about 2.5% of subscribers took advantage of mental health benefits. These persons were paid between 7% and 8% of health benefits in this program in 1978.[18] These figures are consistent with data from CHAMPUS (the Civilian Health and Medical Program of the Uniformed Services), which in 1975 showed utilization rates of from .7 to 3.9%,[19] and from HMOs, where utilization is consistently under 5% of services provided.[20]

Another issue is that of long-term outpatient treatment. Many insurers resist covering these services because of fears of skyrocketing costs. They cite, for instance, statistics showing that for the Washington, D.C., Blue Cross and Blue Shield Federal Employees Health Benefits Program in 1971, 1972, and

1973, 2.3% of those seeking psychotherapy exceeded outpatient costs of $10,000 each per year, one-fourth of the total annual psychotherapy dollar. Another study of the Medi-Cal case load demonstrated that "the dollars follow not the need but the number of psychiatrists practicing within a county."

Two explanations are commonly given for these costs. First, as in the Washington area, many persons are in analysis and often for training purposes. Thus, not allowing payments for psychoanalysis is seen as one logical cost curb that would also benefit the poor.

Second, some patients are "interminable." "Once they begin psychotherapy they seemingly continued with no indication of termination." In a 5-year study of the Kaiser–Permanente Plan, 5.3% of patients were in this category. Efforts to control costs by more intensive therapy led to increased utilization and emotional distress. The clinical solution was to see these patients only at spaced intervals of 2–3 months.[21] Translating this clinical solution into a financial limit would be difficult. One way out might be benefits up to a certain limit (e.g., 30 sessions), then a high copayment thereafter. The fact is that most clients are seen for fewer than 30 sessions at a time. At Kaiser–Permanente, 84.6% were seen for fewer than 15 sessions (mean 8.6%), and 10.1% were seen in "long-term therapy (mean 19.2%)." Commonly, clients stay for fewer than 5 sessions yet still feel that they have benefited from the experience.[18,21]

Peer review can also reduce costs and assure that only appropriate care is paid for. For instance, following a scandal in 1974 involving misuse of psychiatric benefits in the CHAMPUS program, Select Committees on Psychiatric Care and Evaluation (SCOPCE) were inaugurated. These committees controlled costs and utilization on a case-by-case basis rather than through a fixed number of days or visits. At a review cost of $100,000, this system saved $5 million.[18,21] Following this model, particularly for institutional settings, might be far more cost-effective and generally equitable than arbitrary caps. It is unclear whether it could be applied to private practitioners. Federal or state limits or required utilization review might therefore be more appropriate for these clinicians.

The caps on mental health services are arbitrary. They are inequitable and based upon cost fears that are not proven and that, if demonstrated, could probably be controlled in other ways.

Long-Term Care

The limitations on long-term care in NHI proposals has been pointed out. While this limits appropriate treatment for many citizens, the chronically mentally ill, retarded, and physically handicapped persons are particularly discriminated against. Mechanic[22] has summarized their situation and the great difficulties in resolving the problem:

[Given] the intractability of the conditions, they will frustrate physicians and will suffer stigmatization by both medical and nonmedical personnel. Moreover, these patients require a sustained community approach in addition to whatever medical and drug treatment they receive, and it is unlikely that an unspecialized medical context can effectively organize such services.

Whatever efforts are made to extend mental health benefits under NHI must now overshadow the needs of the severely impaired patients who require services organized independently of the traditional medical sector. Moreover, such services will have to be provided largely by nonmedical personnel who may not be covered under NHI. Services for these patients must include diagnosis and assessment, appropriate medical care, sheltered care and preparation for limited employment, aggressive monitoring and training for community living, and continuing social supports. Although a variety of viable modes have been developed in demonstration projects, we have as yet failed to develop any sustained way of financing these efforts on a continuing basis. Even under the best of conditions, such programs are difficult to organize and maintain. Without financial stability they have little chance to become established.

The initial hope that community-based care would be far less expensive than that in institutions has not been borne out by experience. The debate on this goes on, but at this point, while it may be more humane if adequately provided, it is not necessarily less costly and often is more so than traditional modalities. Thus, the shift to community treatment has not provided the financial magic that many early advocates expected.

What *is* clear is that the current forms of financing contribute to the problems. First, financing for long-term care is fragmented. A recent survey, for instance, counted 19 distinct federal programs, each of which finances at least one alternative to institutional care for the elderly. Second, the form of financing creates problems. Funds are channeled through a multitude of local agencies with mazes of varying eligibility requirements and regulations. A third problem is the fragmentation of the coordination task itself. Channeling programs that can supervise treatment and procurement of funding from a variety of sources are only beginning to be organized nationwide. The Community Support Program of NIMH is one such effort that is still small and currently being evaluated. Finally, current insurance programs still reinforce inpatient care. Many restrictions are placed on monies for community care, even when that form of treatment is most appropriate.

These problems demonstrate that this area is one where mental health and health care share common concerns. Problems in long-term care and the treatment of the chronically mentally ill show more similarities than differences.

Once again, the primary stumbling block is a lack of monies. But this is reinforced by poor organizational arrangements, the unwillingness to finance home care or services by families or paraprofessionals, and the still prevailing stigma that is attached to being disabled.

National health insurance cannot be expected to resolve all of these problems. If designed carefully, however, it can encourage a continuum of treatment models and facilities, permit monies to follow the client rather than be scattered in myriad inaccessible programs, and support corporate and volunteer efforts to collaborate with public projects.

Expanding Providers

Whether or not to expand the settings and practitioners that can be reimbursed raises similar issues in discriminatory practices and fervent debate in the field. While providers are limited in both health and mental health, the impact is greater upon the latter field because in it (a) a larger percentage of nonphysician providers can give care and (b) a larger percentage of clients can appropriately receive treatment from these persons. Thus, restrictions in insurance plans discriminate more heavily against mentally ill citizens.

Medical Limitations

The less "liberal" NHI bills sharply limit payments to nonphysician caregivers. Further, many bills restrict payments to new forms of health settings such as neighborhood health centers and long-term care facilities. Since nonphysicians tend to provide these noncovered services and work in these less-reimbursed settings, the bills continue to support a physician-dominated system.[24]

Their approach is in contrast to the Dellums, Corman, Kennedy, and some of the broader catastrophic bills. In these proposals, physicians would still remain in control of the medical system. But growth and usage of other medical professions would be encouraged. In addition, by supporting more long-term care, these bills would facilitate the development of community-based facilities other than hospitals.

HMOs are the exception to this continuum. All ranks of NHI proponents from Kennedy to Enthoven believe that their numbers should grow. Although they are still few in number and their cost savings are a cause of some debate, they are supported in either formal or informal ways in nearly all bills.[25]

Another exception is coverage for chiropractors, where the special workings of the political system show themselves in this profession's ability to be included even when opposed by most physicians. The nonpsychiatric mental health practitioners could do well to understand the chiropractors' political techniques.

Mental Health

There are strict limitations (secondary to funding restrictions) on services that can be provided in HMOs, CMHCs, and other similar locales. Few of these limits exist for inpatient facilities such as hospitals. In addition, even many "accepted" mental health professionals (such as psychologists, clinical social workers, and psychiatric nurses) are restricted from practicing in many settings. These reimbursement limits contrast sharply with the actual locations of mental health services and the persons who provide this care. In 1975 24% of persons treated in the specialty mental health sector were seen in federally funded CMHCs, 22% in free-standing outpatient clinics, 14% in general hospital psychiatric units, 19% by private practice psychiatrists and psychologists, 12% in state and county mental hospitals, and 5% in VA psychiatric units.[8] Roughly equal numbers of psychiatrists, psychologists, and social workers provide mental health services (25,000 of each profession). By 1990 the ratio of psychologists to psychiatrists is expected to grow from 1:1 to 1.84:1.[26]

The argument has already been made that this policy discriminates against the poor. In addition, it often encourages unnecessary hospitalization. Since treatment costs can be covered on an inpatient setting, it is common practice to admit patients who otherwise could not afford outpatient care. This contributes to rising health care costs.

A third problem with this policy is that it discriminates against community caregivers, who, as deinstitutionalization proceeds and federal mental health monies are cut back, are having to cut services and programs even as they are asked to do more. CMHCs have often been criticized for not providing adequate services to the severely ill client. While professional prejudices and poor management have contributed to this problem, low funding levels have also impacted heavily.

Part of the difficulty here is that many persons both in and outside of the mental health profession believe that CMHCs and other community facilities provide lower quality care than do private practitioners. Upton writes in this book that "most persons who can afford it seek treatment from a private psychiatrist when they are suffering from mental illness/emotional problems. They believe they will receive better care on a private basis. Just because they believe this, of course, doesn't make it so, but there is a rationale to back up their point of view."

An opposite point of view can easily be taken. There is a strong case to be made that even when given a choice, some people would prefer care in an organized health or mental health care setting. For example, employees are increasingly given a choice between care in an HMO and the private health care sector. The major example of the organized mental health care system is the Community Mental Health Center (CMHC). Many clients in CMHCs have incomes over $25,000 and presumably could afford private care.[26] CMHCs provide a range of programs under one roof and so might provide more appropriate care or combinations of services than private practitioners. The diversity of staff is also a community setting's strength. This allows a choice of therapists, staff who may be more responsive to different clients' needs, and more opportunities for peer review, supervision, and in-service training.

A fourth problem with limiting provider settings in mental health coverage is that it discriminates against prepaid group plans such as HMOs. This creates several difficulties. First, it reduces the opportunities for mental health and medical personnel to work together, thus reducing quality of care.

In addition, the evidence is growing that prepaid group plans of various types can save costs.[22]

In the Kaiser–Permanente plan, between 1959 and 1979 the rates for mental health services had increased by only 71%, an annual increase of 3.5%. During the same time span, yearly increases in medical costs outside of the HMO averaged between 12 and 20%. The data suggest that HMOs keep all health care costs down and that mental health expenditures rise at a lower rate in these settings than do medical costs.[27]

Studies are now also beginning to show that mental health care, particularly when utilized in a setting such as an HMO, can reduce medical utilization and cost. Thus, the Kaiser Plan determined that patients after brief psychotherapy (2–8 sessions) reduced their utilization of medical services in the 5 years following their therapy by 75%. Group Health Association of Washington, D.C., found that in the year after psychiatric referral medical visits dropped by 30%. Blue Cross of Western Pennsylvania showed that medical surgical days decreased by 54% after outpatient psychotherapy.

Finally, research demonstrates the value of corporate mental health programs in improving productivity. The Equitable Life Assurance Society's Emotional Health Program has led to a $3 return in recovered productivity for every $1 invested. The INSIGHT program at Kennecott Copper Company over 1 year led to a 55.4% reduction in hospital, medical, and surgical costs (compared to 1.5% for nonparticipants), a 52% reduction in absenteeism (compared to 6.3%), and a reduction in nonoccupational accident and insurance costs of 74.6% (38.5% for nonparticipants).

In sum, as the Task Panel Report[10] states,

> These reports of positive indications of health economic benefits achieved through mental health intervention are provocative. Each study individually must be interpreted conservatively. But, as a group, this research is striking. Research from health maintenance organizations (HMOs), from industrial programs, and from regular health insurance plans suggests that providing outpatient mental health services can reduce overall health services utilization and overall health costs.

Thus, there is increasing evidence that expanding the settings eligible for reimbursement might improve the quality of care, help control costs, and increase the nation's productivity.

Expanding Practitioners

Whether to expand the types of practitioners eligible for reimbursement is at least as controversial an issue as whether to expand settings. In medical care, despite increasing pressures to broaden the roles and privileges of nurses and physician's assistants, physicians will continue to play the leading role in service delivery. In mental health, whether this will occur or even should occur is a hotly debated issue. This fact raises serious questions about a financing system that reinforces a narrow medical model of care in mental health.

Dr. Upton, in this book, despite his attempts to be fair, still spends much of his paper justifying the primary position of the psychiatrist in mental health. Few persons will disagree that medical aspects of psychiatric care are the province of physicians, and that a close consultative relationship needs to be maintained between psychiatrists and other mental health professionals. However, a variety of studies confirm that the majority of mental health tasks can be performed by most mental health practitioners and are generally provided by these persons.

These include core functions such as receiving new clients, crisis intervention, planning and referral, administration, and therapy. Further, there is considerable substitution of psychologists and social workers for psychiatrists, particularly in community-based settings.[26]

The findings on psychotherapy effectiveness also raise serious questions about a narrow provider definition. Bergin and Lambert,[28] Frank,[29] Parloff et al.,[30] Smith et al.,[31] and Kisch and Kroll[32] all agree that while psychotherapy is effective, the type of treatment used affects outcomes in only marginal ways for most problems. Further, the profession, education, and experience of the clinician cannot be definitely shown to have differential impacts. This raises the disturbing possibility that even limiting reimbursement to the core four groups (psychiatrists, psychologists, clinical social workers, psychiatric nurses) may be dictated more by political pressures, arbitrary though perhaps necessary limits, and expediency than by research evidence. Frank's[29] description of factors necessary to success, though as yet empirically untested, makes much more sense:

> . . . all therapists, independent of school (or, we add, profession), provide their patients with a common set of non-specific elements: an emotionally charged relationship with a helping person, the opportunity to use the therapist's personal qualities to strengthen the patient's expectations of help, a plausable explanation of the causes of the patient's distress, techniques and procedures based on a rationale acceptable to the patient, and some experience of success with new ways of behaving and feeding.

If this point of view is accepted, then the arguments of Smith, Glass, and Miller[31] for pluralism in mental health practices may be applicable to the professions as well:

> Pluralism means that each school of psychotherapy should be allowed to train its next generation of practitioners, conduct its research, and advance itself as a profession. The policy, or even the attitude, that excludes one school or another of psychotherapy from the academy, the mental health center, or the journals may arise from deep personal conviction, authoritarianism, or politics, but it is unwarranted by a fair comparison of demonstrated efficacy.

This argument is not a new one. We are reminded of a paper presented by one of us,[33] which stated that:

> what we are questioning is the identification of any one set of skills or conceptual preferences with any professional discipline . . . the argument over which is the "best model" may not be the most productive way to get at the real problems. Arguments over the best model may often be the least illuminating in terms of future development. For example, the issue of who should or should not perform psychotherapy will not be settled by polemics and antipolemics or even by discussion and debate alone, but rather in the market place of demand for human services . . . when the challenge is the meeting of human needs and the enhancement of human potential, let freedom ring.

In Conclusion

The chapters in this book have highlighted the many mechanisms through which mentally ill persons are discriminated against in the health care system. Current national health insurance proposals would reinforce this two-tier system of financing care. The authors in this book have wisely argued for legislative changes to remedy these problems.

Many mental health professionals, however, are guilty of similar discriminatory behavior. Those who favor strict limitations on providers of care-settings and/or professions are supporting a service delivery system that will be unable to adapt to the clinical realities of the 1980s. Growing populations of elderly, physically handicapped, and multiply disabled persons will require services by a variety of caregivers as well as closer collaboration between professionals and improved linkages among service settings. The present financing system does not foster such changes.

The dynamics of discrimination against mentally ill persons are deep and not easily removed. They are seen in history from the devil theory of medieval times to the current practices of mentally disturbed individuals being treated as unworthy ill. The national health insurance debate is currently carried out through arcane methods such as reimbursement and benefit mechanisms. The reality that we must be concerned with is whether effective and humane care is available.

Appendix

This Appendix contains summaries of the major health insurance proposals. Each is in two parts: (a) general approach and (b) mental health benefits.*

*The general approach section excludes mental health coverage. Thus, e.g., "unlimited physicians services" does not necessarily mean "unlimited psychiatrists services," which should be verified in the mental health benefits section.

Data were gathered from several sources. The key ones were (1) "Bulletin #109," Public Affairs Information and Action, Mental Health Association, November 8, 1979. The format of this report was adopted for this paper and the PAIA summaries were used for those bills they covered (denoted by P on bill summaries); (2) "Summaries of Selected Health Insurance Proposals and Proposals to Restructure the Financing of Private Health Insurance," Subcommittee on Health and Environment of the Committee on Interstate and Foreign Commerce, U.S. House of Representatives, February 11, 1980. This is the most complete summary to date of the various national health insurance proposals. Bills included in this are denoted by H on summaries; (3) "Background Material on Health Insurance," Committee on Finance, U.S. Senate, June 14, 1979. This is a good summary of those bills it covers and is denoted by S on summaries; (4) all hearings on national health insurance held during 1979 and 1980; and (5) review of each of the bills.

For details of these bills, the reader is referred to the above sources.

A Classification of NHI Bills
(ordered by degree of government control of health care)
1. HR 2969 (Dellums)—total federally run and provided care
2. HR 21 (Corman)—old Kennedy, Corman
3. S 1720, HR 5191 (Kennedy, Waxman)
4. S 1812, HR 5400 (Ribicoff, Rangel)
5. HR 16 (Dingell)
6. S 350 (Long/Ribicoff), #351, HR 3276 (Long/Talmadge, Walgren)
7. S 760 (Long)
8. S 1014 (Hart)
9. S 748 (Dole, 3-D bill)
10. S 1590 (Schweiker)
11. HR 6405 (Martin, old Ford bill)
12. HR 3974 (Martin, Jones)
13. HR 3943 (Jones, Martin)
14. HR 5740 (Ullman)
15. S 1968 (Durenberger)
16. HR 7527 (Gephardt, Stockman, Enthoven proposal)
Note: Numbers 1–3:   Comprehensive Public Service
      Numbers 4–12:   Catastropic Variations Regulated Utility
      Numbers 13–16: Restructuring the Financing of Private Health
                     Insurance Free Market

HR 2969, Dellums, March 14, 1979

General Concept and Approach.   The bill would establish a U.S. Health Service, which would provide free medical, dental, and mental health care, and additional supplemental services to all individuals while within the United States and its territories. The Health Service Act would be administered by a four-tiered system of national, regional, district, and community health boards, all composed of two-thirds health care users and one-third health workers. The program would be financed by a special health service tax on individuals and employers and by general federal revenues. Services would be provided by salaried health workers in facilities established and maintained by the Health Service.

Coverage.   All individuals in the United States would be covered.

Benefits.   These would include inpatient and outpatient care, occupational health services, dental care, home health services, long-term care, drugs, appliances and equipment, child care and homemaking services, health promotion and education, and preventive health services.

Administration.   Population areas of between 25,000 and 50,000 persons would set up boards to plan service delivery systems. District, regional, and national health boards would complete the planning tier.

Financing.   A new "annual health service tax" would be based on income, estates, and trusts, with an excise tax of 4.5% of wages to be paid by employers. General revenues would be equal to 40% of the above totals.

Mental Health Benefits.   These would include inpatient and outpatient care, mental services, long-term care, rehabilitation services, provisions of drugs, preventive health service, and counseling and social services assistance. No limitations are described, nor are there any direct costs to clients. However, a graduated tax structure is set up for all to pay for these services, with the range being 1% of taxable income where it is less than $6000 to $660, plus 14% of excess income over $1200.

Mental health services are considered to include "psychological and psychiatric counseling."

HR 21, Corman, January 15, 1979

General Concept and Approach.   The proposal would establish a health insurance program covering the entire population for a wide range of services. The program would be financed by a federal payroll tax on employers and employees, a tax on unearned income and self-employment earnings, and by federal general revenues. A Health Security Board, appointed by the president, would be established within the Department of Health, Education and Welfare to administer the program. The proposal contains certain provisions intended to reorganize and improve the delivery of health services and to develop community home care programs for the chronically ill.

Coverage.   All United States residents would be covered.

Benefits.   No payments would be required of patients. Benefits would include general hospital inpatient and outpatient care; physician, optometrist and podiatrist services; dental services; home health services; a variety of support services; drugs; medical appliances.

Administration. HEW would administer it using regional offices and various advisory councils. There would be no involvement of private health insurers.

Financing. This would entail a "Health Security Trust Fund" supported by payroll, wage, and income taxes and federal general revenues.

Mental Health Benefits. These would include the following categories:

Inpatient. Coverage would provide 45 days during the benefit period (this term to be defined in regulations).

Skilled Nursing Homes. Coverage would provide 120 days per benefit period, which might be extended for nursing homes that are part of hospitals or for all homes if funds are available.

Outpatient. Coverage would provide 20 visits per benefit period, except when services were provided through group practice organizations, hospital outpatient departments, community mental health centers, or certain other mental health clinics, in which case there is no limitation on number of visits.

Physician Only. No other mental health practitioners are mentioned.

"Mental Health Day Care Service." Sixty days per benefit period would be covered if provided by a hospital, but the benefit would be unlimited if the service were provided by a group practice organization, community mental health center, or mental health day care service under special agreements with the Health Security Board.

Medications. For participating groups, these must be chosen from a list of permitted drugs. Other groups could be reimbursed based upon a list of permitted diseases and conditions and drugs that are allowed to be used to treat these.

Supporting Services. Including psychological services, social work, and health education, they would be covered if part of institutional services or if they were furnished by a group practice association, individual practice association, or certain (unspecified) public or nonprofit agencies.

Alcoholism and Drug Abuse. In addition to reimbursement for above services, these could also receive outpatient treatment in a "free-standing ambulatory center."

S 1720, Kennedy, September 6, 1979 (P,H) (Same as HR 5191, Waxman, September 6, 1979)

General Concept and Approach. This bill provides for a national health insurance program covering the entire population, financed through employer/employee wage-related premiums, Medicare payroll taxes and premiums, state payments for the poor, and federal general revenues. It would be administered primarily by certified private health insurers and HMOs, with the federal government continuing to administer Medicare. A national budget would be established for all services covered under the program, with increases limited to rates of increase in the Gross National Product. Reimbursement fees to providers are negotiated between providers and insurers within given geographic areas.

Coverage.   All U.S. citizens would be covered, with a continuation of Medicare provided. AFDC recipients and residents of state institutions would be covered under private plans, with premiums paid by states. SSI recipients and residents of federal institutions would be covered under private plans and premiums paid by the federal government. Employees would be covered under employers' plans, self-employed through private plans.

Benefits.   These include hospital inpatient and outpatient coverage; physicians' services; 100 days per "spell of illness" at skilled nursing facilities; a variety of preventive services; outpatient physical, speech, and occupational therapy; diagnostic tests and X ray therapy; various medical equipment; dialysis items.

Administration.   A federal national health insurance board would establish policies and standards, set national and state budgets, certify insurers, and negotiate premiums with them. State health insurance boards would implement details on the state level. Day-to-day administration would be handled by private insurers and HMSs grouped into four national consortia.

Financing.   This would be based on wage- and income-related premiums, employer contributions (70–75%), and state and federal payments for certain populations.

Mental Health Benefits.   These would comprise two sections.

Medicare (as Amended).   The coverage would be as follows: (a) *Inpatient* would pay for 150 consecutive days of hospitalization per spell of illness, 60 days between spells of illness. (b) *Outpatient* would pay 80% of the fee equivalent of 20 psychiatric visits, fee to be determined by periodic negotiation within the geographic area. (c) *Partial hospitalization* would pay for day care, with each day counted as ½ day of inpatient care. (d) *CMHCs* would be recognized as providers. (e) *Other mental health professionals*—psychologists, psychiatric social workers, and "counselors"—would be recognized when in CMHC or under "other qualified provider as determined by National Health Board." (f) *Drugs* appearing on an approved list as needed for chronic conditions would be paid for.

Employer Plans.   These would be required to provide, as a minimum, the same benefits as Medicare except that inpatient coverage could be limited to 45 consecutive days per spell of illness.

S 1812, Ribicoff, September 25, 1979 (P,H,S) (Same as HR 5400, Rangel, September 25, 1979)

General Concept and Approach.   The bill would provide for (1) a federal insurance program (to be known as Health Care) including comprehensive coverage of aged, disabled, and poor, and offering insurance against major medical expenses to other individuals and their families through approved private insurance plans. Health Care would incorporate Medical and acute-care portions of Medicaid.

Coverage. Health Care would cover persons currently under Medicare, additional low-income persons, and individuals or employers who chose to purchase it. The mandated employer plan would cover all full-time employees and their families.

Benefits. These would include inpatient, physician services, 100 days/year at skilled nursing facilities, 200 visits/year of home health service, outpatient physical therapy, chiropractors' services, diagnostic tests and X-ray therapy, various medical equipment, dialysis items, and pre- and postnatal and infant care.

Administration. Health Care would be similar to Medicare; employer plans would be administered by private health insurers and HMOs with federally certified minimum standards.

Financing. Health Care would be financed by a combination of Medicare payroll taxes, premiums, and federal, state, and local subsidies. Premium payments would support the employer plans, with employers paying at least 75% of the cost.

Cost Sharing. For the elderly, the disabled, and persons with renal disease the share would be the same as for Medicare, but to maximum of $1250/person; there would be none for low-income persons. For those who buy into Health Care and employer plans there would be a $2500 deductible per family, but none on prenatal and infant care.

Mental Health Benefits. These would again be divided into two sections.

Health Care (Replaces Medicare). The coverage would be as follows. (a) *Inpatient* would pay for up to 30 days per calendar year. (b) *Outpatient* would pay 80% of physician's charges up to a maximum annual reimbursement of $1000 after $60 deductible. (c) *Partial hospitalization* is not mentioned, nor is (d) *CMHC provider status* or (e) *other mental health professionals.* (f) *Drugs,* i.e., those administered in physician's office or included in physician's bill, would be covered. (g) *Catastrophic* coverage would be unlimited after $1250 out-of-pocket expenditures by an individual during calendar year indexed from October 1980. However, mental health expenses in excess of limits noted above could not be counted toward the $1250. That is, costs of any inpatient care for mental health beyond 30 days or costs of any outpatient treatment for mental health beyond $1000 could not be counted toward the $1250.

Employer Plans. These would be required to provide, as a minimum, the same benefits as Health Care except that under catastrophic coverage "family" would be substituted for "individual" and "$2500" for "$1250."

HR 16, Dingell, January 15, 1979 (H)

General Concept and Approach. The Dingell bill would establish a health insurance program for all persons who are employed, self-employed, or on Social Security. Medicare persons would be eligible only for services not covered by Medicare. The program would be federally financed and run by the states.

Coverage.   The plan would cover employees and self-employed persons, social security beneficiaries and their dependents. Arrangements (unspecified) to be made to cover recipients of public assistance and the unemployed. Medicare continues with recipients eligible for additional services not currently covered.

Benefits.   These would provide 60 days/year inpatient (could be extended if money permitted) physician, dentist, podiatric, and home nursing services; optometrists' services; lab services and X rays; physical therapy and related services; medical appliances; certain drugs.

Administration.   The program would be administered at three levels of government—federal, state, and local—with the major operating responsibility falling to the state and local jurisdictions. Each state would evaluate its health resources and capabilities and, in accordance with national guidelines, would develop a state health care plan. The state plan would be submitted to the National Health Insurance Board (created under the bill) and, if it were approved, the board would contract with the state for the administration of the program within the state.

Financing.   A federal "Health Services Account" would give funds to the states. Sources of these monies are not specified but it appears that they would come from federal payroll taxes and federal/state general revenues.

Mental Health Benefits.   This would be provided as follows:

Inpatient.   Thirty days per benefit year would be covered, but limits could be extended if funds were available.

Outpatient and Medications.   Outpatient physician services would be covered, but no specific mention is made of mental health outpatient or other noninpatient services. Prescription drugs would be covered.

S 350, Long/Ribicoff, February 6, 1979 (H,S) S 351/HR 3276, Walgren, March 27, 1979

The latter two are identical to S 350 except that they exclude provisions establishing a new medical assistance program for low-income persons. (S 350/51 was later replaced by S 760.)

General Concept and Approach.   Both bills would provide catastrophic health insurance through (1) a federally administered public plan for the unemployed, welfare recipients, the aged, and persons who do not opt for private insurance coverage, or (2) a private catastrophic plan allowed as an option for employees and self-employed. S 350 also establishes a uniform national program of basic benefits for low-income persons and families.

Coverage.   All residents would be entitled to catastrophic benefits under either a public or a private plan. S 350's additional plan would cover all Medicaid-eligible persons and other families below certain income levels.

Benefits. Institutional benefits (hospital care, 100 days of past hospital services, home health services) after hospitalization for 60 days in 1 year, medical benefits (similar to Medicare, Part B) after $2000 in expenses by a family for these would be provided. S 350's additional program would include a 60-day hospitalization/benefit period, home health care, nursing homes and intermediate care facilities, physician services, lab and X ray services, physical therapy, medical supplies, and a variety of services to children.

Administration. HEW would administer the public plan and private insurers the HEW-approved private plans. S 350's plan would be administered by HEW using private carriers as fiscal intermediaries.

Financing. This would be provided by a 1% tax on employers and on the income of self-employed persons, with 50% of this allowed as a tax credit. No employee contribution would be allowed.

Mental Health Benefits. These would be the same as in S 760.

S 760, Long, March 26, 1979 (P,H,S)

This bill replaces S 350/351.

General Concept and Approach. The bill contains provisions related to catastrophic health insurance, medical assistance for the poor, and certification for private health insurance similar to those in S 350 except for some modifications in the catastrophic health insurance program. In lieu of the 1% payroll tax levied on employers under S 350 to finance a catastrophic program, this proposal would require all employers to provide catastrophic health insurance protection to their employees and family members. Employers with payrolls of $250,000 or less in a year would have the option of taking either a tax deduction for their premium costs or a 50% tax credit for those costs. Public and nonprofit employers, regardless of size, and uncovered individuals would also be eligible for the option of a 50% tax credit. Employers' plans would have to be certified by HEW. The secretary would be required to offer a catastrophic policy in states in which approved plans were not actually and generally available. The bill would permit dependent children to remain under a parent's policy until age 26.

Mental Health Benefits. These would comprise three categories.
Medicare (as Amended). The coverage would be as follows. (a) *Inpatient* would be the same as other illness coverage but with a 190-day lifetime limit. (b) *Outpatient* would pay 80% of physician charges up to a maximum annual reimbursement of $400, after $60 deductible. (c) *Partial hospitalization* is not mentioned, nor is (d) *CMHC provider status* or (e) *other mental health professions.*

(g) *Drugs,* when administered in the physician's office or included in the physician's bill, would be covered.

Medicaid (as Amended). The coverage would be as follows. (a) *Inpatient* would be unlimited. (b) *Outpatient* would be unlimited when provided by CMHC. It would be limited to five visits to a private psychiatrist during a 12-month period unless more are needed to prevent institutionalization. (c) *Partial hospitalization* would be unlimited in a hospital or CMHC. (d) *CMHCs* would be recognized as a provider. (e) *Other mental health professionals* are not mentioned. (f) *Drugs,* when on an approved list and if necessary to prevent institutionalization, would be covered.

Medical Assistance Plan for Low-Income Persons. This would cover inpatient hospital services, including active mental health treatment for 60 days per benefit period.

S 1014, Hart, April 25, 1979

General Concept and Approach. This bill sets up (a) a separate national program of health care services for children and pregnant women (similar to CHAP) and (b) catastrophic coverage of 50% of expenses for services between 10 and 20% of income and 100% of expenses over 20% provided by private insurance companies through contracts and CHHS.

Coverage. The plan would cover all U.S. citizens if arrangements are made through the program.

Benefits. These would be as above—covering hospital, surgical, medical and dental services; medical equipment; other supplies and services deemed to be appropriate (thus, largely determined through regulations).

Administration. Federal contracts with carriers in insurance pools, under federal guidelines, would implement the program.

Financing. Appropriations from federal general revenues would cover the plan, along with repeal of income tax deductions for medical and health insurance expenses.

Mental Health Benefits (Catastrophic Provisions). Services eligible for the above coverage would include hospital and medical services, prescribed drugs and medicines, and other medical supplies and service as the secretary "shall determine to be appropriate for the provision of full and complete physical and mental health care." Thus, the secretary would have great freedom to expand or limit mental health coverage.

Neither CMHCs or ICFs are mentioned. The secretary could determine qualified providers and health care practitioners, thus having much freedom to determine who will provide service.

S 748, Dole, March 26, 1979 (P,H,S)

General Concept and Approach. This bill would create a system of catastrophic health insurance protection by (1) amending Medicare to provide for catastrophic benefits; (2) establishing employer-based private catastrophic health insurance plans; (3) giving aid to those who did not come under any other type of insurance plan to purchase insurance through private companies and setting minimum levels of coverage for this insurance; (4) requiring state Medicaid programs to provide catastrophic coverage equal to that of the residual plan in item (3) or to buy into the plan in item (3).

Coverage. Current Medicare beneficiaries would be covered. There would be employer-based catastrophic plans for full-time employees and families. A residual catastrophic plan for all those not covered under the above would be established.

Benefits. Medicare catastrophic benefits would be provided for Part A services by ending copayment requirements for hospital and skilled nursing home care and durational limits on hospital services. For Part B, 100% would be paid of covered services once expenses of $5000/year were reached or an individual had paid 20% of that deductible out of pocket for these services. The employer plan would be similar, with institutional expenses covered after an individual or family had been hospitalized for 60 days. Part B type services would be covered after expenses of $5000. Residual would be the same except that full coverage could also begin after 5% of income was spent.

Administration. HEW would administer expanded Medicare. Private insurers would administer employer and residual plans with approval by HEW and through insurance pools if desired.

Financing. Medicare would be financed as at present. Employer plans would require employer/employee and employee contributions, with employee share limited to 25%. For the residual plan, individual and family premiums and subsidies for low-income persons through federal general revenues would be required.

Mental Health Benefits. These would be covered as follows:

Medicare (as Amended). (a) *Inpatient* would be the same as other illness coverage but with 190-day lifetime limit. (b) *Outpatient* would pay 80% of charges for a "reasonable number of visits" (to be spelled out in regulations) up to a maximum annual reimbursement of $750, after $60 deductible. (c) *Partial Hospitalization* is not mentioned. (d) *CMHCs* would be recognized as providers. (e) *Other mental health professionals* are not mentioned. (f) *Drugs,* as approved by a national formulary committee, would be covered.

S 1590, Schweiker, July 26, 1979

General Concept and Approach. The Schweiker bill provides a minimum level of catastrophic insurance utilizing a combination of (1) additional prerequisites for tax-deductible employer-based insurance plans, (2) state-administered insurance pooling arrangements, and (3) increased medicare benefits. Minimum catastrophic coverage is defined as complete coverage, without copayments of medical expenses incurred annually by an individual and his family in excess of 20% of the family's adjusted gross income.

Coverage. There would be catastrophic for employees and families. Employees of small employers (under 50 persons), uninsurable risks, self-employed, and those without private or government insurance would be covered through state-administered private insurance pools. Medicare would be slightly expanded.

Benefits. For the employer plan and the pool plans, current Medicare provisions would be followed, but without benefits for skilled nursing home care. At least one of the variety of private plans offered by employers would require employees to pay 25% of hospital costs until they exceeded 20% of income. Under Medicare, all limits on days of hospital care would be eliminated, but beneficiaries would have to pay 20% of costs of hospital care up to 20% of income. Preventive benefits (child care, hypertension screening) would be required under all plans.

Administration. Employers would be required to offer at least three different private plans. Insurers would be required to join in state pools for catastrophic coverage in order to participate in federal health programs. Employers not offering three plans would lose their deductions for premiums.

Financing. For employer-based plans, employer and employee would contribute premiums (not over 25%). For state pools there would be premium contributions.

Mental Health Benefits. Services are defined under Medicare but exclude long-term nursing home care. For catastrophic illness, the patient would pay 20% of expenses until this reached 20% of income when 100% of services are covered, with no maximum day limits at any point.

HR 6405, Martin, February 4, 1980 (H)

General Concept and Approach. This bill would establish a Catastrophic Automatic Protection Plan (CAPP), which would begin reimbursing for catastrophic medical expenses when they reached a certain percentage of income. Copayments would be required until a "stop-loss" limit was reached, whereby CAPP would pay in full for covered services. (2) Employees' tax-free payments to programs and employers' business expense deductions would be modified unless the plans qualified by covering certain services when employees had over $2500 in out-of-pocket expenses. (3) Hospital coinsurance and limits of hospital days under Medicare, Part A would be ended and some (nonmental health) preventive care would be permitted.

Coverage. Medicare coverage would continue for persons under that program and employees would continue to be covered under employer insurance plans. Medicaid beneficiaries would be eligible for CAPP benefits to the extent that they extended state benefits. CAPP would largely serve those with little or no insurance protection—working poor, self-employed, unemployed, and their dependents.

Benefits. These would be essentially those of Medicare, with the same limitations, as well as prenatal and well-baby care. They would be provided for all programs. Cost sharing would be determined by the method shown in Table 1. After an income-related deductible was paid, CAPP would pay for covered benefits, with families paying coinsurance of differing percents. Once a stop-loss limit were reached, CAPP would pay all. Employers' contributions to plans would be modified. Plans would have to provide full payment for CAPP services once $2500 in expenses were reached. (See the House report[10] for more details of this complicated system.)

Administration. HHS would administer CAPP and determine qualified employer plans.

Financing. The program would be CAPP-financed through general revenue funds. Medicare and Medicaid would remain the same. Employer plans would be financed through existing arrangements but with new requirements.

Mental Health Benefits. These would be provided in two ways.

CAPP. Inpatient coverage would be the same as Medicare except that the 190-day lifetime limit would be replaced by a 45-day yearly limit for inpatient psychiatric services. Reimbursable prescription drugs would have to be chosen from a list developed by the secretary.

Partial hospitalization, other provider, and CMHCs are not specifically mentioned.

Employer Programs. These would provide the same coverage as CAPP. "Physically or mentally handicapped" could deduct expenses from their taxes when these exceeded 3% of income.

HR 3974, Martin/Jones, May 7, 1979

General Concept and Approach. The bill would provide for a system of protection against the cost of catastrophic illness by means of federal income tax credits for excessive medical expenses. The proposal would allow persons to claim as credits against personal income taxes amounts equal to (1) 85% of

Table 1. Cost-Sharing Determination

Family income	Out-of-pocket deductible	Coinsurance rate (percent)	"Stop-loss" limit
Not over $4000	$300	10	$500
Over $4000 but not over $10,000	$300, plus 20% of income over $4000	15	$500, plus 25% of income over $4000
Over $10,000	$1500 plus 20% of income over $10,000	20	$2000, plus 25% of income over $10,000

those medical care expenses (not compensated for by insurance or otherwise) that exceed 15% of "modified adjusted gross income" (as defined in the bill) but do not exceed 25% of such income, plus (2) 100% of medical care expenses paid by the taxpayers that exceed 25% of modified adjusted gross income. The tax credit would ordinarily be claimed on the regular income tax return.

Coverage. All persons with taxable income would be covered. Persons without taxable income would be eligible for refundable tax credits upon application.

Benefits. Medical care expenses included for purposes of tax credits would be the usual, customary, and reasonable amounts paid for (1) the diagnosis, cure, mitigation, or prevention of disease for the purpose of affecting any structure of function of the body [except as limited in item (3) below]; (2) transportation primarily for and essential to medical care; (3) 50% of the amounts paid for domiciliary and intermediate care facilities; or (4) insurance (including Medicare Part B premiums) covering such medical care.

Other existing programs would not be changed.

Administration. This would be done by the IRS.

Financing. Funds would come from federal general revenues. Present medical expense deductions would be repealed.

Mental Health Benefits. Medical care is defined as care "for the diagnosis, cure, mitigation, treatment, or prevention of disease or for the purpose of affecting any structure or function of the body." It is unclear whether mental illness qualifies. If it does, it would be covered as above.

For persons in "domiciliary and intermediate care facilities," 50% of costs would be covered.

HR 3943, Jones/Martin, May 5, 1979

General Concept and Approach. The bill would amend provisions of the Internal Revenue Code pertaining to employers' business expenses deductions for contributions toward employee health insurance plans. Employers would no longer be allowed to claim as a business expense for federal tax purposes contributions toward employee health insurance covering inpatient hospital care unless the insurance contract required the following: (1) that the beneficiary pay or personally obtain insurance for 25% of the cost of insured inpatient hospital care, and (2) that total beneficiary copayments for hospital care insured under the plan be limited to $2000 per year, or 15% of the beneficiary's average adjusted gross income for the previous 3 taxable years, whichever would be less. Employer contributions on behalf of employees to a health maintenance organization plan would not be subject to these requirements.

Administration. The Internal Revenue Service would be responsible for determining whether the business expense deduction would be allowed.

Mental Health Benefits. No change from current law would occur.

HR 5740, Ullman, October 30, 1979 (H)

General Concept and Approach. The bill limits the amount of the employer's contribution to a health care plan that is tax-free to the employee. If the cost of a plan exceeded a trigger point "of $75/month/family, plans would have to follow certain payment and service guidelines including limiting employee costs to $2000."

Coverage. This plan applies only to employed persons.

Benefits. If costs of a plan exceed $75/month/family, the plan would have to offer inpatient, outpatient, and physician's services; related services and supplies; diagnostic, X ray and lab services; 100 home health visits; prosthetic devices. Also, copayments, deductibles and coinsurance would have to be limited to $2000/year/employee.

Administration. Plans would be administered by insurance carriers or other private entities. Treasury would determine if plans met criteria.

Financing. There would be no changes.

Mental Health Benefits. These are potentially limited by not requiring "diagnosis or treatment of a mental condition" to be included under the service guidelines. They could be included but they would not have to be.

Partial hospitalization, CMHCs, and other mental health professions, are not mentioned.

S 1968, Durenberger, November 1, 1979 (H)

General Concept and Approach. This bill limits the amount of an employer's contribution to an employee's health benefits plan that is tax-free to the employee. For an employer with over 100 covered employees, at least three options must be offered, each providing (1) minimum benefits covering at least the same types of services as are covered under Medicare and (2) catastrophic benefits paying 100% of the costs of services after nonreimbursable expenses exceeded $3500 in any year.

Equal Contribution Requirement. The bill contains a provision referred to as the "equal contribution requirement." For any employer, regardless of size, offering more than one coverage option, the amount of the employer's contribution would be the same regardless of which option the employee chose. If an employer's contribution amount exceeded the actual cost of the particular option selected by the employee, the employee would be entitled to receive a rebate equal to the difference.

The rebate would be returned to the employee either in cash or in another form of compensation or benefit. The bill specifies that the employee would have the option of receiving the rebate in cash. (Such rebate would be taxable to the employee as income but would not be subject to social security, railroad retirement, or unemployment tax.)

Administration. Plans would be administered by insurance carriers or other appropriate carriers with regulation by HEW and Treasury.

Mental Health Benefits. None are specified. For employers with over 100 employees, Medicare coverage plus catastrophic coverage, as above, would be required.

HR 7527, Gephardt/Stockman, June 9, 1980

General Concept and Approach. The bill would provide coverage by (a) excluding from income employer contributions toward premiums of qualified plans, and giving refunds to employees who choose plans costing less than their employer's excludable provision; (b) giving tax credits to self-employed workers; (c) giving aged and disabled a direct contribution in the form of a voucher to purchase membership in a plan if they chose not to continue to receive present Medicare benefits; and (d) providing a contribution in voucher form to the poor equal to the average health care expenditure in the area they reside in.

Coverage. All Americans would be covered under one of the provisions.

Benefits. These would be for inpatient and outpatient care, drugs, medical equipment, well-child care and eye examinations for children (but not eyeglasses, hearing aids, or dental care), home health or nonhospital institutional care for 100 days/illness spell. It is unclear whether long-term care is included since "inpatient, outpatient, and other institutional health services at appropriate levels of care" might include it.

Administration. The Health Benefits Assurance Corp. in the Department of the Treasury would review private plans and send them to HHS for approval. Plans each year would send brochures describing their services to HHS, which would distribute them. Plans would be required to have open enrollment each year. Premiums would be set by HHS unless states exercised their option to do so.

Financing. This would come from existing sources. A provision requires the repeal of Medicare if over 50% of eligible persons choose the voucher plan instead.

Mental Health Benefits. "Items and services related to mental or emotional illnesses or conditions" and "treatment for chronic chemical dependency" would be excluded.

Additional Provisions. Sec. 306 ends PSROs, uniform reporting, capital expenditure limitations, and much of current health planning and limits federal involvement in HMSs.

References

1. English J: Statement, February 12, 1979, House Subcommittee on Health of the Committee on Ways and Means. Serial 96-91.
2. Harris P: Testimony, November 29, 1979, House Committees on Interstate and Foreign Commerce and Ways and Means. Serial 96-88.

3. Waxman H: Statement, November 29, 1979, House Committees on Interstate and Foreign Commerce and Ways and Means. Serial 96-88.
4. Davis K: National Health Insurance, Benefits, Costs, and Consequences. Washington DC, The Brookings Institution, 1975.
5. Russell LB: Medical care, in Pechman, JA (ed): Setting National Priorities: Agenda for the 1980s. Washington DC, The Brookings Institution, 1980.
6. Congressional Quarterly, Inc: Health Policy—The Legislative Agenda. Washington DC, Congressional Quarterly, Inc, 1980.
7. US DHEW: Health United States—1979. Washington DC, US Department of Health, Education and Welfare, Public Health Services, Office of Health Research, Statistics, and Technology, 1980.
8. US DHEW: The Alcohol, Drug Abuse, and Mental Health National Data Book. Washington DC, US Department of Health, Education and Welfare, Public Health Service, Alcohol, Drug Abuse, and Mental Health Administration, January 1980.
9. Keisler CA: National Health Insurance, Testimony, November 14, 1975, in Kreisler, CA, Cummings, C, VandenBos, GR: Psychology and National Health Insurance—A Source Book. Washington DC, American Psychological Association, Inc, 1979.
10. Task Panel Report on Cost and Financing: The President's Commission on Mental Health: Task Panel Reports, Volume II, Appendix. Washington DC, US Government Printing Office, 1978.
11. Flax JW, Wagenfield, MO, Ivens, RE, Weiss, RJ: Mental Health and Rural America—An Overview and Annotated Bibliography. Rockville Md: US Department of Health, Education and Welfare, Public Health Service, ADAMHA, National Health Institute of Mental Health, Division of Mental Health Service Program, 1979.
12. Enthoven A: Health Plan. Reading Mass, Addison-Wesley Publishing Co, 1980.
13. Marmor T: Rethinking National Health Insurance. *Public Interest* 46: 73–97, 1977.
14. Robbins H: Statement, February 21, 1980, Subcommittee on Health of the House Committee on Ways and Means. Serial 96-91.
15. McSweeney AJ: Including psychotherapy in National Health Insurance. *Am Psychol* 32: 722–730, 1977.
16. Crowell E: Redistribution aspects of psychotherapy's inclusion in National Health Insurance. *Am Psychol* 32: 732, 1977.
17. McGuire T: Statement, February 21, 1980, Subcommittee on Health of the House Committee on Ways and Means. Serial 96-91.
18. Brown B: Critical concerns—National Health Insurance. *Psychiatr Q* 50-1: 24, 1978.
19. Wilkins J: Colorado Medicare study—A history. *Am Psychol* 32: 746–749, 1977.
20. Cummings NA, Follette WT: Psychiatric services and medical utilization in a prepaid health plan setting: Part II. *Med Care* 6: 31–41, 1968.
21. Cummings NA: The anatomy of psychotherapy under National Health Insurance. *Am Psychol* 32: 711–719, 1977.
22. Mechanic D: Consideration in the design of mental health benefits under National Health Insurance. *Am J Public Health* 68-5: 482–488, 1978.
23. Pollack W: Long-term care, in Feder J, Holahan J, Marmor T, (eds): National Health Insurance: Conflicting Goals and Policy Choices. Washington DC, The Urban Institute, 1980.
24. Robyn DL, Hadley J: New health occupations—Nurse practitioners and physicians assistants, in Feder J, Holahan J, Marmor T (eds): National Health Insurance: Conflicting Goals and Policy Choices. Washington DC, The Urban Institute, 1980.
25. Luft HS, Feder J, Holahan J, Lennox KD: Health maintenance organizations, in Feder J, Holahan J, Marmor T (eds): National Health Insurance: Conflicting Goals and Policy Choices. Washington DC, The Urban Institute, 1980.
26. McGuire, TG: Markets for psychotherapy, in VandenBos GR: Psychotherapy and Practice, Research, Policy. Beverly Hills, Sage Publications, 1980.
27. Keisler C, Cummings NA, VandenBos GR: Introduction, Chapter 4, in Keisler C, Cummings NA, VandenBos GR (eds): Psychology and National Health Insurance: A Source Book. Washington DC, American Psychological Association, Inc, 1979.

28. Bergin AE, Lambert MJ: The evaluation of therapeutic outcomes, in Garfield SL, Bergin AE (eds): Handbook of Psychotherapy and Behavioral Change: An Empirical Analysis. New York, Wiley, 1978.
29. Frank JD: Persuasion and Healing: A Comparative Study of Psychotherapy, rev ed. Baltimore, The Johns Hopkins University Press, 1973.
30. Parloff MS, Wolfe B, Hadley S, Waskow E: Assessment of Psychosocial Treatment of Mental Disorders: Current Status and Prospects. Rockville Md, Clinical Research Branch, NIMH, February 1978.
31. Smith ML, Glass GV, Miller TI: The Benefits of Psychotherapy. Baltimore, The Johns Hopkins University Press, 1980.
32. Kisch J, Kroll J: Meaningfulness versus effectiveness: Paradoxical implications in the evaluation of psychotherapy. *Psychother: Theory Res Practice* 17-4: 401–413, 1980.
33. Brown BS, Long SE: Psychology and community mental health: The medical muddle. *Am Psychol* 23-5: 335–341, 1968.

Robert L. DuPont

The 1980s may prove to be the decade we rediscover the old adage "There is no such thing as a free lunch." The fact that, as a nation, our "benefits" and "entitlements" cost us as individuals seems clearer with each passing day. It is hardly surprising that the dominant issue in the field of mental health is money—since that appears to be the dominant issue in most fields. More remarkable to me is the fact that during the past two decades mental health professionals have taken for granted that our services should be covered by health insurance. This has been true even as our definitions of our roles have expanded almost without limit during these years, and even as the category of "providers" (a revealing description of the dominance of the financial transaction involved in our services) has exploded. Now we find, to our discomfort, that the one who pays the piper is being more visibly seen to call the tune. Many of us do not like it. The first reaction for many psychiatrists has been to pull the medical cloak more snugly around us: Let's save money by excluding the "nonmedical" providers. Next to go is "long-term intensive" psychiatric outpatient treatment. Will this process end with coverage for mental illness restricted to the physician prescribing psychotropic medications on "brief office visits" coupled with hospital-based inpatient care? Those, after all, are the final defensive positions.

My own perspective on these issues is shaped by over 10 years of work in the drug-abuse field. Drug abusers are shunned not only by society at large but by most mental health professionals, so I view the professional paranoia of many of my mental health colleagues with some ambivalence. It is fine, and fully justified, to rail against discrimination—I have done more than my share of that over the years in advocating the needs of the nation's millions of drug-dependent people. Satisfying as this complaining is, I believe there is a more effective strategy: Take advantage of the discrimination to build your strength. The difference between successful coping and dysfunctional stress reaction, after all, has less to do with the nature of the stressor than it has to

Robert L. DuPont • Clinical Professor of Psychiatry, Georgetown University Medical School, Rockville, Maryland 20852.

do with the *meaning* of the stress and the *techniques* used to cope with it.

In the drug-abuse field we have had more than our share of internecine battles—drug-free versus methadone, outpatient versus inpatient, public versus private, middle class versus the poor. We have also developed a clearer understanding of the goals of treatment, which are relatively simply communicated and measured (reduced drug use being primary, with secondary goals of increased work productivity and decreased criminality). We have also spent much energy calculating the costs and benefits of treatments as measured by treatment follow-ups. I do not want to overstate the successes of these efforts. They are still being developed and we have more questions than answers. Despite the success the drug-abuse field has had, we are still the first "coverage" the cost-conscious health insurers cut. But we have come a long way in a decade toward legitimacy, and the prospects for data-based arguments for effectiveness at reasonable costs have brightened.

Will such arguments make a difference when the primary decisions about what services will be covered by health insurance, as Dr. Upton clearly shows, are being made on nonrational grounds? I do not know. I do believe the chances are better that they will make a positive difference. I also believe the mental health field will be better for the effort to justify its expenditures. My own not-so-secret hope is that this nondefensive, hard-nosed approach will not only have an effect on the health planners and politicians but that it will lead to a more thorough review of all medical expenditures. Why should it be that only the psychiatrist should be accountable for the cost-effectiveness of his interventions? When was the last time you heard about cardiologists or orthopedists being asked to justify their charges on the basis of "results?" I am convinced that once the same questions are asked across the "health" spectrum, the mental health field will stand out strong and tall. For that dream to come true, however, we will have to complain a bit less and work a bit harder to show just what we do well (and perhaps, not so well).

Meanwhile, we can stick to the strong position that mental health and drug abuse and alcoholism coverage should be as generous (or as limited) as the coverage of any other "illness" and that the same limits on who is an acceptable "provider" should be applied in the mental health area as in other areas. (After all, it is not only psychiatrists who are finding the competition growing from medical practitioners—consider the "wellness" movement and the emergence of nonmedical healing for all illnesses from cancer to multiple sclerosis.) In all this struggle, we can be sure that the same forces that have led to health insurance being a national entitlement—and by this I mean the "public" demand for services—will continue to operate powerfully (although ambivalently) to support the growth of the mental health field.

Henry A. Foley

This commentary will briefly describe several of Dr. Upton's central themes and the evolution of mental health coverage and problems associated with that evolution as supportive evidence to Dr. Upton's central theme, it will critique several provocative notions in Dr. Upton's book, and it will provide a conclusion about what may be ideal and what is realistic about expanded coverage for psychotherapy.

In 1978 the President's Commission on Mental Health called special attention to the psychiatric needs of children and youth, the elderly, minorities, the chronically mentally ill, and other underserved populations.[1] In 1980 the Select Panel for the Promotion of Child Health endorsed the notion that mental health services be fully available and adequately valued as major components of health services directed at child health promotion. The panel recommended to the Congress and the Department of Health and Human Services that hospital-based and ambulatory mental health services, long-term psychiatric care, counseling, and crisis intervention be made available to children and adolescents.[2] Despite the evidence for the need for psychiatric services, the efficacy of some mental health services has been question in the media and among professional groups. A specific mental health service, psychotherapy, has been reviewed by the Office of Technology Assessment of the United States Congress (OTA). OTA has reviewed the studies on the efficacy of psychotherapy and has accepted the notion that psychotherapy for certain illnesses seems efficacious and should be promoted and further studied.[3] So, the timeliness of Dr. Upton's defense of the coverage of psychotherapy in outpatient settings is clear. Its cogency may not be.

Henry A. Foley • Institute for Health Policy Studies, University of California, San Francisco, San Francisco, California 94143.

Upton's Themes

Dr. Upton calls for full and complete coverage for mental health care under National Health Insurance (NHI)—controlled and limited by careful, professional monitoring rather than by public law. He attempts to show that broad coverage is affordable to society and that comprehensive mental health care will actually reduce the overall cost of medical care. He challenges the current limits for mental health care coverage that are based on the cost of service rather than the need for service. He stakes out the position that there should be coverage for persons with clinically recognized needs. Specifically, Upton argues that psychotherapy should be available to patients to address their clinical needs and not to enhance the general quality of their lives. Thus, he alerts his audience (primarily planners and lawmakers) that treatment is linked to diagnosis of illness and not to the education of a client. He rejects the notion that the concern about the cost of medical care should be the major stumbling block for National Health Insurance coverage. However, his definition of clinically recognized needs is too loose and may be too broad for insurers. Upton's major contribution is to challenge the current framework for considering mental health coverage. As a clinician, he appropriately takes the position that care should be based on need and not on cost considerations only. He believes that the current debate about National Health Insurance and current proposals before Congress will lead to excessive restrictions on the level of expenditures for mental health care.

Upton's argument raises these basic questions: Should psychotherapy be covered under insurance? Can a case be made that psychiatrists and other mental health care providers may in fact provide psychotherapy for clinical needs and not psychoanalysis directed primarily to improve the quality of life for the client? These questions are best viewed against the evolution of mental health care coverage.

The Evolution of Mental Health Coverage

Over the past 25 years, health insurance companies have expanded the coverage for the care of the mentally ill. For example, contracts negotiated by the United Auto Workers and the AFL-CIO include mental health care coverage. Further, 100% of the Blue Cross plans in this country cover in-hospital treatment of mental illness. In general, the major medical policies of the commercial insurers provide coverage, unless there is a specific written exclusion for psychiatric treatment, either on an inpatient or on an outpatient basis.

Notably, the federal government through the National Institute of Mental Health has pushed for and obtained mental health coverage in several of its programs, primarily the Federal Employees Health Benefit Plan (FEHBP) and the Civilian Health Medical Program of the Uniformed Services (CHAM-

PUS). In contrast, government has provided minimal mental health coverage in the Medicare program.

The impact of expanded coverages has been to make psychiatric medicine available to private practice outside the walls of state and county institutions. At the same time, insurance coverage of mental health services exposes psychiatrists and other mental health service providers to the increased level of fiscal oversight now experienced by other medical specialists. Although relatively late to the reimbursement table, psychiatry must abide by the rules of the innkeeper. The innkeeper is the insurance industry. It does not single out psychiatrists for special treatment, but it expects them to accommodate to peer review and to accept payment for treating medical disorders and, perhaps, for defined emotional problems.

In any case, both private insurers and the federal government have had some negative experiences with mental health coverage. Specifically, on the private level, insurers found that coverage for psychoanalysis for improving the quality of life or promoting patient self-actualization was too expensive. On the federal level, officials in the Washington community saw many of their staff and colleagues utilizing psychoanalysis to improve the quality of their lives and not necessarily for clinical needs.

This inappropriate utilization of a health insurance benefit detracted from the positive experience with overall utilization, specifically in the FEHBP Blues plan. Since the early 1970s, the percentage of the total health dollar paid for psychiatric treatment by the Blues plan has remained stable at the range of 7 to 7.7% of all benefits. This relative stability challenges the notion that mental health problems are less predictable and riskier to insure than are physical health problems. About 1.1% of the total covered population utilized their mental health benefit in any year.[4] In the FEHBP, it has been found that new enrollees use far fewer inpatient services but more outpatient services than the total enrollment. This finding is favorable to Dr. Upton's position.

In addition, the Congress found that during the first half of the 1970s the CHAMPUS program lacked sufficient oversight in the review of the utilization of mental health services. Members of Congress questioned particularly the modalities provided in long-term residential care settings for children and adolescents. Mechanisms for clearer determinations of appropriate treatment, cost containment, and quality assurance were needed.

For corrective purposes, the Defense Department secured the assistance of the National Institute of Mental Health. The latter developed an independent, authoritative quality-control system for CHAMPUS-financed residential treatment services. On a case-by-case basis, an interdisciplinary team of mental health experts reviewed the troubled child beneficiaries under psychiatric residential treatment. The number of children in treatment under CHAMPUS dropped from 3000 to about 200 in 3 years. Through the establishment of this peer review mechanism, children were assured of appropriate treatment, and the taxpayer was protected against the expensive abuse of the CHAMPUS benefit by charlatans. This experience illustrates that liberal coverage of mental and nervous disorders need not result in overutilization, waste, or fraud if there is an effective peer review mechanism.

The Current Debate

The aggressive responses to correct abuses in FEHBP and CHAMPUS should be underscored because some planners and lawmakers are not convinced that such abuses will not occur with broader mental health coverage. Many of these officials have been drawn into the debate on what should be the extent of coverage for mental health services under a national health insurance program. Some of these officials face even more immediate decisions on the extent of coverage in existing insurance programs. It is instructive that the Senate Defense Appropriations Subcommittee has indicated that it will limit coverage in 1982 if the current peer review program fails. Public officials, elected or appointed, can support health programs if their activities are efficacious and benefit the taxpayer, and if they are efficiently run and if waste for unnecessary services is eliminated. If officials fail to insure that programs meet these criteria, these same officials run the risk of losing office. Within this political context, they assume that psychiatric treatment is directed toward clinical needs.

Throughout the last 20 years, coverage for in-hospital treatment for mental illness has expanded. Upton points out that it is precisely in this area that the reimbursement system is skewed. Under many health insurance programs, coverage for outpatient mental health care is minimal, and it is often absent in others. This result makes it difficult for psychiatrists to expand their practice to provide mental health care for outpatients.

Reinforcing the pattern of care in inpatient settings is the fact that the VA system is, in effect, a hospital-based psychiatric system and has minimal coverage for its beneficiaries in outpatient settings. Some argue that coverage is so minimal that it is ineffective.

However, while psychiatrists face extreme difficulty in obtaining payment for outpatient services, they are not alone in dealing with a reimbursement system that is primarily hospital-based. Internists, family practitioners, and pediatricians all experience the same reimbursement effects. By its reimbursement mechanisms, it is possible that the American health care system is so locked into inpatient care that future expansion of coverage for outpatient care will be marginal.

The difficulty with current National Health Insurance proposals is not, as Upton suggests, that they will probably decrease total expenditures for mental health care. Rather, because the proposals are based on hospitalization they will tend to increase the cost of health care. As we have seen recently, hospitals are likely to expand the psychiatric sections of their hospitals as they experience a decrease in the need for obstetrical and gynecological beds. The failure of current proposals, especially those oriented toward catastrophic illnesses, is that they do not sufficiently expand outpatient coverage, and so reduce the need for extensive hospitalization and thereby shift the locus of care away from expensive hospitalization. One hopes that the data on the experience of various plans provided in Upton's paper will be used to persuade health planners and lawmakers to reconsider current proposals.

It is important to recall that in the early 1970s advocates of mental health care coverage—within and without government—faced the difficult task of getting their foot in the medical door for some minimal level of coverage. They successfully demonstrated the need for mental health care services. Unfortunately, in attempting to propose a reasonable benefit package to a Republican administration and a Democratic Congress, they used, as a basis for the package, utilization of the early 1970s drawn from private insurance plans, prepaid groups, or the experience of the Community Mental Health Centers program. The upper levels of average utilization became limits in various National Health Insurance proposals. Even though the planners may not have intended this result, the "average" that made sense for most of the population covered in these plans became "limits." That an average patient might utilize 20 visits a year, or 10 or even 5, was not an adequate reason to create limits that would exclude the patient who is not within the average but may need more than 5 or 10 or 20 visits.

Planners also faced the perception that the peer mechanism for utilization review was not adequate to avoid potential abuse. However, progress has occurred in the past 6 years. Peer review of psychiatric treatment has been expanding, and it insures that treatment is therapeutically necessary. Recent experiences of the Aetna project for federal civil service employees and of the CHAMPUS project for dependents of members of the armed services appear to prove that peer review is an effective way to manage costs. Both the American Psychiatric Association and the American Psychological Association established, and now supervise and guide, these retrospective peer review systems. Major insurance companies are negotiating with both associations to expand their own peer review activities.

The review system as stated tends to support advocates like Dr. Upton who desire the clinical evaluation and clinical treatment of the mentally ill, universal coverage, and clients free to choose from services provided either in private practice for a fee or in organized settings in the public and private sectors.

In defense of his position that there be coverage of psychotherapy for clinical needs in outpatient settings, Dr. Upton also draws upon various studies of health programs that describe a concomitant reduction in utilization of other medical care services when mental health care services are instituted. Dr. Upton overstates the case about savings, however. The possible cost saving of psychiatric care on general health care utilization is inconclusive, but most studies clearly show that despite some offsets, psychiatric coverage costs more than no coverage under existing plans. Through offsets, psychiatric costs may be reduced somewhat, but not total health costs incurred by a health program. More appropriate care ensues, however, such as when unrecognized health problems are treated in a timely way.

Coverage in the United States for mental health care services has expanded in the private sector as well as in the public sector. The efficacy of psychotherapy for some clinical needs is becoming accepted. Descriptions of the basic packages for mental health care for the total United States are now discussed in the United States Congress.

Distractions to Upton's Case

The case for coverage for psychotherapy is not well served by several of Upton's approaches. His approaches may be provocative, but they may detract from his theme and, in a few instances, politically polarize parties to the debate. While he points out that mental health coverage under Medicare is minimal, he does not state the fact that Medicare has not changed because seniors do not request mental health coverage and because psychiatrists, by and large, don't treat older persons. As always, most psychotherapy is used by college-educated, upper-middle-class white persons. As a consequence, there is little incentive or organizational movement to change the reimbursement system. It is not sufficient to have advocates within the federal government, be they within the National Institute of Mental Health or the Health Care Financing Administration, pressing for expanded coverage for Medicare if no outside negotiating pressure is sufficient to induce the Congress to change the Medicare system—a system that is primarily hospital-based, even for physical medicine.

Upton attempts to argue that the helmsman of the mental health team should be the psychiatrist, due to his training as a physician and his unique knowledge concerning medication and the psychological processes of humans. However, he recognizes that a critical characteristic needed for effective treatment appears to be a high quality of personal interaction between therapist and patient. Upton does not deny that such a high quality of interaction can be found in relationships between patients and health and mental health providers other than the psychiatrist. The helmsman of the mental health team might preferably be one who has the ability to coordinate the other members of the team—physicians, psychiatrists, psychiatric social workers, psychiatric nurses, and clinical psychologists—and to effectively involve "significant others" in the individual's life—the spouse, family members, clergy, and self-help and self-care groups, which lie outside the net of formal caregivers. Upton's assumption that knowledge gained from the biomedical model is determinative for leadership has been challenged in the last few years by thoughtful critics within and without medicine. In fact, some of the past training of physicians has led to their ignoring nutritional needs, ignoring psychological realities facing their patients, and ignoring the whole person interacting with his environment. The helmsman could be any person knowledgeable about the expertise of each member of the team and knowledgeable about when that expertise should be appropriately utilized. The notion of the psychiatrist as helmsman, or for that matter, the physician as helmsman, is too prescriptive and would probably further exacerbate pecking-order problems in the health field. Such a notion is not essential to make the case that psychiatrists should be reimbursed for psychotherapy. In fact, it is counterproductive.

The number of psychiatrists is decreasing. The decrease might be attributed to the fact that the reimbursement system is not sufficiently remunerative for those who charge for units of time rather than for units of procedure. Until the reimbursement system is changed to eradicate these disincentives, it is unlikely that we will see the number of psychiatrists increasing, and yet, persons become ill, some remain ill, and some need psychiatric services. Payment to other qualified mental health providers who are willing to accept the current payment system may be a realistic necessity and desirable. Nonphysician providers who offer a range of mental health services have been competitive to psychiatrists. Such competition may have deflated increases of prices and the incomes of psychiatrists in the 1970s.[5]

Again, in relation to the helmsman concept, Upton argues that the psychiatrist is in the best position to treat the patient who experiences psychological pain from being in the hospital. He does not, however, entertain the notion that the patient might be better treated outside the hospital and that his stay in the hospital could be shorter than it is now. Both approaches may obviate psychological difficulties experienced by treatment in a hospital or occasioned by the hospital environment itself.

Upton questions the effectiveness of public programs, such as the Community Mental Health Centers program, and he argues that the client should be free to choose practitioners in the private sector as well as in the public sector. The option is acceptable if there is appropriate control of utilization in the private sector and the costs equate with those experienced in organized settings, especially prepaid groups. The critique that community mental health centers and perhaps some of the prepaid groups have not reached older persons or the chronically mentally ill is also true of those who practice in the private sector. It is not clear that inadequate payment for services is the major deterrent to the provision of care for these populations. It may very well be that mental health providers—physicians and nonphysicians—find these types of patients extremely difficult to treat and consequently less rewarding than other types of patients afflicted with mental illness.

It is also not clear what Upton means by early intervention. If he means consideration of a clinical condition that has not yet become severe, early intervention would certainly be encouraged. If he means intervention modeled after annual physical examinations, it should be pointed out that with the exception of childhood checkups, there is no evidence of efficacy in this area sufficient to encourage such intervention. In fact, intervention might be intrusion and overdoctoring, leading to further dependency on the part of the population on its health care system and to avoidable expenditures.[6]

Upton would have a stronger case if he did not argue that coverage for mental health care provided under National Health Insurance would reduce the cost of health insurance in general. Canada experienced an expansion of the utilization of health care services when private psychiatrists, under their Medicare plan, began to treat lower-class patients who previously had not been treated. The demand for services simply exceeded the supply of psychiatrists. Criteria will have to be very clear to patients, that psychiatrists and other mental health providers would treat clients selectively depending on work load, facilities, and cost.

Desirability versus Reality

Dr. Upton has presented his thesis for coverage under National Health Insurance at a time when there is no National Health Insurance program and little likelihood of one soon. There is now evidence that utilization of psychotherapy need not be exorbitant, that it results in more appropriate health care, and that it is more and more boundaried by peer review mechanisms. Coverage is available in many plans and will become more available if consumers demand it. Some states have legislated that mental health services must be covered, at least as an optional benefit, in all health insurance sold in their states. Paradoxically, some states are considering cutting back mental health coverage to the poor through Medicaid. Such action suggests that mental health coverage for psychotherapy is not considered a basic insurance benefit for all. The value of psychotherapy resulting in more appropriate health care and in less need to hospitalize in either the private or the public sector has been underestimated. Thus, the case can be made for making psychotherapy, as well as other mental health services, available to all in clinical need.

Dr. Upton makes a contribution with his description of the practice of psychotherapy and its relation to the ill and with his list of several successful insurance experiences. He underestimates the potential higher hospital bill for psychiatric treatment contained in current NHI proposals. He detracts from his main point by the introduction of his notion of the psychiatrist as helmsman and thus risks alienating the support of other mental health providers. Indeed, everyone's support is now needed to assure and expand the level of coverage. Psychotherapy is only recently being marketed, and the stigma of mental illness has not left the American scene and continues to block remedial marketing efforts.[7]

Ideally, psychotherapy responsibly provided, effective and satisfying to the consumer, will help those who market such a service benefit before and after the implementation of National Health Insurance. Realistically, more than peer review is necessary to allay the fears about the potential costs of psychotherapy and its effectiveness, as well as about other medical procedures and therapies practiced in the health sector.

References

1. The President's Commission on Mental Health: Report to the President. Washington, DC, US Government Printing Office, 1978.
2. The Select Panel for the Promotion of Child Health: Better Health for Our Children: A National Strategy. Washington, DC, US Government Printing Office, DHHS (PHS) Publication No. 79–55071, 1980.
3. U.S. Congress, Office of Technology Assessment: Background Paper No. 3: The efficacy and cost-effectiveness analysis of medical technology. Washington, DC, US Government Printing Office, 1980.
4. Hustead EC, Sharfstein SS: Utilization and cost of mental illness coverage in the federal employees health benefits program, 1973. *Am J Psychiatry* 135:3, 1978.
5. Sharfstein SS, Clark HW: Why psychiatry is a low-paid medical specialty. *Am J Psychiatry* 137:7, 1980.
6. Illich I: Toward a History of Needs. New York, Pantheon Books, 1978.
7. Sharfstein SS: Third-party payors: To pay or not to pay. *Am J Psychiatry* 135:10, 1978.

Robert W. Gibson

In 1965 the Medicare Legislation (Title 18 of the Social Security Amendments of 1965) opened with the reassuring sentence: "Nothing in this Title shall be construed to authorize any federal officer or employee to exercise any supervision or control over the practice of medicine or the manner in which medical services are provided. . . ." Some 15 years later, not only do we recognize that Medicare and Medicaid have been used to exert enormous control over the practice of medicine and the delivery of services, but all National Health Insurance (NHI) is contingent on extensive regulatory legislative control of the health care system. Indeed, third-party payers, private as well as governmental, no longer apologize about control, especially cost containment, but now consider it an obligation to influence the manner in which services are provided.

It is futile to debate whether the delivery of mental health care will be influenced or even controlled by forces external to psychiatry; it is already happening. The significant questions to be addressed at this juncture are: Who will exercise the control? What techniques will be used to influence mental health care? How will policy decisions be made as to how health care resources are distributed? And a host of related questions related to planning, coordination, cost containment, manpower, licensure, and so forth.

For example, HR 1 of 1973, one of the early NHI bills, began "recognizing that health care is an inherent right of each individual and of all of the people of the United States . . . the Congress finds and declares that health services must be so organized and financed as to make them readily available to all . . . and that it is a function of government to insure that these ends are attained."

Why is there so much emphasis on the control of health care?

In 1965, the last year before Medicare began to have some effect, the total expenditures for health care were approximately $40 billion, accounting for

Robert W. Gibson • President and Chief Executive Officer, Sheppard and Enoch Pratt Hospital, Baltimore, Maryland 21204.

5.9% of the Gross National Product. Now, some 15 years later, the total costs for health care have multiplied by about sixfold, exceeding $200 billion annually and accounting for more than 8% of the GNP. In other words, not only have health care costs escalated, but they have done so at a greater rate of inflation than that experienced in the overall economy. The price tag has become so great that expenditures for health care must compete with other high-priority concerns, such as energy, national defense, pollution, and a host of other vexing problems.

The runaway costs for health care have been so disturbing that earlier assertions that health care is a right have quietly been retracted. For example, in the statement of purpose for the National Health Planning Act of 1974 (PL 93-641) it is stated, "The achievement of equal access to health care at a reasonable cost is a priority of the federal government." Equal access is no longer a right but only a priority. And an extremely important condition has been introduced—"reasonable cost." There can be no objective measure for reasonable cost; at best, it will be a judgment. Reasonable cost will not be a medical judgment. It will be made through the political decision-making process.

Faced by this prospect of increased regulation of the health care system, it is only prudent to study past experiences. In the field of general medical and surgical services, more than 90% of payments have come from third-party payers for many years. Many insurance programs do not cover mental illness, and those that do often have higher deductibles, higher coinsurance, and lesser limits for mental health services. Nevertheless, a substantial part of the cost of in-hospital psychiatric care has for many years been provided by third-party payers. As a consequence, we already have considerable information on the potential influence national health insurance could have on in-hospital psychiatric care.

Medicare is a prominent example of governmental third-party control of medical practice. Despite the sentence disclaiming such intent, much of Medicare's control of in-hospital treatment was purposeful. Other aspects of the control were probably accidental but nevertheless quite significant. Originally, in the King–Anderson Bill of 1965, the plan was to exclude under Medicare all care in psychiatric hospitals. Interestingly, provision was made to cover psychiatric care in general hospitals. Legislators, and their advisors, who had worked on the Medicare legislation, had been told that it was desirable to shift the locus of psychiatric care to general hospitals. Therefore, they wrote legislation that would encourage such a shift. Much could be said on either side of this controversy, but that would take us away from the central issue. The important point is that these early opinions were based on limited information and acted upon with virtually no professional input.

Many individuals and many associations put forward arguments that treatment in psychiatric hospitals should be included. Eventually, these pleas prevailed at least in part. Coverage for treatment in psychiatric hospitals was provided but with a 190-day lifetime limit on coverage; extremely low limits were placed on outpatient psychiatric care. Strangely, no mechanism was provided for coverage in community mental health centers even though the community mental health movement was a strong initiative of the federal government. In effect, legislators covered psychiatric treatment but kept their fingers crossed.

Medicare and Medicaid, which started out as relatively limited programs, have steadily expanded in scope. Those individuals receiving benefits under Social Security for total and permanent disability are now covered by Medicare even though they are under the age of 65. Benefits have been expanded for those suffering from renal disease. Medicaid expenditures have steadily increased at a staggering rate since enactment of the original legislation. The states have had a continuing problem meeting their portion of the Medicaid expenditures. This has led to proposals that the federal government should assume a greater portion of the financial burden for the medically indigent. There has been growing support for federal coverage for catastrophic illness. As government assumes a greater responsibility for financing health care, the political process becomes increasingly influential. Decisions about health services are influenced by the state of the economy, inflation, presidential and congressional elections.

It seems unlikely that National Health Insurance providing comprehensive coverage for all individuals as it was originally conceptualized will be enacted in the forseeable future. But extensions of Medicare and Medicaid linked to mandated employer-financed private insurance will probably continue.

By whatever name, this kind of national health insurance will be used not only to finance health care but, of even greater importance, it will be used to manage the health care system. The traditional techniques of management—planning, organizing, coordinating, staffing, implementing, motivating, and controlling—will in some form be incorporated into the administration of such a national health insurance. In fact, the groundwork has already been laid for such controls.

For example, appropriations to assist health maintenance organizations have been used to promote prepaid organized systems of health care in contrast to individual private practice. The Professional Standards Review Legislation is designed to involve physicians in utilization review activities, which, it is hoped, will reduce length of hospital stay. The Health Planning Act establishes a complex network of citizens groups at the local, state, and national level that are, through State Health Plans, expected to plan, coordinate, and control health care resources. The Health Professions Educational Assistant Act of 1976 is aimed at manpower—the most important of all health resources.

Despite this interest in managing the so-called nonsystem of health care, there is little support for a national health service in which the government would own facilities, hire staff, select the locations for providing services, and pay the costs through taxation. The approach is rather to rely on a "voluntary" participation in which economic incentives and disincentives can be used to shape and run the system. The reluctance to go the route of a National Health Service stems from many sources, but there appears to be a growing skepticism and distrust for governmental intervention not only in health care but in many other human services.

The expenditures for health care have already become so great that management is a vast undertaking. In this situation, the economic considerations are likely to prevail. There is a real danger that the decision-makers will be too far removed from the health caregivers by a series of administrative layers. We have already experienced examples of this phenomenon. In addition to potential dehumanization of health care services, it is recognized that regulation adds to the cost.

The demands frequently take the form of bureaucratic intrusion seemingly to the point of harassment. For example, in 1976 a task force on regulation created by the Hospital Association of New York State to assemble information on the scope of the problem found that no fewer than 164 different regulatory agencies had some jurisdiction over hospitals in the state. Acknowledging that government has the right to regulate hospitals, the task force, in its study of the impact of regulation, wondered why 25 separate agencies must review hospital admitting procedures, why 33 agencies protect patients' rights, and why 31 agencies insure patients' safety. The task force found that during the past 10 years, while the total number of employees in the state health department went from 2000 to 3500, the number of accountants went from 2 to 170, and the number of attorneys went from 3 to 30. But the number of physicians declined from 69 to 60. The state's new austerity budget calls for 568 new regulatory positions in the department!

Most of the regulatory efforts are well intentioned. But unfortunately, the controls overlap, are sometimes contradictory, and add to the cost of care. Preoccupation with these multiple requirements may distract mental health professionals from their main goal: providing high-quality treatment services appropriate to the patient's need. In exasperation, staff protest that it has become more important to document that some arbitrary requirement has been met than it is to do something that will be really helpful to the patient.

Despite the heavy emphasis on reducing length of stay, an October 1976 report commissioned by the Department of Health, Education and Welfare estimated that utilization controls would reduce the cost of additional services under the American Medical Association's national health insurance proposal by $0.3 billion (less than 0.2%) and under the Health Security Bill by $1.4 billion (only 0.7%). Regulation adds to costs through special reports, legal services, requirements for documentation, and the like. Beyond that comes the time of clinicians diverted from patient care, as they are kept busy meeting the requirements. It would not surprise me if these activities added 5 to 10% to the national health care budget. Surely our profession can develop a better system.

In the relatively early days of Medicare around 1971, the Social Security Administration was taken to task because of escalating costs of the Medicare program. Actually, there was little that the administrators of the program could do to control costs, since the program was not designed for that purpose but was rather primarily a means of paying the bills for medical care. In any event when the administration and Congress came down, there was a sharp increase in the denial of claims; there seemed to be a policy of "when in doubt, deny." Eventually, a reasonable equilibrium was again achieved, but in the meantime, many patients had suffered. And the point is that the system was not responding to medical needs or issues of therapeutic adequacy but was being influenced by the economic and political pressures.

A similar experience occurred with the federal employees' health benefit programs (all of which are administered by private carriers). In 1972, when a $60 million deficit was projected for this billion-dollar-a-year program, there was a distinct increase in the denials of claims for psychiatric hospital treatment. To be sure, patients had the option of appealing these denials. As a practical matter, they were in a virtually untenable position. Often, the denial was applied retroactively to prior claims. If a patient elected to continue in treatment while the appeal was in process, he would be adding substantially to a bill that he could not afford to pay out of pocket. Ultimately, many of the denials were reversed when contested, but only a small percentage were contested, and for many patients this meant a premature disruption of treatment.

Obviously, both sides of the issue must be considered. Treatment programs should be clinically sound yet at the same time must be fiscally viable. Administrators may be unfamiliar with clinical matters, but some clinicians refuse to recognize the economic necessities. Errors in judgment by clinicians are likely to err in the direction of supporting high-quality services at the expense of fiscal needs. Errors by nonclinical administrators are likely to err in the direction of placing financial solvency above sound clinical care and humanistic values. There needs to be method for ongoing interplay between these two competing demands.

Thus far, the negatives have been stressed. National Health Insurance can be used to improve mental health services. For example, the Medicare legislation contained a requirement that all psychiatric hospitals must be accredited by the Joint Commission of Accreditation of Hospitals. When Medicare was enacted, less than half the psychiatric hospitals in this country had such accreditation. The carrot of Medicare payment caused a sharp increase in psychiatric hospitals seeking accreditation, and within a few years, almost all had achieved it. In more recent years, the accreditation process has come under some criticism, but this should not detract from the potential for National Health Insurance to improve standards and quality of care.

To date, the most effective method for improving treatment through the setting of standards is to require adequate levels of resources—facilities, staff, dollars. These structural elements for care can require that, at a minimum, facilities must be safe and provide adequate space for living, activities, recreation, and privacy. In addition, standards can be set to assure that there will be personnel in adequate numbers and with adequate training and credentials to provide the services necessary for good patient care. Beyond this, it is reasonable to require hospitals to develop appropriate procedures and policies, to maintain adequate records, to protect confidentiality, and to establish linkages to other community services.

Standards aimed at controlling the process of psychiatric treatment have been tried but with mixed results. Legislation establishing PSROs (Professional Standards Review Organization) was developed to monitor the care of patients paid for by Medicare and Medicaid, but in many instances this has been expanded to include hospitalized patients in general.

The utilization of PSROs to review medical care was a reflection of the increased demand for accountability. Stated in simple terms, the reasoning went: Adequate health care is considered to be a right; this places the responsibility on our society to provide such services; public funds must be used to pay for the services; therefore, the public has not only a right but an obligation to receive an accounting for what is done. PSROs have not been particularly active in psychiatric hospitals, but they have been utilized to a considerable degree in the psychiatric units of general hospitals.

There are many problems associated with the review of psychiatric treatment because of difficulties in evaluating, quantifying, and documenting the efficacy of psychiatric care. PSRO legislation requires that data on treatment be developed through profiles for usual length of stay and appropriateness of treatment. In psychiatry, such information has not been collected systematically. There is considerable question as to just how meaningful such criteria can be. Techniques such as medical audits have had uncertain results. Differing philosophies of treatment, motivation of the patient, and variation in the goals of the treatment may alter the type of treatment to be offered and the length of time that will be required. Heavy emphasis on cost-effectiveness can interfere with the essentially humanistic approach so necessary to psychiatric treatment. It is much easier to count the number of days of hospitalization than it is to assess the subjective relief and improvement in adaptive potential that result from the days in the hospital. No wonder psychiatrists resist the imposition of standards for the practice of their profession.

Even without standards, the practice of psychiatry has been scrutinized by public and private health insurers through the process of claims review. Reduced to its simplest form, the claims review process goes like this: A patient seeks help; a psychiatrist provides treatment; a claim for service is submitted to the third-party payer; either the claim is paid or it is denied. If the claim is paid, the psychiatrist will continue to provide the services in accordance with his best judgment as to the patient's therapeutic needs. If the claim is denied, there are serious consequences both specific and widespread.

When the claim for a particular patient is denied, it is not only disturbing to the physician but it creates a serious problem for the patient. Troublesome as short-term impact on the particular patient may be, the long-term consequences can be even more serious. In a given case, a professional is likely to continue the treatment that is deemed medically necessary despite the difficulty about the payment, or at least make other arrangements. In the long run, however, if claims for a particular type of treatment are consistently denied, it will begin to influence the manner in which those services that are most readily reimbursed are encouraged, while those for which denials consistently occur are discouraged. It is a variant of the behavior modification technique except that it is not simply a matter of tokens at stake; it is the mental health and sometimes the life of the patient.

As a matter of principle, those paying for care are accountable for the payments they make. The payer is responsible for appropriate expenditure of tax dollars in the case of government programs, proper use of insurance premiums in the case of the private insurance companies, and prudent utilization of employee benefits in the case of an employer or a union official. Using this funding mechanism to better organize and improve the health care delivery system is not unreasonable if properly applied. The key is that standards and criteria that are used must reflect the professional opinion of practicing psychiatrists.

Claims review is understandably disturbing to psychiatrists. Professionals who have had many years of training, particularly physicians, expect acceptance of their professional judgments. Indeed, they have become so accustomed to it that they sometimes think of it as a right rather than a privilege. Realistically, professionals can no longer expect to have a total control over their professional activities. External regulation has become so much a part of the current scene that psychiatrists must rely on their national organizations working with government, third-party payers, patient advocates, and other mental health professions.

The American Psychiatric Association has long advocated peer review. In recent years, there has been an effort to blend the concept of peer review with claims review. An outstanding example of that approach has been the APA CHAMPUS (Civilian Health and Medical Program of the Uniformed Services) Review Program. In this program, standards of practice were developed by a national adivsory council of psychiatrists. These standards were designed to meet CHAMPUS regulations as well as accepted psychiatric practice. Procedures were developed so that claims could be referred for review to psychiatrists who had been selected by APA district branches. Psychiatrists reviewing claims utilized broad guidelines established by the national advisory committee but relied upon their own personal judgments based on clinical experience and training. Although not bound by these decisions, the CHAMPUS fiscal intermediaries have come to rely heavily on the recommendations of the professional reviewers.

The CHAMPUS program has caught the attention of private insurers. Several large insurance companies have expressed interest in contracting with the APA to utilize a comparable system for the review of claims by their subscribers. In this process, there is an interest in control of expenditures, but in addition, emphasis has been placed on maintaining treatment procedures and practices that are accepted by professional leaders.

It can be assumed that any program of national health insurance will have to utilize some form of claims review to control costs and to maintain quality care. If such claims review is conducted exclusively by the third-party payers, there will be many disadvantages: (1) Financial pressures may unduly impact on clinical care; (2) third-party payers are likely to utilize clinicians not in active practice; (3) insurers rather than practicing professional leaders will establish the standards and criteria; (4) review by the third-party payers will not be open to public scrutiny; and (5) third-party payers are likely to use their findings to modify contract agreements for financial advantage.

In short, the emphasis of claims review when done by the third-party payers is on cost control and not on improvement of the health care system.

If psychiatrists are a central part of the claims review system, as has been done under the APA CHAMPUS Program, the consequences will be quite different: (1) Clinical judgments will represent the current thinking of psychiatric practitioners; (2) there will be adequate numbers of practicing psychiatrists to conduct the clinical reviews; (3) professionals will establish and refine standards and criteria on an ongoing basis; (4) there will be an opportunity for widespread professional input into the standards and criteria; and (5) the findings of such reviews can be used to improve the level of psychiatric practice and even to control abuses that occur.

In establishing benefits, it would be most desirable if we could simply state that a patient will receive whatever treatment is necessary. It is unrealistic to expect such a blanket coverage. It would be quite difficult to get complete agreement from a group of professionals as to what is adequate and necessary in a given case. With such a degree of uncertainty, the third-party payer is at a loss to justify payments, particularly in a highly inflationary environment. Perhaps a greater problem is the uncertainty of the costs that would be involved in such a program. Presumably, National Health Insurance would involve substantial if not complete underwriting through taxation. Funds must be available to pay for the treatment, and these have to come through finite appropriations on a year-by-year basis. In CHAMPUS, there has in the past been an open-ended benefit package. In several instances, the program exhausted funds before year's end and had to seek emergency appropriations. At times, such appropriations were not forthcoming so that payment could not be made for the services rendered. Having a better defined package of benefits offers a greater opportunity for predicting costs.

There is a serious concern, however, in setting such limits in that they have a tendency to become fixed. For example, despite repeated efforts, the Medicare and Medicaid limits on psychiatric inpatient and outpatient treatment have not been significantly changed. Ideally, there should be ongoing review of benefits based on studies to determine what impact any changes might have on treatment. Recognizing hazards for setting limits, I will nevertheless make a proposal for a starting benefit package.

Even with limited benefits, National Health Insurance should have virtually no financial obstacles to treatment along the following lines: emergency and crisis intervention services with emphasis on preventing inappropriate hospitalization; outpatient services including diagnosis and treatment with a minimum of 20 outpatient units of service (the usual 50-minute interview might be 1 unit, a 20-minute interview ½ unit, and group therapy ⅓ unit); inpatient hospitalization up to 45 days, with each day of inpatient hospitalization counting as 1 day and each day of partial hospitalization counting as ½ day.

A second set of benefits should be available once it has been determined that further treatment is needed and that the condition could reasonably be expected to respond to treatment. Such determination should be made by qualified professionals. Under this second set of benefits, there should be no limit to the number of outpatient services, particularly if there is evidence that failure to receive such treatment might lead to hospitalization. Additional inpatient partial hospitalization benefits equal to the first set of benefits should be available.

Beyond these benefits, there should be available to individual patients a broader range of mental health services. Mental health education should be included to encourage the use of the benefits of the program. It is frequently found that through ignorance or fear, persons suffering from mental disorder do not seek treatment to which they're entitled. Actually, it may be necessary to encourage greater utilization to overcome this reluctance, particularly in the disadvantaged groups, which may have less understanding of the services. Some resources should be especially allocated for pilot programs that can be used for the high-risk groups and those that are currently underserved, such as the young, the aged, and the minority groups.

Insurance coverage, particularly for hospital and partial hospital care, must go further. National Health Insurance should not ignore the problems of the chronically ill and those in need of long-term care. There must be provision made not to shift patients from the acute treatment facilities to those that provide longer-term care. There has evolved a whole spectrum of services offering care at varying levels of intensity. As yet, these have not been sufficiently supported economically, and they need to be under National Health Insurance. And even beyond this, we need some provision for research and demonstration projects to assure that advances can be made in the treatment of the chronically ill.

To assure that National Health Insurance provides adequate coverage for mental illness, psychiatrists must participate actively in designing the program and in carrying it out. Unfortunately, most psychiatrists have not been trained in the kinds of administrative, management, and political skills that are now needed to influence the processes that are determining the future of mental health care. Training and experience in the professions and the selection process lead the professional to prize his autonomy and to resist encroachment at all costs. Psychiatry is not as much a part of the organized system of health care as are some other segments of medicine. Some physicians even have a gut feeling that, as professionals, they should stay out of the political process.

But the plain facts are these: Health care is a significant political issue and the responsibility of government. In fulfilling this responsibility, federal and state governments will become increasingly involved in the financing of health services and will expect the right to manage and control the system. The funding mechanism will be the main tool used to administer and reorganize the system. Policy decisions about health care will impact on the parameters within which psychiatrists can provide mental health services. Beyond this, we must assume that administrative decisions will have a direct impact on the doctor–patient relationship. As a profession, psychiatry has an obligation to seek a meaningful role in setting policy, in administration, and in the governance of the treatment of patients.

Milton Greenblatt

National Health Insurance is now a vital topic awaiting action at the highest level of government. In one sense, the concept of National Health Insurance gets its validity from the earliest promise of the Declaration of Independence, which noted that all men possess the inalienable rights of life, liberty, and the pursuit of happiness. Implicit within this promise, to many people, is the right to health, for without health, happiness is elusive, liberty is constrained, and life itself may be in peril.

The promise of the Declaration of Independence remained essentially silent for generations. However, in recent times there has been a gradual but definite shift in the people's attitude toward health. Health, formerly a privilege granted to those robustly endowed by nature, or to those capable of affording proper medical care, has gradually attained status as a right. Illness, formerly a misfortune visited upon the individual, too often with catastrophic consequences, has become a concern of the body politic and of industry, including in particular the insurance industry. Now state and federal governments spend billions to assure the health of the people, to support health service systems, to control pollution, and to provide hospitalization and treatment, especially for the mentally ill and retarded. The national contribution for research and development, for the exploration of innovative programs, and for training and manpower has indeed been enormous.

Since the 1930s the health insurance industry has grown by leaps and bounds, *pari passu* with a dramatic, almost revolutionary change in the care of the mentally ill. Formerly, the vast majority of the seriously mentally ill had been taken care of in state, county, and federal facilities, but since World War II, inspired particularly by the Kennedy administration, a great deinstitutionalization movement has taken place. A new public health orientation to

We are indebted to Evelyn Myers for help in developing this commentary and in particular for her excellent review of health insurance and psychiatric care.[1]

Milton Greenblatt • Neuropsychiatric Institute and Department of Psychiatry and Behavioral Sciences, University of California, Los Angeles, California 90024.

the delivery of psychiatric services has arisen. Most mental institutions have experienced a dramatic phase down in population, and a few have been phased out altogether. A more or less satisfactory phasing up of a broad spectrum of community alternatives has also occurred, together with a great mobilization of citizen interest, training of many paraprofessionals, and a greatly increased effort to render outreach community care to the under-served, the poor, and minority groups. At the same time, an enormous increase in private practice of psychiatry has taken place.

This great movement has demonstrated that most of the mentally ill do not have to languish in custodial hospitals but that they possess a potential for rehabilitation—if vigorously treated by psychopharmaceuticals, social therapy, community programs, or office psychotherapy—formerly not fully appreciated. Further, patients newly admitted to hospitals often do not have to be legally committed; the vast majority can be treated as volunteers, eventually returning to the community at varying levels of functional adequacy. It became possible to predict with some degree of accuracy the outcome of various kinds of mental illness under specified conditions of therapeutic intervention.

At the same time as psychiatry was going through this remarkable development, insurance coverage was changing rapidly, too. In 1940 only about 10% of the American public had protection against the costs of hospital care. By 1975 about 80% of the civilian population under age 65 had some coverage under private insurance. (Individuals over 65 had achieved coverage for hospital care through Medicare and Medicaid.) Even outpatient coverage increased substantially, with approximately 64% of the civilian population under 65 having some private insurance for office care. The skyrocketing costs of health care made the public eager to seek insurance, and the insurance companies, as well as the federal government [Medicare, Medicaid, CHAMPUS, (Civilian Health and Medical Program of the Uniformed Services)], responded.

In the 1970s a number of bills were introduced into the Congress aiming to extend health insurance to all citizens not otherwise taken care of. In particular there was concern for the damaging effects on the patient and his family of "catastrophic" illness. The major issues, as argued in committees, centered around overall costs, level of coinsurance, and duration of coverage, including number of outpatient visits allowable. Discussion also centered around whether National Health should proceed piecemeal on a progressive basis, or whether the nation should attempt to embrace the challenge of providing health coverage to all citizens at once. With regard to mental illness, much of the negotiation centered about establishing parity in coverage between mental illness and other medical disorders. David Upton's plea in this volume has been for universal coverage within fiscal realities.

Data from the National Center for Health Statistics for 1974 tell us that about 31% of Americans under 65 have no private coverage (some have government-financed insurance). What we need to know are the projections as to how many who have no coverage or are inadequately covered today, but need and want coverage, will in fact be covered in the future by the expanding insurance industry. Thus can responsible public officials plan for the scope and costs of a future National Health Insurance program.

The American Psychiatric Association's Role

From the beginning, the posture of the American Psychiatric Association (APA) has been one of strong support for National Health Insurance, with particular empahsis on equal coverage for mental illness. Under the guidance of Dr. Walter Barton, medical director, the APA let it be known to the public that mental illness was being treated far differently, and much more successfully, than 25 years ago. Many more people were being treated on an ambulatory basis, in offices and clinics, and those who needed hospitalization were often treated in general hospitals or private psychiatric hospitals. The obvious logic of the case was to make available to the patient with mental illness the same kind of health security that was available to the patient with appendicitis or diabetes.[2]

A landmark change in the history of insurance for mental illness stemmed from the negotiations of the APA, as represented by Dr. Daniel Blain, with United Auto Workers, which eventually led to a generous package of ambulatory care benefits for 4.2 million auto workers in 1966. This contract required no initial payment by the client.

Studies were then carried out to focus on pre- and postutilization patterns and costs, and to clarify important conceptual problems, such as the definition of mental illness, the accepted forms of treatment, and the feasibility of insurance coverage for the various treatment modalities.

The APA also worked actively to insure that psychiatric benefits were included in Medicare and Medicaid, and it was able to make a strong case for inclusion of substantial psychiatric benefits in any National Health Insurance plan. Evelyn S. Myers and Patricia L. Scheidemandel, staff members of the APA, worked with Louis S. Reed, a leading health economist, to establish a reliable data base for planning health insurance systems. Psychiatric support and consultation were supplied over the years by Walter Barton, Howard Rome, Perry Talkington, Robert Gibson, Stuart Gould, Harold Visotsky, John Donnelly, Leonard Ganser, and many others.

Present Coverage for Mental Disorders

A 1969 study estimated that more than 63% of the civilian population had some private insurance coverage for hospital care of mental illness, and 37% had some coverage for out-of-hospital care. There was significantly less coverage for mental illness than for other illnesses—that is, fewer days of hospital care, limitation on the number of outpatient visits, ceiling on chargeable fees, limitation on diagnosis covered, and higher level of copayments. As general hospitals have accepted more mental patients for treatment, as both inpatients and outpatients, insurance coverage has broadened, and as length of stay in public hospitals has decreased and more efforts have been expended to lower costs in these hospitals by collection from patients and third parties, insurance companies have shown greater willingness to cover hospital patients.

Benefit payments to mental patients account for less than 10% of costs of all benefits for health insurance.

Utilization data suggest that there is higher utilization of benefits among the affluent and educated, but that this is changing as the lower socioeconomic groups overcome their resistance to seeking care for mental and emotional problems. Although utilization in general has increased over time, a plateau phenomenon has been noted in recent years. Thus, the initial fear that services for mental illness would invite endless costs has been largely quelled, and present indications are that mental illness coverage *per se* would not necessarily break the bank. However, the fact that services may be utilized more by the affluent raises a serious concern. Will National Health Insurance become one more vehicle for discrimination against the poor and underserved? And, what forms of education or outreach must be developed to make certain that reasonable equity is achieved in health care coverage?

Not only are mental health coverage costs within a feasible range, compared to total costs for all insurance, but it would appear that appropriate treatment for emotional disorders may reduce utilization, and therefore costs of services, for other medical disorders. This saving is not inconsiderable, estimated to be in the neighborhood of 20%.

Yet anxieties over the potential costs of mental health coverage in a national program of comprehensive coverage are not totally eliminated by the above consideration, for estimates of the need for mental health care in the general public are alarming. The recent presidential commission estimated that 15% of the population requires mental health care now—and the probability is that this estimate is on the low side. Although much depends on how we define mental illness/emotional disorder, the 15% figure cited refers essentially to individuals who are suffering acutely and whose performance in important spheres of life is seriously impaired. They would presumably be included even in a narrow definition of mental disorder. If alcoholism, drug addiction, and emotional problems of children and the elderly are included, and if disorders now classified under behavioral medicine aberrations are also included (sleep disorders, eating disorders, smoking addiction, etc.), costs could escalate. In the long run, it will be difficult to justify exclusion of behavioral aberrations from insurance coverage because of the great part they apparently play in both health and longevity.

VA Exclusion from National Health Insurance

A recent statement by Donald L. Custis,[3] chief medical director of the Veterans Administration, has this to say about the VA's relationship to National Health Insurance:

> . . . political and economic developments appear to have eliminated, for the foreseeable future, the prospect of any meaningful national health insurance legislation. Of even greater importance is that both the V.A. Congressional Committees have now taken the position that the veterans medical care system must be exempted from any such program.
>
> These moves signal the close of over a decade of V.A. concern with national health insurance. Any further pursuit of management options anticipating a medical service module at variance with that of an independent V.A. system, under direct authority and allotment from Congress, places at risk our credibility with veterans service organizations and serves no productive purpose. Provision of third party reimbursement has been dropped from the FY '82 budget.

Later the same message states: "We must resolve to maintain the independence and vitality of a separate system of health care." Thus, the political power of the massive veterans' lobby appears to have prevailed over attempts by some National Health Insurance advocates to embrace the VA health system in a national health plan.

Today the VA operates 172 hospitals, at least 1 in each state, and treats approximately 1.2 million inpatients per year with an average daily census of 78,000. More than half of these patients are psychiatric cases. Outpatient and ambulatory care visits passed the 16.4 million mark in fiscal 1975.[4] Thus, the VA in essence provides health coverage for a very large number of service-connected and non-service-connected veterans, from whom actually very little or no financial contribution is expected. In effect, the VA extends health insurance to veterans through its own health service organization, probably the largest health service organization in the world. That this large organization has held together over the years is a great administrative triumph. However, the fundamental question always remains as to the quality and adequacy of health care provided to individual veterans under such a system. It is also fair to ask of any health care system meant to serve such a large population whether its services are utilized adequately by various community subgroups, particularly by veterans from minority cultures. In turn, when veterans from minority cultures do receive services, it should be determined if the services are as adequate and satisfactory for them as they are for veterans of the majority culture.

Since a National Health Insurance plan cannot but result in a huge new bureaucracy with far-flung service components, centralized in its management and financing, and monitored by the federal government, we are naturally interested in the success of this kind of very large endeavor. Some commentators have envisioned the VA system as a prototype for the expansion of national health care. Perhaps the VA system itself, they say, could be expanded to include the millions of potential clients that would receive benefits under a national insurance plan.

Fortunately, we have data from a recent 4-year study in Los Angeles of health care services to a sizable sample of veterans of both Anglo and Hispanic origins.[5] The findings regarding veterans' attitudes toward VA services and their satisfaction with such services are disappointing. Only 10% of veterans would utilize VA services if they had the option to go elsewhere. The VA is used as a last resort. Further, approximately 25% of veterans, whether Anglos or Hispanics, view care they received in VA facilities as unsatisfactory, citing lack of personalized interest, routinization, lack of "humaneness," or, in the case of Hispanics, actual discrimination against them as minority persons. To be sure, the complaints were registered more against lower-level personnel who presided over the entry procedures than against higher-level professional caregivers, but the overall view of this 25% was negative. It should be noted that the younger Vietnam veteran was generally more critical than the Korean War or World War II veteran. He expected a higher standard of health care and was more vociferous in stating his criticisms.

If veterans tend to shy away from VA health services, using them only when no other options are available, and if approximately 25% are not satisfied with services rendered, it is difficult to claim huge success for this method of health care coverage for a large population. Does this experience cause one to question whether any large, governmentally centralized health organization would be likely to suffer from similar bureaucratic deficiencies? How would it affect the development and the quality of American medicine, which today depends so much on individual initiative and inspiration? Those of us who have had experience with state and federal health organizations have cause for concern that the quality of patient service may be seriously compromised by the very bureaucracies erected for the ostensibly humanitarian purpose of giving health care to a large number of deprived people.

Who Should Be Paid?

The question of who should receive reimbursement for services rendered is now one of the most nettling problems in the whole field of insurance for mental illness. When coverage applied mainly to hospitalization, physician services seemed quite naturally to qualify for reimbursement, but when ambulatory outpatient treatment for mental illness burgeoned, and allied professionals such as psychologists, social workers, and nurses began to take primary responsibility for patients, the situation became more complicated. The thirst for independent reimbursement has become a heated issue. In Canada, essentially only the physician is reimbursed, but in the United States, nonphysicians have qualified in various states for independent reimbursement status. We are faced with a number of incontrovertible historical facts that make organized psychiatry's opposition to nonphysician reimbursement increasingly difficult to uphold.

First, these allied professionals (especially psychologists) are well organized, have gained recognition as practitioners in many states, have their own board-type certification, run their own training programs, and are settled into independent practice in many communities.

Second, in institutional practice, in health maintenance organizations, and in many new federally funded community mental health centers, they are highly respected members of the mental health team, often taking primary responsibility for establishing therapeutic relationships with patients, though they may be guided by physicians. Indeed, we learn that most of the therapy provided in community mental health centers is provided by nonphysician mental health professionals, with psychiatrists functioning as consultants and/or taking responsibility for prescription of drugs.

Third, as long as in the present state of our knowledge it has not been demonstrated that nonpsychiatric professionals are ineffective, or vastly less effective than psychiatrists, the valid issue can be raised that the use of nonpsychiatric professionals may be more cost-effective than the exclusive use of psychiatrists. Here, the great qualitative difference between treatment of mental illness and treatment of physical illness comes sharply to the fore: In mental illness there is great stress on the "therapeutic use of the self," whereas in ordinary physical disease therapeutic results rest more on technical knowledge and procedures. Many nonphysician professionals—indeed, many nonprofessionals—have intuitive, or learned, capacities to relate to mentally disturbed persons with positive clinical effects, sometimes to the chagrin of highly trained, credentialed professionals who may have failed in the very task.

Because the physician rightly believes that the treatment of the mental illness of the person cannot easily be separated from the treatment of the whole individual, and is fearful that the nonphysician will miss the full implications of signs and symptoms that have possible dangerous consequences for the patient, a great deal of controversy has been engendered among mental health professionals. The following options for reimbursement, therefore, are being considered: (1) Provide reimbursement for services *only when supplied by a physician;* (2) reimburse psychologists (social workers, nurses) only when services are under the *supervision of a physician;* (3) reimburse psychologists (social workers, nurses) only when services are *authorized by a physician;* (4) reimburse psychologists (social workers, nurses), in addition to physicians, *as members of the mental health team;* (5) reimburse psychologists (social workers, nurses) *as independent practitioners.*

Psychologists have received recognition as independent providers under CHAMPUS, in federal health benefit plans since 1975, and in some states. Social workers and nurses have not yet met with similar success but are intent upon gaining recognition. The obvious next question to face any proponent of National Health Insurance would concern what professional groups should be included, or excluded, and under what conditions. For example, should rehabilitation experts, pastoral counselors, clinical pharmacists, practitioners of transactional analysis, etc., be independently reimbursed for their particular contribution? One hopes that decisions on these sensitive issues will be facilitated when definitive research clarifies the relative therapeutic efficacy of intervention by psychiatrists vis-à-vis other nonphysician professionals.

What About Reimbursement for Psychoanalysis?

Only a small proportion (about 5% or less) of individuals seen in psychotherapy are under treatment by conventional psycholanalysts, using conventional psychoanalytical techniques—i.e., patient treated on a couch, three or four times or more per week over extended periods. Conventional psychoanalytic therapy as practiced is used primarily for the educated, for the affluent, for the further training of professionals going into the mental health field, and for a relatively narrow set of problems such as obsessive-compulsive neurosis, chronic incapacitating anxiety, and chronic borderline psychoses that have proved refractory to other therapies. The psychoanalytic method is hailed as a great and effective clinical modality by some, and as a cost-ineffective, mainly investigative and research instrument by others.

The question whether National Health Insurance should reimburse for classical psychoanalytic treatment obviously hinges on its cost and its effectiveness. Cost can be very great, and since it is probably most applicable to individuals with a high degree of verbal and psychological sophistication (a capacity for what has been called "interception"), its use would not necessarily encourage an equitable deployment of National Health Insurance resources.

Proponents of psychoanalysis as a modality to be covered by National Health Insurance argue that its efficacy is validated by the large number of reports from practicing analysts. At any rate, it is claimed that its efficacy is as well established as that of nonanalytic psychotherapy, already covered by innumerable insurance companies.

The whole issue, however, may be mooted by the fact that in almost all bills introduced into Congress for a National Health Insurance program, definite limits to the number of outpatient visits (as well as hospitalization days) have been included. The recent national emphasis on controlling inflationary medical costs and balancing the budget, and the generally unstable economy, make it unlikely that these limits will be removed. Indeed, in the last few years the possibility of enactment of a comprehensive form of National Health Insurance *per se* appears to have been fading.

National Health Care in Other Nations

In Canada, the federal law sets forth the principles upon which the health services of the provinces are based. These principles include universality of coverage without discrimination, setting of a maximum payment that can be expected from each subscriber, setting of a floor of payment to the physician, and transferability of coverage from one province to another. The federal government, the provincial government, and the insured person contribute to the national health service program. The subscriber contributes on a monthly basis from his salary, but if he is unemployed, allowances are made and his coverage is unaffected.

Under this plan, hospitalization is unlimited, and office care is unlimited. The subscriber has a choice of doctor but must go first to a general physician who also does some surgery. If the subscriber wishes to go initially to a specialist, he must personally pay for the services. Psychiatric coverage, whether hospital or office care, is on the same essentially unlimited basis. There is no independent reimbursement of psychologists, nurses, or social workers.

The Canadian people seem to like their National Health plan. However, physicians do complain that their income from National Health is not adequate and that it may indeed be declining. However, younger physicians are assured of an income as soon as they go into practice. There is no significant waiting period for the public to discover them, as is the case in the United States.

In Great Britain, emergency care is covered for every person in the British Isles, in a National Health Service organized and administered by four Regional Health Councils, appointed by the government. Although there was considerable difficulty and dissatisfaction expressed particularly by physicians when the plan first started, much of the turmoil has settled down.

In the British system, every person is registered with a district general practitioner and has no other choice (unless he goes the private route). The district practitioner is family-oriented, makes home calls, and performs minor surgery. He in turn may refer complicated cases to a consultant, who also sees the patient either in his office or at home. Indeed, there is extra reimbursement for home visits. Each general practitioner is related to a community hospital, which in turn may feed into a regional hospital and then to a university hospital, for specialist care and treatment. Outreach from the community hospital to the sick person is via district nurse and social worker, who work closely with the general practitioner.

The individual subscriber contributes to the system through his salary, but if he or she is not working, the government picks up the tab. There is no discrimination in the British system between the rich and the poor; however, the rich often use the private route to go to their consultant of choice.

The average citizen of middle or lower class seems to like the National Health Service. However, a common complaint is that there is a long waiting list for elective surgery. The British general practitioner is assured of a good stable income. The consultant, since 1972, is permitted to have a part-time private practice without limit on how much he can earn.

Without going into further details of these systems, it is obvious that broad coverage for illness, both physical and mental, exists in the two English-speaking countries, and that the public as a whole is probably better served in these countries than in the United States. The amount invested in health care each year depends on allotments made at the national level, but apparently the national budget is not bankrupted by the plan. We do not hear that the people of either country clamor for a return to the free-market health system. These countries (and others) seem to have achieved for their citizens what the United States has been arguing about for decades.

In view of the apparent success of the National Health system in a number of other countries, why has the United States lagged in its adoption of such a program? Some of the reluctance stems from fears of huge costs that will overburden the nation's budget, especially during a period of uncontrolled inflation and growing national deficit. Some of the hesitancy doubtless stems from the reluctance of physicians to give up their independence, and with it possibly some of their income as well. The powerful American Medical Association lobby is very protective of the physician's autonomy in practice, and with it his incentive to deliver quality care according to the highest standards. There is great concern that at the private level the physician–patient relationship will deteriorate, and at the national level the high achievements of U.S. medicine in research and education will be blunted. American physicians are extremely proud of the claim that American medicine is the best in the world. Finally, in many parts of the nation the lower classes receive excellent care in university-sponsored hospitals, and indeed, coverage for health care through the initiatives of private and public insurance has been spreading rapidly, slowly closing the gaps in care that existed only a few years ago.

National Health Insurance and the Growing Edge of Psychiatry

If and when the nation gets a National Health plan, will that plan be current with advances of modern psychiatry? Thus far, most insurance companies have failed to cover partial hospitalization, although partial hospitalization was included as one of the essential services under the original community mental health legislation. Researchers strongly endorse partial hospitalization for a great many mentally ill patients. Indeed, only a small minority of patients cannot be treated as effectively, or more effectively and at a lower cost, in a Day Hospital Treatment Center than in the hospital. Inclusion of coverage for partial hospitalization would encourage the spread of this modality to many more places where it is sorely needed.[6,7]

Several other new modalities have shown their merit and should be included, particularly since they have utility for the neglected chronic population. We recommend for inclusion under a National Health plan, at a minimum, the following: sheltered rehabilitation (workshops) for mentally ill patients seeking skill enhancement or new skill development of relevance to the work-a-day world, halfway houses,[8] cooperative apartments,[9] community lodges,[10,11] home treatment (prevention of hospitalization),[12] training in community living,[13] and foster home surrogate family living.[14]

Each of these have proven their worth in terms of clinical effectiveness and cost-efficiency. Further, it is imperative that the practicing clinician have available to him a number of options, so that he may select the modality that is most promising for his particular patient, or shift to another modality if one has failed. I think the reader would be pleasantly surprised, in view of the uncertain results of research on efficacy of individual psychotherapy, to learn how efficacious these methods are, particularly for some long-term patients. It is imperative that advances in community psychiatry, including crisis intervention therapy, should not be neglected in any insurance coverage plan.

Finally, experience over the last 20–30 years has left a strong impression, namely, that the mental health of the nation should no longer be governed by the two principles that have been the standbys of the past: (1) Hospitalize those who have come to public attention because they are seriously mentally ill, are dangerous to themselves or others, and/or are unable to provide for their food, clothing, or shelter; and (2) treat those less seriously ill in private offices, provided they recognize their malady and seek appointment.

It is all too apparent now that these strategies have led to the care and treatment of only a fraction of the population that needs help. Those who disturb the peace, take the initiative to seek treatment, or trust establishment-blessed treatment systems are receiving attention. The poor, the minorities, the less-educated, and those who are unskilled in the game of entry into, or manipulation of, treatment systems tend to be neglected. The recent presidential commission recognized that despite all the community mental health legislation of the past, the nation has let slip away its obligation to reach out to the underserved, poorly served, and nonserved—the minorities and the hard-to-reach chronic mentally ill population.

The process of outreach to the neglected mentally ill can only reach an effective level if and when policy-makers support a public health view of psychiatry. That view maintains that care and treatment of the mentally ill must not end with the treatment of those who come to attention in conventional ways, but that conscientious planning for all the mental health needs of a defined geographic population must be the dominant theme of the next decades. Just as the public health orientation in medicine has been responsible for eradication or control of many diseases such as smallpox and syphilis, and has been involved so successfully in food sanitation and pollution control, so psychiatry's future should be intertwined with measures to understand and enhance the mental health of the entire citizenry. This will involve, among other things, a massive development of epidemiological research, the delineation of belief systems and cultural modes of subpopulations, mobilization of support systems, and reeducation of people to healthier life-styles.

Research

Provision of health care via any federally or privately funded system requires a broad base of knowledge concerning consumer needs and demands and their utilization patterns in relation to type and cost of services offered. Basic information is needed as to what are the most appropriate and effective service systems and what are the effects of new or modified systems on client and provider morale, on quality of care, and on the whole caregiving organization. For example, will a National Health Insurance program of a given type encourage or discourage prospective students from entering the field of medicine (nursing, psychology, social work) and will it change the quality of students who apply to the health professions, or their enthusiasm and creativity in the field of choice? These questions are not as yet fully answered, and some are hardly considered. Fortunately, the quietus between the high enthusiasm for National Health Insurance of the early 1970s and the present caution based on fiscal and economic conservatism allows for a period of study and research on such vital questions.

The Rand Corporation of California was recently awarded a grant from the Department of Health and Human Services to study some of these questions. The project has been under way since the fall of 1974. The reader is referred to numerous documents supplied by the Rand Corporation relative to their progress to date. A review of health insurance study publications by Joseph P. Newhouse and Rae W. Archibald, 1978, scans the literature in the field and makes evaluative comments based on critical analysis.

The Rand study enrolled experimental families in Dayton, Ohio, and Seattle, Washington, and in Massachusetts and South Carolina. The objectives of the study are several: (1) to estimate how alternative cost-sharing arrangements affect the demand for health care services; (2) to assess the impact of raising the cost of health services on the health status of the individual; (3) to determine whether (and by how much) cost-sharing arrangements affect poor families more than higher-income families; (4) to ascertain how the ambulatory care system can accommodate to varying levels of demand or stress; (5) to gain familiarity with the difficulties of administering health insurance plans that place a ceiling on out-of-pocket payments; (6) to learn how the quality of medical care differs among individuals who have various insurance plans; (7) to compare utilization, quality of care, health status outcomes, and consumer satisfaction in an existing prepaid group practice with the fee-for-service program.

Let me add to these important questions, some concerns of mine already voiced. (a) How adequate will health coverage be for the American citizen 5 and 10 years from now if no National Health plan is adopted? (b) What is the relative efficacy of mental health services provided by psychiatrists vis-à-vis other nonpsychiatric professionals? (c) How can we insure that an equitable proportion of the national expenditure for health under a National Health system will go to the poor, the minorities, and other populations hitherto underserved?

References

1. Myers ES: Health insurance and psychiatric care, in Kaplan HI, Freedman AM, Sadock BJ (eds): Comprehensive Textbook of Psychiatry, ed 3. Baltimore, Williams and Wilkins, 1980, ch 56 pp 3182–3197.

2. Reed LS, Myers ES, Scheidemandel PL: Health Insurance and Psychiatric Care: Utilization and Cost. Washington DC, American Psychiatric Association, 1972.
3. Custis DL: State of the Department Message. Washington DC, October 29, 1980.
4. Veterans Administration History in Brief. VA Pamphlet No. 06–77–1, May 1977.
5. Becerra RM, Greenblatt MG: Hispanics seek health care: A study of 1,088 veterans of three war eras, Report submitted to Veterans Administration Central Office, 1980.
6. Herz MI: Partial hospitalization, brief hospitalization, and aftercare, in Kaplan HI, Freedman AM, Sadock BJ (eds): Comprehensive Textbook of Psychiatry, ed 3. Baltimore, Williams and Wilkins, 1980, ch 32 pp 2368–2381.
7. Kramer BM: Day Hospital: A Study in Partial Hospitalization in Psychiatry. New York, Grune and Stratton, 1962.
8. Budson RD: The Psychiatric Halfway House: Multiple Systems and Individual Programs. Pittsburgh, University of Pittsburgh Press, 1979.
9. Chien C, Cole JO: Landlord-supervised cooperative apartments: A new modality for community-based treatment. *Am J Psychiatry* 130(2):156–159, 1973.
10. Fairweather GW, Sanders DH, Tornatsky LG: Creating Change in Mental Health Organizations. New York, Pergamon Press, 1975.
11. Fairweather GW, Sanders H, Maynard DL: Community Life for the Mentally Ill. Chicago, Aldine Publishing Company, 1969.
12. Weiner L, Becker A, Freidman T: Home Treatment. Pittsburgh, University of Pittsburgh Press, 1967.
13. Stein LI, Test MA: Training in community living: One-year evaluation. *Am J Psychiatry* 133(8):917–918, 1976.
14. Polak PR, Kirby MW: Follow up evaluation on an inpatient alternative program. *Am J Psychiatry* 133(8):916–917, 1976.

Zigmond M. Lebensohn

In the early 1930s I heard a lecture in which a University of Chicago philosopher tried to describe George Santayana's then current ideas about the existence of a Deity. Santayana, who was born a Spanish Catholic, had become, at that period of his life, something of an atheist. The lecturer tried several times to catch the essence of Santayana's beliefs and finally emerged with the following summation: "Santayana," he said, "is one of those curious philosphers who believes there is no God but that the Virgin Mary is his mother!"

In a similar vein, Dr. Upton seems to be afflicted by the same fatal ambivalence. On the one hand, he believes there should be no arbitrary limits on psychotherapy; on the other hand, he recognizes that we must reduce the cost of care without affecting the quality of care. Dr. Upton tells us that the psychiatrist must refuse to be rushed into setting standards or protocols for the duration or frequency of psychotherapy, yet he sets standards himself when he suggests that certain conditions such as "chronic symtomatic maladjustment" (the neuroses) will require intermediate to long-term psychotherapy. "By this," continues Dr. Upton, "I mean, on average, 50 to 400 treatment visits over roughly 1 to 4 years." Dr. Upton vigorously and commendably champions the cause of "full coverage" for the treatment of mental illness/emotional problems, yet he warns that psychiatric treatment cannot mean "a process to enhance the quality of life."

This warning (with which I wholeheartedly agree) is weakened a bit when he goes on to say that in psychiatric treatment "the psychiatrist . . . seeks to point his patient in the direction of achieving satisfaction and fulfillment in terms of the way he (or she) leads his life." Although I agree that this often occurs as an added benefit in the course of successful long - term psychotherapy, this position does not differ very much from efforts to "enhance the quality of life," which Dr. Upton specifically excludes from his concept of allowable psychiatric treatment under NHI.

Zigmond M. Lebensohn • Chief Emeritus, Department of Psychiatry, Sibley Memorial Hospital, and Clinical Professor of Psychiatry, Georgetown University School of Medicine, Washington, D.C. 20009.

Of course, it could be argued that *all* good medical and/or psychiatric care, if successful, "enhances the quality of life." I have the strong feeling, however, that what Dr. Upton really objects to are efforts to help people who are vaguely dissatisfied with their lot in life to "fulfill their potential" or something of that sort. Such a pursuit, of course, is not at all objectionable and may even be laudable if pursued on a personal, fee-for-service basis. Psychoanalysis or any other long- term process of "transformation" may be used, provided the recipient pays for the services himself. However, this type of service (i.e., efforts to help people fulfill their unspecified potential) is hardly compatible with the aim of any NHI plan I have ever known.

It must be freely admitted, however, that the task of setting fair standards that will benefit patients with real distress yet not be subject to abuse by MHPs (mental health professionals) or their "clients" is most difficult indeed. Yet the exigencies of the situation require that psychiatrists, who see these problems every day of their professional life, cut the Gordian knot and give legislators proper direction. Oh, for those halcyon days when all therapy of any kind, for whatever reason (and who could afford it), were not hampered by any limitations or regulations except those set up between the therapist and his "client."

But we are no longer living in those halcyon days and no amount of wistful wishing will bring them back. Dr. Upton is properly concerned when he points out that the most liberal NHI plan now under consideration would authorize only 20 full outpatient sessions per year. Such token coverage works a very real hardship on thousands of patients throughout the country who desperately need more than token help, and furthermore, it cruelly discriminates against psychiatric patients. Even current Medicare practice (now limited to $250 a year!) provides the most meager and inadequate coverage of outpatient psychotherapy for those of our citizens over age 65 whose needs for such therapy are perhaps greater than those of any other age group. Dr. Upton's observations are particularly pertinent when we consider our ever-growing older population.

In spite of the fact that Dr. Upton doesn't seem to resolve his major conflict (that is, the need to *remove* limits vs. the need to *set* limits on mental health care), his paper is full of cogent warnings that future legislators would do well to heed if they wish to avoid disastrous inequities in any future form of NHI legislation. Many of Dr. Upton's observations and warnings are not new, but in his book we find them all in one place, expressed clearly and coherently with factual backing wherever such backing is possible.

Early in his paper Dr. Upton uses the term *mental health professionals* (MHPs) to refer to psychiatrists, licensed clinical Ph.D. psychologists, and social workers with a master's degree (M.S.W.s or above). In his proposals, Dr. Upton includes rather than excludes these MHPs as treatment providers. I am in complete accord. Any experienced psychiatrist with an awareness of the magnitude of the problems facing us in America will agree with his estimate. As long ago as 1962, while reflecting on the same issue and contemplating future efforts to provide mental health care to those who needed it, I concluded my Kober Lecture[1] with a similar plea:

> Inherent in this great effort will be the ever-increasing use of large numbers of nonmedical personnel such as psychologists, social workers, nurses, administrators, ministers, and lay therapists. To some this may pose a serious threat to the integrity of psychiatry as an important part of medicine. *However, the task is far too great and far too important to be accomplished by any single discipline* [italics added]. The challenge is clear. We must mobilize a total effort, interdisciplinary in nature but medical in its direction. To this end it will be more important than ever for the American psychiatry of the future to remain an integral part of American medicine. For it is the essential harmony between psychiatry and medicine that offers the best promise of scientific progress against the mental illnesses of our time.

It is ironic to note that there has been a phenomenal growth in the number of nonmedical MHPs (much greater proportionally than the increase in the number of psychiatrists), but each of the various disciplines has tended to go off on its own. They have shown considerable reluctance to place the psychiatrist "at the helm" of the mental health care delivery system, as Dr. Upton correctly recommends. Whether this reluctance is based on parochial loyalties or smoldering distrust of the medical model is not clear. Psychiatrists must examine themselves objectively and mercilessly to discover where the fault lies and correct it. For unless the "essential harmony" is restored (or established), our efforts will be for naught.

In this connection, Dr. Upton recommends that all qualified nonmedical MHPs be included on the "treatment wheel" but sensibly adds that psychiatrists should be "at the hub." He makes clear that the *psychiatrist* (and when he uses this term, I assume he means the general psychiatrist) "is especially well qualified to evaluate and treat persons with mental illness/emotional problems." It is the general psychiatrist—not the psychoanalyst, behavior therapist, biological psychiatrist, or any other subspecialist—who is freer of bias and better equipped to evaluate any given mental illness/emotional problem and refer the patient to the most appropriate therapist.

In an article some years ago,[2] after reflecting for a long time on this dilemma, I suggested a model that I called the Radial Concept of Psychiatric Services to replace the time-worn "Linear Path Downward" (Figure 1). In the first of these models the patient, instead of being a helpless object pulled by gravity to ever lower levels, is conceptualized as being in the center of a circular pattern (together with an experienced psychiatrist to guide him), free to select any one of a wide variety of psychiatric outpatient or inpatient treatments based on what is best for him at that particular point in his illness.

> The various treatment modalities are thus not seen in a hierarchical order (as they are in the Linear Path Downward) with any one method considered intrinsically better than the one below it, but rather as a wide range of modalities, any one of which may be just right for a particular patient at a given time. . . . It is often difficult to determine what is best for a particular patient at a given time. But therein lies the art and skill of the psychiatrist. This specific art and skill (triage) has never been sufficiently stressed in psychiatric training or practice. Thus, many psychia-

trists emerge from training with a shockingly constricted overview of the rich assortment of treatment modalities available even in their own communities.

Dr. Upton seems to agree with the need to place the psychiatrist in a front-line position where he can practice "triage" and referral. But this need seems not to be felt in our CMHCs (Community Mental Health Centers), even in those few that have a psychiatrist "at the helm." The usual practice is to insist that the new patient first struggle past a clerk, and then (if his residence happens to be in the proper catchment area for that CMHC) he is passed on to

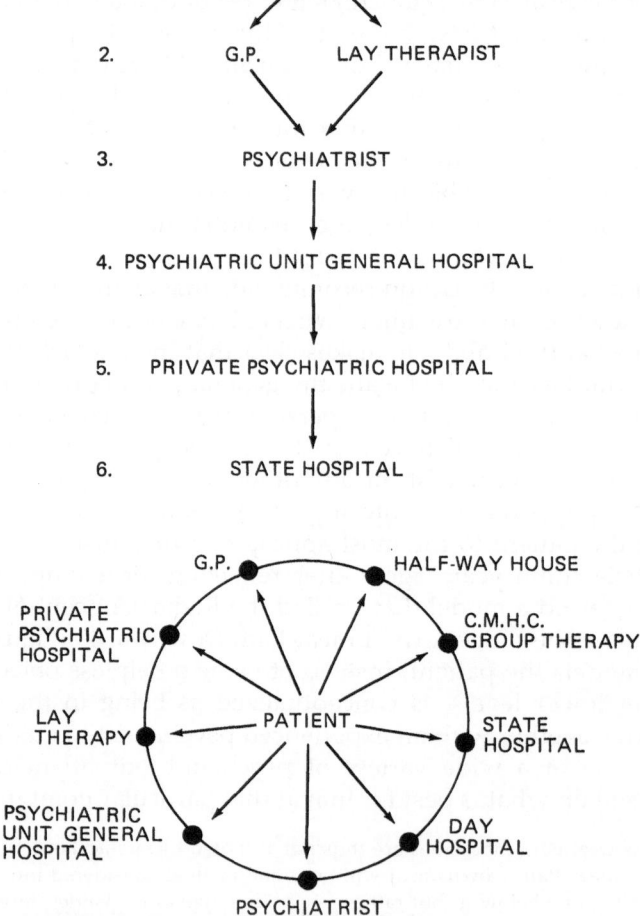

Figure 1.   (Top) Pilgrim's Progress or The Linear Path Downward; (bottom) Polybelted Radial Concept of Mental Health Services. The Radial Concept should be modified by placing the general psychiatrist or the personal physician in the center of the treatment wheel to guide the patient in selecting the most appropriate treatment.

an intake social worker. From there he may be referred to a clinical psychologist for testing or evaluation. Finally, after several days or weeks of waiting and masses of paper work, the psychiatrist may enter the case. But this does not necessarily mean that he actually sees the patient. In most instances it may only mean that the psychiatrist presides over a clinical conference in which a multitude of reports are read and a treatment plan is worked out. No wonder, Dr. Upton reports, that there are only 5.3 visits per patient to CMHCs per year, whereas there are 38 visits per patient per year to private psychiatrists. The huge dropout rate suggests widespread patient dissatisfaction with the current procedure. From the patient's point of view it would be infinitely better, wherever possible, to reverse the usual sequence. Why not arrange for the psychiatrist to be the first MHP to interview the patient? This, of course, is the procedure followed with great effectiveness in the private practice sector.

Although it may be more stressful for the psychiatrist at the CMHC to serve on the front line and be the first to see the patient, this new approach would be far better for the patient and, in the final analysis, a source of great pride and satisfaction to all the MHPs involved.

In an attempt to gain some idea of the cost of psychiatric care under NHI, efforts have been made to compare the cost of 1 hour of therapy in the CMHC with the cost of 1 hour's therapy in the private practice sector. Although it is fairly easy to get reliable data on fees charged by psychiatrists in private practice, it is surprisingly difficult to arrive at an accurate estimate of the cost of 1 hour of therapy in the CMHC. Dr. Upton quotes some earlier NIMH reports showing that "the unit cost per psychiatrist treatment hour is actually higher at the CMHC than it is in the private sector ($45 vs. $37)."[3]

Although Dr. Upton refers to this as an "oddity" because it is the reverse of what one would expect, this finding could hardly be considered an "oddity" by any psychiatrist who has had firsthand experience with costly government bureaucracy and its inevitably heavy overhead. Although the study quoted is now out of date, it is my impression that even then the authors of that study underestimated the cost of 1 hour of psychiatric care in a CMHC. In view of all of the countless conferences and salaries paid to staff members whether they were treating or not treating patients, plus overhead, etc., I think that the cost in the CMHC would be closer to $75 per psychiatrist treatment hour than the $45 estimate arrived at.[4]

In addition, it should be pointed out that the psychiatrist who charges $50 or more per treatment hour pays local and federal taxes on his income, which then go to support a wide variety of public services, including, of course, the community mental health centers. There is no such payment of taxes by the community mental health center itself, so that in the final analysis, the cost to the country is even greater. Unfortunately, many people, including those who should know better, are overly concerned by the high fees of psychiatrists and who feel that treatment in a CMHC costs much less. These people fail to reckon with the hidden costs that must be paid by the taxpayers.

At this point the reader should probably be warned that this commentary is written by a psychiatrist who has been in the active private practice of general psychiatry in Washington, D.C., for over 40 years. I have thus had ample opportunity to see or treat almost every conceivable type of psychiatric disorder and to use psychotherapy, chemotherapy, electrotherapy, and hospitalization on the psychiatric unit of a general hospital whenever indicated. I have done my share of teaching, writing, and consulting. Since I practice in the nation's capital, I have had ample opportunity to observe at close hand the psychiatric problems faced by government officials and have a healthy respect for their efforts to resolve them. From the extensive experience of over 40 years I have, by now, a reasonably good idea of what works and what doesn't work in psychiatry. Thus far I am sorry to say that the CMHC system is not working and its orientation has shifted so much that, in my opinion, it is no longer capable of dealing effectively with the serious psychiatric disorders that plague our communities. Our poor experience with the CMHCs has important bearing on what might easily happen to psychiatry under any form of NHI. The reasons for the failures of the CMHCs are numerous and complex, but a major reason, it seems to me, is the tendency of most CMHCs to place almost exclusive reliance on the psychosocial model and their failure to use the medical model.

It should be made clear that I am *not* recommending sole reliance on the biomedical model. My concern about the dangers of the exclusive use of any one model in psychiatry was amply expressed in one of my recent papers, in which I stated, "Just as there is no single cause for mental illness, so is there no single treatment method. There is no justification to be smug about any one approach in psychiatry. The medical model, that most ancient, honorable and useful model, has come under heavy attack in recent years, particularly from those who do not really understand it. Although other models may be useful from time to time and in certain instances, no other model can be as broad or all-inclusive and as subject to scientific scrutiny as the medical model."[2]

Kety[5] has defined more exactly what is meant by the medical model. Because it has an important bearing on the quality of psychiatric treatment that citizens should be receiving under any future NHI plan, it might be well to repeat his definition here.

> The medical model of an illness is a process that moves from the recognition and palliation of symptoms to the characterization of a specific disease in which the etiology and pathogenesis are known and the treatment is rational and specific. That progress depends upon the acquisition of knowledge and may often take many years or centuries. Numerous medical disorders and one or two mental illnesses have moved to the final stages of understanding, but many are still at various points along the way. After the recognition of symptoms, there comes the realization that some symptoms occur in fairly regular clusters, which are then described as syndromes. These may ultimately turn out to represent one or several etiological and pathogenetic components, the nature of which may be obscure at earlier stages of knowledge.

The evolution of a medical model from symptoms through syndromes to diseases with specific pathology and, ultimately, with definitive etiologies and rational
treatment is an excellent example of the scientific method applied to the alleviation
of human suffering. It involves careful observation and study, the generation,
sharpening, and testing of hypotheses, and the elucidation of underlying mechanisms, all pointing toward prevention and effective treatment. In many instances
throughout medicine, this process has been successful and there is justifiable concern that the fruits of this knowledge are not available to all the population.

Although I am personally convinced that the rational practice of scientifically oriented, medically based psychiatry represents the most effective
approach to most cases of mental illness/emotional problems, I must admit
that there still remain many disorders that simply do not respond to any
treatment method currently available. Psychiatry has often been accused of
making excessive therapeutic claims and raising false hopes, which were later
dashed on the rocks of grim reality. We are now going through a period in
which psychiatry is on the defensive. We are being asked to provide proof of
the safety, efficacy, and appropriateness of our treatment methods, just as if
we were launching a new drug on the market that had to be assessed by the
FDA. In late 1978 a Senate finance committee held hearings in an attempt to
determine how much to pay for psychotherapy under Medicare and Medicaid. In 1980 a Senate bill was introduced that would establish a commission
to evaluate various types of therapy in regard to their safety, effectiveness,
and appropriate use. A 6-year controlled study of five different therapies for
severe depression is already underway at NIMH. A third study on the effectiveness of psychotherapy is planned under the auspices of the Alcohol, Drug
Abuse, and Mental Health Administration (ADAMHA).

Thus, I am understandably concerned when Dr. Upton makes the flat
statement, "Many persons who display the antisocial personality can be
helped by mental health care; their behavior can be controlled." Unfortunately, there are no references to substantiate this claim. Certainly my own clinical
experience with antisocial personality disorders (in fact, with the whole
gamut of personality disorders) leaves me rather pessimistic as to how effective psychiatry alone can be in coping with these "malignant" problems.
Persons afflicted with severe personality disorders rarely, if ever, reach out
for help, even though they may cause intense emotional trauma to members
of their family, their employers or their colleagues. Most often they are referred for treatment by the courts after having been apprehended for some
antisocial act. But they themselves are not "hurting." Therefore, they do not
reach out for help as does the anxiety- or guilt-ridden patient who wants
relief. Without this type of motivation, successful therapy is well-nigh
impossible.

The above reservations also apply to Dr. Upton's plea for more MHPs in
our correctional system—in our prisons, jails, and courts. Psychiatry's track
record in this area is not one to write home about. To be sure, the past
support for such services has been niggardly at best and recruitment of top

professionals has been difficult. It is already very difficult to recruit good MHPs to staff our large state mental hospitals. The paucity of professional satisfactions has made the problem of staffing our correctional institutions even more difficult. Nonetheless, Dr. Upton's concern is real and laudable. Whether corrective action will be taken is a question of political and economic priorities. However, I agree with Dr. Upton that the MHP "should not be involved in the actual process of determining the guilt or innocence of the defendant." If the MHP could be relieved of this thankless and inappropriate task, then he might have more time to devote to therapy.

In addition to the political and economic issues, the moral issues involved in limiting coverage under any type of NHI are particularly painful. Dr. Upton labels any attempts to limit or spare appropriate medical care as "immoral," whether the condition being treated is physical or mental. This position, which, on the surface at least, is most appealing from the humanitarian point of view, implies that all citizens should have a right to health care. Not all students of the problem agree with this point of view. There could be many potential and undesirable complications if medicine in general, and psychiatry in particular, were to succumb unequivocally to the clamor for a *right* to health care. Mark Siegler, in a most thoughtful article,[6] repudiates the notion that there should be a "right to health care" but adds, "I believe a good society ought to provide certain forms of health care to its population but should do so for reasons other than citizens' claims of a right to such services." Dr. Siegler then goes on to delineate these reasons and suggests what appears to be the essence of what takes place in the private practice sector when he says, "I believe every citizen should have a principal physician who would be responsible for guiding the patient through the maze of the health care bureaucracy, to obtain services needed for optimal care." This is somewhat similar to my Radial Concept of Psychiatric Services, previously discussed on p. 243.

In this connection Dr. Upton also considers the care provided by the MHP practicing in the private sector to be superior and more effective than the care available at the CMHC. Although I am in private practice and have long been one of its staunchest advocates, even I am somewhat embarrassed when I am told that the MHP in private practice, working without constraints, cannot only alleviate the presenting problem but can also change the patient's personality so that "crises do not repeat themselves ad infinitum." Would that this were always so! Later in his text Dr. Upton repeats his argument: "Management of symptoms often can only be arrived at through personality change. . . ." Such a statement flies in the face of the successful experience in the behavioral therapies that are focused on symptom removal without necessarily requiring a concomitant personality change. Although Dr. Upton's objectives (namely, to effect a personality change during therapy to prevent a recurrence of symptoms) are indeed commendable, they are infrequently attained in clinical practice.

The usual sequence of events following the relief of acute symptoms is continuation of therapy, supportive in nature, over a long period of time, sometimes for years, until the condition is stabilized. Although the patient may continue in therapy for some years, the total cost need not be great since, in many instances, treatment sessions may be as infrequent as once every month or two.

It is the *continuity* of care and not its *frequency* that really matters. This represents what psychiatrists may call supportive or maintenance therapy following resolution of the acute symptoms. It represents what Siegler[6] calls "The process of caring." He adds, "I have argued previously that a major deficiency of modern medicine has been its overemphasis on its curing potential and its relative disregard for its greatest asset, the caring function." Medicine, more than any other profession, has the tradition of caring and taking the responsibility for the welfare of another person seeking help—the patient.

To return for a moment to the subject of mental health care costs, Dr. Upton is correct in pointing out that medical and surgical care is often far more expensive. He states, "Indeed it is a myth that mental health care is more expensive than other forms of health care." He refers in the course of his paper to several studies illustrating, he claims, that private-based outpatient mental health care is cost-containable.

But later on, Dr. Upton cautions us: "Despite the fact that private-based mental health care seems affordable on the broader scale, we cannot call for unlimited coverage for such care under NHI without examining the cost of psychoanalysis, a generally open-ended form of treatment that most of the public erroneously considers typical of psychiatric care. Psychoanalytic treatment of mental illness/emotional problems is in the distinct minority; however, when employed it is expensive." A 1973 Joint Information Service (JIS) study[7] cited data by Reed that revealed that only 2% of patients insured under the Blue Cross and Blue Shield Plan for Federal Employees incurred charges greater than $5000 in 1973 for outpatient therapy, most of it presumably for psychoanalytic therapy. But these expenses accounted for 17% of *all* outpatient psychiatric benefits paid out under the plan. Dr. Marmor, the senior author of the JIS survey, added, "A heavy burden of responsibility devolves upon the advocates of such therapy to justify so disproportionate a cost."[7]

This leads us to ask, what is likely to be the future for psychoanalysis under NHI? In my own commentary on the same JIS survey,[8] I, too, was concerned about the inequity of any publicly financed mental health plan that paid such a disproportionate percentage of its funds to such a small segment of the population. I concluded with the following observation:

> It is most unlikely that classical psychoanalysis as it once existed will be covered by any form of national health insurance. It should also be recognized that classical psychoanalysis has become increasingly rare. Psychoanalysis has unquestionably had a profound influence on American psychiatry. Indeed, it has influenced it to such an extent that most of its useful and valid concepts have already been incorporated into the body of psychiatric theory and practice. What is not so generally recognized, however, is the extent to which general psychiatry has influenced the

practice and theory of psychoanalysis. This Joint Information Service Survey simply confirms what many of us have long suspected has been occurring in psychoanalysis, namely, that most analysts see a substantial number of their patients in nonanalytic psychotherapy. An increasing number of analysts are using psychoactive drugs when indicated, and many more have joined the staffs of psychiatric units of general hospital where they can readily admit and treat their patients when they need hospitalization. Thus it appears that there is a discernible movement back to the medical model, a movement which should bode well both for medicine and for psychiatry.

Is psychoanalysis really the culprit in regard to increasing the overall cost for outpatient psychotherapy? Dr. Upton arrives at no firm conclusions, but he confronts the issue squarely and challenges psychoanalysis on several grounds, including cost-effectiveness. Although cost-effectiveness of psychoanalysis was not a national issue during his lifetime, Freud himself would probably have been astounded (and perhaps troubled) by the current widespread overuse of psychoanalysis as a *treatment method* in this country. He considered the treatment function of psychoanalysis as being of lesser importance. Writing for the Encyclopedia Britannica in 1929, Freud[9] stated, "The future will probably attribute far greater importance to psychoanalysis as the science of the unconscious than as a therapeutic procedure." Little did he dream that the overapplication of psychoanalysis might become a national socioeconomic issue.

Since frequency of treatment sessions is a key issue in determining the cost of psychotherapy, Dr. Upton allows Dr. Marmor (a psychoanalyst with highest credentials) to answer in part the question that opens the above paragraph. Dr. Marmor feels, as do I, that it is not the frequency of sessions but how long they go on that is of greatest importance. Thus, a patient seen once or twice a week for several years may do better than one seen four or five times a week for a shorter period. Although there should be no discrimination against psychoanalysis as a treatment method, there is a real need to set realistic limits on frequency. It is my firm conviction that fewer sessions will not impair the health or the progress of the patient.

Dr. Upton adds a disturbing footnote in regard to the APA's peer review program for a large insurance company, which, he states, appears to be biased in favor of psychoanalysts as opposed to psychiatrists who are not analysts. If his observations can be confirmed, this would be a serious miscarriage of professional judgment. It would even appear to be self-defeating for organized psychiatry to give preferential treatment to psychoanalysis, if Dr. Upton's description of it as "the most expensive and often least effective, in my opinion, of all long-term intensive outpatient treatments" is true.

Dr. Upton goes on to say: "Organized psychiatry must be willing to air the possibility that psychoanalysis may be unnecessary, in addition to being cost-ineffective, for many, but certainly not all, patients." I would go even further and suggest that organized psychiatry also consider the possibility that psychoanalysis, inappropriately applied, not only may be unnecessary but may do actual harm. This is not stated as a criticism of psychoanalysis as a treatment modality. The same *caveat* may be issued in regard to any psychiatric treatment method. The old maxim that any treatment with the power to do good has also the power to do harm applies here. Take penicillin, for example. Thousands of people owe their health, even their lives, to this remarkable antibiotic. Yet each year scores of patients die due to allergic reactions to penicillin. There is no doubt that psychoanalytic treatment has improved the lives and the mental health of innumerable people, but when used inappropriately, it, too, may do serious damage. The same caution applies to other types of psychotherapy and to chemotherapy as well.

I agree wholeheartedly with Dr. Upton that guidelines are desperately needed for setting the optimal frequency of treatment sessions in psychotherapy, difficult though this task will be. But if Dr. Upton is correct in his assessment that "organized psychiatry," perhaps influenced by those analysts who hold positions of leadership, has chosen to present a "united view" endorsing the viability of all treatment methods currently practiced, including psychoanalysis, then treatment guidelines will continue to develop on a *laissez-faire* basis. I question whether it is realistic to expect any agreement on treatment guidelines regarding the optimal frequency of treatment sessions unless and until the psychoanalysts on the decision-making commission abandon their parochial rigidities and take a more global view of the problem.

Some of Dr. Upton's fears regarding the reluctance of insurance carriers to foot the bill for outpatient psychotherapy are already being justified. For example, he refers to a study of the Blue Cross/Blue Shield FEHB plan under which the patient is allowed "unlimited treatment visits to private providers of psychiatric care, the insurance covering 80% of the cost of treatment after a $100 deductible fee is paid by the patient." This *was* indeed true at the time of the study on which Dr. Upton reports. Since then, as Dr. Upton notes, the benefits have been reduced from 80% to 70%, presumably to permit adding dental care benefits. Although proponents of this change point out that it represents only a 10% reduction in psychiatric benefits, it really represents a 50% *increase* in what the individual patient must pay. So we see once again that outpatient mental health care is being discriminated against.

I am glad that Dr. Upton encourages the increased use of self-help groups such as Alcoholics Anonymous, *et al.* I would add to his list Recovery, Inc., an organization that has had a remarkably good record of enabling patients and former patients to help each other and, while so doing, help themselves.

Up to now, I have tried to point out some of the strengths and some of the weaknesses of Dr. Upton's arguments for equal coverage for mental illness under NHI. Although I, too, support the concept of equal coverage, I recognize that there must be some control when a third party is paying the bill. But these controls should be similar to those that apply to medicine and surgery and should not discriminate against patients in need of psychiatric care. In 1975 when the results of the JIS survey on the private office practice of psychiatry were published, I was pleased to note that the average frequency of treatment (combining data from both analysts and nonanalysts) was one visit per week. The data provided by this survey confirmed my own experience that most cases can be and are treated at the frequency of one session per week. Therefore, when I suggest that any viable NHI plan should pay for a maximum of 50 sessions (1 hour each) per year, I do not think we are setting unrealistic standards. Special situations that might require more frequent sessions could be settled by peer review.

I am painfully aware that the establishment of maximum limits is often subject to abuse. The maximum very quickly tends to become the minimum. Nonetheless, we could treat a far greater number of patients with our limited mental health manpower if we adopted these reasonable limitations.

In addition to recommending payment for 50 full outpatient visits a year, I would also recommend that there be no limit to the overall length of psychotherapy. This may startle some, buy my recommendation is based on many years of practice and close observation of patients in therapy. Even those who are paying for all or a substantial part of the cost may still need long periods of supportive treatment after the acute symptoms have subsided, in order to prevent relapse or the development of substitute symptoms. Sometimes therapy may last as long as 3 or 4 years, and in some cases even longer. To prevent any open-ended abuse of this provision, it would be relatively simple to require all cases remaining in therapy over 3 or 4 years to undergo peer review.

Dr. Upton has rendered America, and especially the countless thousands of its citizens who would benefit by mental health care, a great service by pleading their cause with rare eloquence. If he has overstated his case at times, it is not for the sake of the mental health professionals but for the benefit of the thousands of patients who suffer from mental illness/emotional problems.

References

1. Lebensohn ZM: American psychiatry—Retrospect and prospect. Med Ann DC 16(7):392, 1962.
2. Lebensohn ZM: Pilgrim's progress, or the tortuous road to mental health. Compr Psychiatry 16(5):415–426, 1975.
3. Sharfstein S, Taube CA, Goldberg ID: Problems in analyzing the comparative costs of private versus public psychiatric care. Am J Psychiatry 132:29–32,1977.
4. Lebensohn ZM: Balancing clinical needs and legal rights. Paper delivered at APA Annual Meeting, Toronto, Canada, May 5, 1977.
5. Kety SS: From rationalization to reason. Am J Psychiatry 131:959, 1974.
6. Siegler M: A physician's perspective on a right to health care. J Am Med Assoc 244(14):1591, 1980.
7. Marmor J, Scheidemandel PL, Kann CK: Psychiatrists and Their Patients. A National Study of Private Office Practice. Washington DC, Joint Information Service of the American Psychiatric Association and the National Association for Mental Health, 1975.
8. Lebensohn ZM: Commentary on psychiatrists and their patients, in Marmor J, et al: A National Study of Private Office Practice. Washington DC, Joint Information Service, 1975, p.174.
9. Freud S: Psychoanalysis—Freudian school. Encyclopedia Britannica, ed 14. New York and Chicago, vol 18 p 674.

Judd Marmor

Dr. Upton's paper is a timely and important contribution to the clarification of the most pressing issues facing our nation in the years ahead. Mental and emotional illness imposes an enormous economic drain upon our economy, even more so if untreated. The simple truth is that ignoring it does not cause it or its consequences to disappear.

The age is long past when we, as a nation, can afford to forget or disregard the many millions of Americans who are affected, directly or indirectly, by the destructive impact of mental illness. Providing mental health services for our mentally and emotionally disturbed citizens, who make up no less than 10% of our population, does not constitute a luxurious self-indulgence on the part of our society. We can appreciate the fiscal restraints that make legislators reluctant to add or increase such services in legislative proposals. However, failure to provide such services inevitably reflects itself, as Dr. Upton points out, in higher costs of other medical services. It is well known that more than half of all patients who consult other physicians because of physical symptoms have substantial mental or emotional problems contributing to their complaints. More often than not, no organic basis can be found for their symptoms, but their use of diagnostic tests, in-hospital studies, and even occasional unnecessary surgery adds substantially to the cost of medical care. Moreover, in the absence of the indicated psychiatric treatment, it can be a recurring cost year after year.

Failure to provide such needed mental health services is also reflected in other significant indirect costs to society that are incalculable but nevertheless real. Without assuming that mental illness is the only, or even the major, factor in such social problems as juvenile delinquency, crime, violence, work inefficiency, and job absenteeism, there is no doubt that it does play a significant contributory role and that its indirect cost to society in these areas can be enormous. Add to this the cost of long-term mental hospitalization, which can often be prevented by early psychiatric treatment and aftercare, and it

Judd Marmor • School of Medicine, University of California at Los Angeles, Los Angeles, California 90024.

becomes clear that providing adequate mental services is not an indulgence but a wise investment.

It is worth noting in this context that psychiatry has made notable advances in the treatment of mental disorders in the past few decades—a fact that the public at large, as well as some of our legislators, seem to be unaware of. To mention just several—there are fewer patients in mental hospitals today than there were 15 years ago, despite the fact that our population has increased by 20 million during that period. The length of mental hospitalization has been dramatically shortened by the introduction of new and potent psychopharmacological agents; the development of group techniques have made psychotherapy available to greater numbers of people at lower costs; and techniques of individual psychotherapy have become more effective, utilizing fewer visits to accomplish comparable results. The average annual number of office visits to all psychiatrists, excluding only long-term intensive psychoanalytic treatment, has been shown to be not more than 39[1]—a figure that we believe is actuarially quite feasible in any national health insurance plan.

In recent years the vast majority of legislators on Capital Hill have come to recognize that adequate provision for treatment of mental illness is both necessary and desirable. Unhappily, however, when they are faced with the pressure of so-called political realities, this laudable objective tends to be sidetracked. For example, in the 97th Congress, the major health insurance proposals (all based on a "competition" model) either explicitly or implicitly restrict or eliminate altogether coverage of psychiatric illness. The Gephardt/ Stockman bill eliminates *per se* the coverage of psychiatric disorders from the minimum benefit package. Senator Durenberger's bill, on the other hand, takes Medicare as its basic benefit package and, while not eliminating psychiatric treatment *per se*, would limit services to the same arbitrary and discriminatory $250 per year outpatient and 190-day lifetime inpatient levels dictated by Medicare. In addition, proposals for catastrophic insurance introduced in the 96th Congress (1979–1980) did not provide satisfactorily for the treatment of mental illness as a catastrophic illness. In the Long–Ribicoff proposal, a family outside of the federally assisted category cannot qualify for catastrophic insurance if a member of the family is mentally ill, because nothing over $500 incurred for the outpatient treatment of such illness can be counted toward the $3500 expenditure that is required to qualify for such catastrophic coverage. This means that such a person, or family, would have to be treated for a "physical" illness for the next $3000 of expense in order to then be able to qualify for catastrophic insurance for further outpatient treatment. This almost forces the practicing physician to find some physical justification for the patient's disability in order to obtain relief for a suffering patient and his family. Public policy should not force the physician into such an untenable dilemma. Limiting psychiatric coverage *per se* does not cut costs because treatment for the psychiatric disorder tends to go on anyway, but under such circumstances it is rendered by a nonpsychiatric physician and is then covered under general benefits for physician service. Thus, the consequences of limiting mental health services coverage is simply to push patients toward practitioners who are less well trained and less qualified to treat the particular problem. In short, if serious mental and emotional illness is ignored on the basis that it will cost too much to treat such people, we will often unwittingly create additional economic burdens for society and lessen or eliminate such individuals' ability to carry on as productive members of society. We treat people every day in our practices who are maintained through some minimal type of psychiatric and supportive treatment that keeps them on the rolls as taxpayers and producers rather than as wards of the state. In the long run, this represents a saving to the state rather than an additional expense.

A similar problem exists in the limitations for the treatment of mental and emotional illness in Medicare. Restricted psychiatric outpatient benefit in Medicare tends to force these patients into inpatient treatment. This not only is more expensive but runs counter to the current philosophy of trying to treat patients on an outpatient basis within the community and to prevent hospitalization wherever possible. This emphasis on outpatient treatment is consistent with the report of the Committee on Ways and Means in HR 17550 in 1970 "to create incentives to encourage outpatient services and disincentives for long stays in institutional settings."

Still another inequity in the Medicare system that will not work in the long run is the 190-day lifetime limitation for treatment of mental illness in psychiatric hospitals, although there is no such limitation for similar treatment in general hospitals. Actually, the cost in general hospitals is more expensive generally than in psychiatric hospitals and, moreover, it is usually antitherapeutic to force a patient to shift from one institution to another in the middle of his illness.

In recent years progress has been made in various legislative proposals introduced in Congress with regard to comprehensive National Health Insurance. Many leading legislators have come forth with support for nondiscriminatory treatment of mental and emotional illness in a National Health Insurance program. The American Psychiatric Association has strongly supported this position as a matter of basic principle.

At the same time, the American Psychiatric Association clearly recognizes and strongly emphasizes the importance of accountability to make such a program workable. It has been placing great emphasis on peer review as an integral part of a National Health Insurance program, with review of both inpatient and outpatient treatment by local committee of peers. Its model of psychiatric peer review calls for concurrent review at the beginning of treatment, again at an established median point of treatment for that specific condition, and again at twice the median if the patient still requires treatment beyond the second point of review. Such a second level of review would involve detailed examination by the Peer Review Committee, which would then authorize a longer period of treatment only if clearly indicated.

Still another aspect of the American Psychiatric Association's position on

National Health Insurance is its opposition to deductibles and coinsurance in the treatment of the mentally ill, if such copayments are not part and parcel of the entire health care system. The inclusion of such copayments under mental health services is not opposed if they are part of the total system, but it is the association's position that with regard to mental health services such copayments should not be required until after the first 10 outpatient visits. The reason for this is that copayments before the first 10 visits would tend to discourage the early psychiatric intervention that is so essential to the treatment of mental illness. After the first 10 visits, coinsurance ought to be on a sliding scale based on ability to pay, or else limited to 20% of the charge.

The American Psychiatric Association is dedicated to the goal of insuring excellence of care to psychiatric patients to the fullest extent that is humanly possible within our present limitations of knowledge. It would like to see ended, once and for all, the discrimination that exists in the treatment of the mentally ill. We know that many people urgently need psychiatric treatment and are unable to avail themselves of it for economic reasons. Living as we do in a technologically highly advanced nation, rich in natural resources and deeply steeped in humanistic traditions of freedom and equality, we cannot afford to deny to substantial numbers of our fellow citizens the right to such treatment simply because of their inability to pay for it. It is high time to make this important social objective a reality.

Reference

1. Marmor J, Scheidemandel PL, Kann CK: Psychiatrists and Their Patients: A National Study of Private Office Practice. Washington DC, Joint Information Service, 1975.

Philip R. A. May

David Upton's thoughtful and comprehensive discussion of national insurance for mental health care is timely and everywhere to the point. Even where one might not agree, it must be admitted that the issues raised are valid and important for public debate and informed decision. If we may not achieve an ideal system, let us at least try to learn from our own previous mistakes and to avoid those that have been made in other countries. This commentary will focus on two major concerns—care for the elderly, and care for psychotic (mentally ill) patients.

Dr. Upton's onslaught on the mistakes of Medicare correctly depicts "how easily inadequate health insurance can be legislated and instituted" and how the elderly have been systematically discriminated against by placing arbitrary limitations on their care if they are not likely to recover to full functioning—precisely when one would have thought that humanitarian and compassionate concerns would require skilled care.

To the list of serious Medicare mistakes, I would add that there is a major flaw in payment procedures. The Medicare system permits, even condones, what can be described, at best, as unthinking delay and underpayment to patients and, at worst, as flagrant cheating of patients out of their rights. Elderly persons and the mentally ill often accept with silent resignation insurance companies' arbitrary and unjust decisions not to pay their claims. Timid, uncertain, confused and bewildered, unable to fully comprehend the wording of the policy and the booklets, ignorant of medical terminology, cowed by the authoritarian reasons for the denial, beset by impressive and demanding forms, weakened by illness, alone and unaided, they have neither the will nor the capacity to stand up for their rights and pursue vigorously the correction of an unjust denial. Such claims are paid only if their cause is championed by a determined and knowledgeable friend or relative—or by an attorney.

The plain facts are that insurance companies are in business to make money. They make more if claims are delayed or denied, and it costs them

Philip R. A. May • Neuropsychiatric Institute, Center for Health Sciences, University of California, Los Angeles, California 90024.

nothing if claims are subjected to interminable review and grueling paper work—the cost is passed on to the taxpayer or the insured. We cannot therefore expect the insurance companies to help the elderly and the mentally ill to assert their rights. Nor can we reasonably expect busy doctors and office staff to assume the task of investigating unpaid claims. There is a need for a system to monitor, review, and audit all claims denied to such persons to insure that their rights are protected, that claims are not denied when they should be paid, and that they are not taken advantage of by the insurance companies. And the system should contain severe penalties for companies that willfully deny claims, or obstruct the process by self-serving paper work.

This is a special need and it needs special action. The Veterans Administration has representatives who help veterans get the benefits that are their due—we need a similar service for the elderly and the mentally ill. There are already "advocates" who watch out for the rights of the mentally ill in respect to informed consent to treatment and participation in research, their activities might be expanded to include vigorous pursuit of patients' insurance rights. Better, however, to have an *independent* system with the full legal right to audit and monitor the insurance companies' records.

Turning now to Dr. Upton's thesis that a restricted definition of what is medical care could be costly and self-defeating. One of the greatest needs of the elderly and the mentally ill is for rehabilitation and social support services. In these respects, current care is, at best, fragmented and erratic; at worst, it is a disgrace. It is no good setting up a "health care" system for this group unless steps are taken to insure adequate rehabilitation and social support services such as home-finding, homemaking, shopping, social services, transportation, telephone, meals, recreation, etc. Keeping people alive is one thing; at least equally important, I think, is the need to do something about their quality of life. As Dr. Upton points out, medical technology is fantastically expensive. There must be hard thinking as to whether it is better for patients and their close ones to fund costly high-powered prolongation of life or to spend the money on improving their quality of life while they are still able to enjoy it.

Finally, Dr. Upton calls for the preservation under National Health Insurance of the existing dualistic public and private health delivery systems. I think it particularly important here to avoid the British mistake of fostering a split between public and private care. If a person can afford it and wants to pay for some or all of his own care privately, that should be seen as a blessing and as a relief to the load on the system. But it should not be allowed to reduce a person's entitlement to public services when the services in question are not available or not affordable privately. Private patients and private practitioners should have full access, without discrimination, to the entire range of social support and rehabilitation and special psychiatric services that are available in the public sector. The revolving door that Dr. Upton refers to does not revolve exclusively because of failure in the medical system; it revolves at least as much due to failures in social support and rehabilitation.

By contrast, Dr. Upton gives little space to the potential role of the public hospital. Perhaps he is realistic; perhaps there is indeed no escape from their vicious cycle of scandalous neglect and underfunding. I would not, however, wish to be so pessimistic. As I see it, many of the real advances in the treatment of severe mental illness have started in such hospitals—and the staff there are at least willing to take on the task of treating chronic mental illness, which is more than can be said for some of those at CMHCs (Community Mental Health Centers). The time has come when hospitals should be allowed—nay, encouraged—to compete with CMHCs for program funding, with the decisions made on the basis of merit for the patient, rather than by ideology. There might even be funding for two alternative systems, hospital-based and CMHCs. Let the system that is best for the patient win in healthy competition.

This in no way detracts from the force of Dr. Upton's observation that it is important and cost-effective to fund outpatient treatment, and not to follow the old system of prolonging inpatient care. Excessive cost can be avoided, however, only if the right patients are treated in the right way by the right people. The urgent need is to provide outpatient care for chronic disabling disorders as an alternative to hospitalization, not to provide outpatient care for some other group that has no immediate need for hospital care and whose future need for such care is problematic.

Mildred Mitchell-Bateman

I find it very hard to write this commentary without being redundant, because so much of what Dr. Upton has written expresses and supports my views on the philosophical issues surrounding the financing of mental health care. Since this is the case, perhaps my best contribution to the usefulness of Dr. Upton's white paper would be to highlight, reemphasize, and editorialize upon the crucial points. One hopes that Dr. Upton's paper and the commentaries in this book will undergird the work of those who will be formulating policy on mental health care coverage under National Health Insurance.

The phrase "too little, too late" best expresses the nature of the care too many emotionally disturbed and mentally ill persons receive. How often do we struggle to help a fractured family reconstitute itself after a teenage member serves as the focal point for eruptions and disruptions that thrust the family into a maze of police, courts, lawyers, and social and psychiatric areas of care? As the tangled family relationships become teased out, it begins to be clear that the teenager, and probably family members at some point in their development, failed to receive appropriate professional attention at the appropriate time. When early symptoms of mental illness or emotional problems appeared in the teenager, he (she) received no professional attention or, at best, very little attention—resulting in an incomplete resolution at his symptoms. Even as the teenager's symptoms became more flagrant, the treatment he received, if any, remained superficial and temporizing in character. Finally, and only after a very serious or tragic event, did the teenager receive the "full attention" of a mental health professional. Of course, by this point, the teenager and perhaps other family members, required intensive mental health care and perhaps other social services as well—with great expenditures of time and effort from helping sources.

Financing of mental health care is traditionally not designed to encourage or assist with the delivery of early and appropriate professional care. As a matter of fact, extensive coverage for mental health care often becomes avail-

Mildred Mitchell-Bateman • Department of Psychiatry, Marshall University School of Medicine, Huntington, West Virginia 25701.

able only when a "problem" has become so severe that a person has to be hospitalized for treatment. On the other hand, we now face the situation where in many instances even the availability of hospital care for mental illness will be in short supply. It is likely that it will be increasingly more difficult to convince utilization review committees that inpatient care is appropriate for a given patient.(For example, when a patient demonstrates even the slightest ability to "live" outside the hospital, he may be denied inpatient treatment.) Furthermore, the fact is that even when coverage for hospital care is available for a given patient, it is often limited. The treating physician (psychiatrist) must always be mindful of the 20- or 30-day limits on coverage for treatment of mental illness that many patients face. Often, since the psychiatrist wants to spare the patient a loss of coverage for another acute episode of mental illness, he is forced to discharge the patient prematurely. The result is that the patient receives inadequate care. It isn't any wonder, therefore, that some patients become chronically mentally ill, or at least chronically dysfunctional. Comprehensive mental health care, including inpatient care when it is necessary, is simply not available to them. Consequently, many patients suffer acute, severe, and numerous recurrences of their illnesses. The outlay of professional services for such patients escalates and eventually becomes highly expensive. But such outlays must really be categorized as "too late."

I shall now return to the task of commenting on the very timely white paper that Dr. Upton has prepared.

As one reads the Overview of Dr. Upton's paper, it soon becomes clear that Dr. Upton has carefully analyzed the inadequacies of (1) coverage for mental illness under existing health care plans and insurance, including Medicare, Medicaid, and Health Maintenance Organizations (MHOs), and (2) mental health care coverage in current proposals for legislation that would establish National Health Insurance (NHI). As a result of Dr. Upton's analysis, the reader can easily come to the conclusion that if current plans for NHI are an indication of what may eventually be enacted as NHI legislation, there is a real danger that mental health care under NHI will have serious limitations. These limitations, as Dr. Upton states, could "result in a rigid, monolithic clinical approach to most patients in contrast to a more diversified approach where each patient is treated according to his or her unique, specific needs."

The overriding question, of course, is why it is that mental health care is consistently low on the totem pole for its appropriate share of health dollar expenditures. The President's Commission on Mental Health noted in its report that the percentage of persons requiring some type of mental health care is closer to 15%, rather than the 10% estimate relied upon for so long. Yet expenditures for mental health care have consistently remained at 12% of the total health care dollar.

While a little progress has been made in expanding private health insurance coverage for care of mental illness, such coverage still remains limited when compared to coverage for physical illness. In addition, the unwholesome features of poor coverage for outpatient mental health care services and alternatives to inpatient (hospital) mental health care have been retained—even when coverage for mental health care has been expanded.

While the president's commission did fail to provide a detailed model for NHI legislation, it did enunciate principles and recommend certain policies relative to coverage for mental health care. Space here does not permit full development of a rationale in support of such principles and policies. In many respects, however, Dr. Upton has done an excellent job in providing the substantive discussion needed to understand them. Further, Dr. Upton has been able to restate and markedly improve upon policy in certain areas (see Chapters 3 and 5).

In Dr. Upton's view, persons should not be excluded from receiving mental health care because they have a condition or a "diagnosis" that makes them ineligible for such care. Rather, Dr. Upton feels that eligibility for mental health care should be based on the degree of pain and disability from which patients suffer. The importance of making *comprehensive* treatment resources available under NHI becomes apparent under this philosophy since many forms of mental illness and emotional disorder require broad-based and multidimensional care.

Dr. Upton's discussion of who should provide mental health care is organized around the roles and functions of "private providers" and "public sector providers." Dr. Upton notes that coverage for mental health care, under plans for NHI, is unlimited at the Community Mental Health Center (CMHC); he also notes that coverage for "private care" is limited under these same plans, with the patient being allowed only a certain number of "visits" for care. The careful analysis in Dr. Upton's paper of the nature of care available in both the public and private sectors draws out the deficiencies and strengths that each of the sectors offers. An additional point I would like to make here is that the patient has no clear way of flowing from one sector into the other in order to benefit from the specific type of care he (she) may need. For example, the "private care" patient now treated intensively on an inpatient basis for a schizophrenic episode would require a much shorter hospital stay if he could have access to a partial hospitalization program as administered by a CMHC. At least two factors have worked to prevent this: (1) Insurance coverage does not usually extend to partial hospitalization, and (2) many patients are reluctant to seek treatment outside of their ongoing "one-on-one" psychotherapy and many psychiatrists are reluctant to encourage their patients to do so.

As we work to improve insurance coverage for mental illness, there are great advantages to be gained by increasing the availability to patients of all modalities of treatment—regardless of the unit under which any particular modality is administered. However, at the same time that we work to correct funding mechanisms for mental health care so that a full range of services are covered, we must also develop quality control measures for mental health care. We should clarify the indications for specific modalities of treatment. This means we must measure the effects of particular treatments on the widest variety of conditions.

I would like to see a really no-holds-barred, in-depth look at that "other part" of the mental health care delivery system that even Dr. Upton has discussed all to briefly in his otherwise very careful and detailed look at who should provide mental health care. While it seems reasonable to assume, as Dr. Upton does, that "under NHI, funding of public hospitals will have to increase from present levels in order to provide responsible patient care," it should be noted that Medicare and Medicaid did increase the level of funding of many state hospitals. It is true that Medicare and Medicaid dramatically raised the quality of care many hospitals delivered. Yet there came a point when legislators and budget administrators started to balk at the rises in *per diem* patient care expenditures in the hospitals. (The state hospital's budget often suffers from too much visibility of the details of the hospital's operation. The "total care" that the hospital seeks to deliver to its patients is insufficiently appreciated.) With the plight of mental patients residing in the community becoming ever more visible, the "obvious" solution seemed to be to shift dollars from hospital to community-based care. This was done in many cases. Unfortunately, however, it often led to inadequate funding of both hospital care and community-based care. In addition, although the CMHC was seen as the new primary locus of treatment for the patient, it was not prepared to handle the chronic mental patient (due to the lack of training of staff and the attitudinal set of staff, as well). Indeed, the CMHC often continued to view the patient as the responsibility of the state hospital. (Reimbursement through Medicaid was not available to the CMHC for long-term care of the chronically mentally ill patient outside of the hospital.)

To recapitulate, when hospital *per diem* rates for patient care began to rise under Medicare and Medicaid, it often happened that hospital budgets were cut without any real awareness that this would seriously hamper the delivery of quality care to those patients who still had to be treated in hospitals. On the other hand, monies "saved" from cutbacks in funding of hospitals did not always find its way into community-based mental health programs. During its public hearings, the President's Commission on Mental Health heard example after example of situations where reductions in budgets of state hospitals did not result in shifts of funds to community-based operations.

Low levels of funding of public hospitals often make it impossible for these institutions to provide their patients with a total approach to mental health care that utilizes multiple modalities of treatment applied over proper intervals of time. (At the moment, such complete, comprehensive care is available primarily only to the affluent through private psychiatric institutions.) Too often the public hospital finds itself in the position of having to say to the patient, "Sorry, never mind what care you need. Since your illness didn't respond to treatment within the time allowed, you'll have to get your care somewhere else." The hospital staff treating this hypothetical, but very real, patient may actually convince themselves that outpatient treatment will be better for him (or her) anyway. They will develop with the patient a rationalization for outpatient care that is in fact therapeutically faulty. The patient may indeed continue to do well on an outpatient basis and thus make the staff happy by relieving their guilt (at having to discharge the patient prematurely and being unable to provide him with the care he needs). On the other hand, the patient's level of "wellness" may turn out to be superficial. Chronic mental illness may begin to grow in him like a cancer.

How, then, can we insure that public hospitals will be able to deliver full and complete mental health care to those persons who require their services? Could public hospitals be converted by administrative fiat to private nonprofit or even for-profit institutions? Could states then convert their current institutional budgets into purchase of service dollars? Would this not allow states to architect better Medicaid programs and vastly improve their own policy and programs for medical care for indigent mentally ill patients? (Currently, such patients are often inappropriately cared for in general hospitals and nursing homes.)

It is conceivable that even the most financially deprived and poorly run state hospital, if given a budget tied into reimbursement dollars as opposed to a fixed budget and freed to generate additional fees for services, could function as a responsive, quality care facility supplying those treatment resources needed by those persons it serves.

Perhaps there are other considerations with regard to how a national health insurance program will affect the delivery of mental health care in the public institutional sector. Unfortunately, we see little being written or talked about with regard to the effect NHI will have on that sector. Indeed, it seems likely that NHI will force many public hospitals into a "reactive position." They will be forced to meet expectations about their role that have not been spelled out and that really may be totally inappropriate. It is not improbable that under NHI, many public hospitals may be asked to "go away—disappear." They may be legislated out of existence. Yet, we are aware of the rather painful and undesirable consequences for many patients and the communities within which they reside when hospital closings have not been planned with a total awareness of the pressures such closings place on both patients and their communities.

I would like to see some thought given within the current health insurance structure to the conversion of public hospitals to private hospitals that I mentioned above. There are many public hospitals that still provide a great deal of acute mental health care. (This factor is often overlooked by those who indiscriminately reduce the budgets of public hospitals.) Projections need to be made as to how much of this function would shift to the private sector if acute hospital care were properly covered by NHI. If it can be ascertained that public hospitals would continue to provide acute mental health care under NHI, then their conversion *now* to private nonprofit institutions might be reasonable and feasible.

A word about the "acceptability" of inpatient psychiatric treatment in the public hospital. Patients' rights legislation and hospital administrative policy designed to insure patients' rights have too often resulted in premature discharge of patients from inpatient care. Longer hospital stays would seem to be indicated for many patients. One wonders if patients of public hospitals, and the communities these hospitals serve, would not be better off if the hospital were to function as a "community operation" rather than "the state or the county" institution.

Shifting from the issue of the public hospital's role and place in the provision of mental health care, Dr. Upton's examination of the functions of the various mental health professionals is quite valuable for its clarity. Most discussions of the roles and functions of the various mental health professionals have shed more heat than light. Dr. Upton helps to pull us in from the extremes in either direction. At the risk of overkill on the subject, I would like to expand upon a few of Dr. Upton's concepts. Dr. Upton states, "We have as yet no precise measuring stick that allows us to judge the quality of psychotherapy the individual mental health professional provides, whatever the particular profession." In this connection, solo practitioners, because they often practice in isolation, are especially vulnerable to the development of "blind spots" in their clinical approach to their patients. For this reason, I believe it would be useful if some mechanism could be developed to check or review the work of all psychotherapists engaged in solo practice. This would be different from "peer review," which takes a more procedural look at the treatment a practitioner delivers to a patient, rather than a look at treatment content, the therapeutic relationship itself, and the quality of treatment outcome for the patient.

I would also note that psychotherapy, as a treatment method, can be harmful to the patient's health on occasion! This can occur, for example, if a particular psychotherapist, in treating a patient who suffers physical symptoms, does not pay sufficient attention to the psychological components of physical illness or to the possibility that mental illness or emotional problems can cause physical symptoms. I should also emphasize here that multimodal approaches to mental health care are indicated for many patients, often including somatic treatment. Therefore, without the psychiatrist's involvement in treatment planning (including periodic review of the actual treatment a patient receives), many patients will not receive appropriate mental health care. It may be said that the patient who is not exposed to a psychiatrist in the course of his care is receiving "psychological treatment" or "counseling," or even health care; however, we should distinguish this from comprehensive treatment and rehabilitation for "mental illness/emotional problems."

In his white paper, Dr. Upton has enunciated what many would agree are the appropriate standards for treating person who suffer mental illness/emotional problems. Yet the fact is that there is a shortage of psychiatrists; there are not enough psychiatrists to adequately staff CMHCs and public mental hospitals. Given this reality, should we continue to ascribe an essential role to the psychiatrist as regards the provision of mental care? Indeed, in many settings, nonpsychiatrist physicians function to prescribe psychotropic medications to patients; in addition, they handle other medical aspects of health care for the particular mental health facility with which they are associated. Still, it cannot be denied that the psychiatrist's presence in a leadership role leads to quality mental health care. (At least, many models of mental health care would promote this premise.) I should stress that even when the psychiatrist functions in a leadership role, care must be taken to integrate those functions with the functions of other mental health professionals.

In our concern for the great shortages in the numbers of psychiatrists and psychiatric nurses, we must not neglect to inform health policy-makers of the importance of maintaining training support for other mental health professionals and paraprofessionals. It will be extremely difficult at best to provide quality mental health care under NHI if we do not promote the training of *all* mental health professionals. We must insure that there are sufficient numbers of mental health professionals and paraprofessionals of all types so that the patient can be afforded a multidisciplinary treatment approach to his illness. (This raises the issue of fiscal support for nonreimbursable costs of all medical care. Under NHI, how will staff educational costs be funded?)

With regard to the costs of mental health care, the reader is referred to Chapter 2, entitled "Mental Illness/Emotional Problems: The Prevalence and the Cost." There is no doubt as to the costliness of treatment for mental illness/emotional problems, but there still seems to be a gross lack of awareness of the greater cost of nontreatment or inadequate treatment.

A lawyer was asked recently on a radio talk show how a jury or court arrives at a monetary award for personal injury. In replying, the attorney stated that in addition to calculating the cost of treatment a persons requires, an effort is made to estimate the injured person's earning capacity over his or her expectant life-span and to consider this in the context of his family role. (For example, is the person the main source of financial support for the family?) This factor, plus the added financial and psychological stress and strain on the family of caring for the injured family member (perhaps on a long-term basis if the person is permanently handicapped) must be taken into account by the court in determining a judgment. In a similar vein, we should consider the cost of mental illness/emotional problems to be not only the cost of treatment for a person over time but also the loss in his potential earning power over time, as a contributing member of society, that results from his illness.

I heartily concur with the case that Dr. Upton makes throughout his white paper for "full treatment" of mental illness/emotional problems. Coverage for such illness/problems should be on a par with that which is accorded for medical illness. Furthermore, we should have a policy of not requiring a patient to pay an initial deductible for outpatient care, or at the least a very minimal initial deductible. This should be a guiding principle with regard to insuring all health care in order to encourage a patient to seek early and appropriate treatment. The requirement of modest copayments on the part of the patient for *all* outpatient care could, under certain circumstances, foster individual responsibility on the part of the patient for appropriately limiting his care. To reemphasize, such copayments, if instituted, should be required for all types of medical care. A policy of limiting outpatient visits for mental health care and requiring larger copayments on the part of the patient for psychiatric outpatient care would be counterproductive. If such a policy was instituted, many patients would delay obtaining timely therapeutic intervention. As a result, many patients would eventually require hospital care for their mental illness/emotional problems.

As we work to remove discrimination in health care legislation against the mentally ill, we must carefully examine all aspects of both federal and state health care policy that would impede rather than foster the development of a mental health care system responsive to the health care needs of all persons.

Morris B. Parloff

From time to time psychotherapy researchers have complained that their findings have not impacted sufficiently on the practitioner or on the policy-maker. We have carped that our voices have not been heard in high councils and that our wisdom has gone unrecognized and unrequited by the government decision-makers. I regret to inform you that those idyllic days are now gone. We can no longer be confident that our papers will be read only by fellow researchers. Policy-makers are reading our reports, and the clinicians are listening.

Some may be cheered, as I am, to learn that our research efforts are being attended to in the real world rather than merely in the cloistered halls and minds of academia. It is my purpose, however, not to dwell on the celebration but to invite the consideration of some of the sobering implications of having even our most tentative and preliminary findings interpreted directly, not by sophisticated, research-wise investigators but by novices. Of particular concern is the potential soundness or unsoundness of the inferences that the policy-maker may draw from research evidence in making decisions that may materially affect the field of psychotherapy. I say "materially" because I mean to include a range of consequences, but especially the crassly material ones—health costs, grant funding opportunities, third-party reimbursements, etc. The policy-maker's decisions may affect clients, patients, practitioners, and researchers today and in fiscal years to come.

This paper, which is in the public domain, was made available for this volume by the author. It was originally presented as the presidential address, 9th Annual Meeting of the Society for Psychotherapy Research, Toronto, Canada, 1978, and first appeared as "Can Psychotherapy Research Guide The Policy Maker?—A Little Knowledge May Be a Dangerous Thing," *American Psychologist* 34, no. 4 (April, 1979). Opinions expressed herein are those of the author and do not necessarily reflect the official position of the National Institute of Mental Health.

Morris B. Parloff • Chief, Psychosocial Treatments Research Branch, Division of Extramural Research Programs, National Institute of Mental Health, U.S. Department of Health and Human Services, Rockville, Maryland 20910

Policy decisions will be made in part on the basis of our research and in part on value judgments regarding need and technical and political feasibility. I anticipate that the researcher need now be preoccupied less with the fear that the clinician will not take his evidence seriously than with the likelihood that the policy-maker will!

I propose here to review the issues that have stimulated this unprecedented interest in our work and to identify the urgent questions that clinicians and policy-makers are addressing to the researcher. I shall then review and anguish a bit about the answers that have recently been made available to them by the report of the President's Commission on Mental Health (PCMH), and finally, I shall offer some recommendations for identifying research priorities and developing mechanisms for providing the decision-makers with carefully evaluated research evidence.

Members of our new audience are raising very pragmatic, prosaic, yet profound questions regarding the efficacy of the wide range of psychosocial interventions currently offered to the public. Clinicians and government officials are experiencing mounting pressures from such not easily disregarded sources as the courts, insurance companies, and national health insurance planners. Third-party payers—ultimately the public—are demanding crisp and informative answers to questions regarding the quality, quantity, durability, safety, and efficiency of psychosocial treatments provided to an ever-widening range of consumers and potential consumers.

As long as the individual was prepared to pay for his own "therapy," it was a matter of considerable indifference—benign and otherwise—to society for what purposes the client sought treatment in the practitioner's office, clinic, classroom, and, more recently, hotel ballroom. It is an individual's inalienable right to seek therapy, self-enhancement, education, enlightenment, and titillation as long as he is willing to pay for it.

Now, however, when society is being asked to pay for psychotherapy, it proposes to exercise its right and responsibility to determine how the terms *health* and *need for services* will be defined, who is qualified to provide such services, and how effective such services are. Society reserves the right to differentiate between those problems that are of public concern—and therefore eligible for public support—and those problems that are viewed as frivolous, "cosmetic," or capriciously "elective."

Particularly in a period when the costs of health care continue to soar, private and public health insurance planners will seek to impose clear and restrictive rules of eligibility on both patient and psychotherapist.

Currently, psychotherapists appear wittingly to treat, manage, and enlighten an increasing range of clients or patients: the disturbed, the disturbing, the demoralized, the disadvantaged, the abused, and the disabused. The aim of normalizing has been augmented by the task of treating the miseries of normalcy, i.e., boredom, stagnation, blocked spontaneity, meaninglessness, and the imperfect sense of personal identity. In addition, the psychotherapist treats the emotional concomitants and sequelae of physical distress and injury. More recently, psychotherapists have responded to calls to use their skills in assisting individuals to control their self-abusive, life-threatening habits of sedentary living, reckless driving, overeating, smoking, drinking, and excessive use of drugs. Currently, too, psychotherapists are asked to "treat" the social problems of crime, delinquency, rape, and racism. Indeed, psychotherapy is viewed as the treatment for all reasons and unreason.

It is currently estimated that 15% of this nation's population may have diagnosable mental disorders per year, although only 3% of the population receives specialized mental health services in any given year.[1] With the expansion of private and public support of health care, it may be anticipated that we will see a sharp increase in the number of patients seeking specialized mental health treatment within the next decade.

The administrator has long been preoccupied with the problems of health services delivery. The aim is to bring community mental health services to the people and the people to the services. This frenetic and costly effort has been predicted on the assumption that the treatments to be delivered have previously been established as useful and effective. Belatedly, the question now being asked is: How effective are these therapies, even under the ideal conditions in which the therapist and patient actually share a common language, cultural background, and biases?

Such questions from policy-makers and administrators are inevitably translated into pressure on the practitioners, who in turn find themselves faced with a related set of questions. Of perhaps the greatest concern to the psychotherapist is the evidence of a growing skepticism regarding the utility of psychotherapy as a treatment approach. Psychotherapists, regardless of their own skepticism about research, are increasingly turning to the researcher in the hope of receiving encouraging and supportive answers to four basic questions persistently raised by the critics of the field: (1) Does the change effected by psychosocial treatments exceed that which may be attributable to the mere passage of time or the individual's own recuperative powers, i.e., what is the role of *spontaneous remission?* (2) Are the effects of psychotherapy attributable to the use of specific techniques clearly differentiable from the influences of so-called nonspecific techniques of suggestion, persuasion, or commonsense advice, i.e., what is the role of *placebo effects?* (3) Does the therapist's effectiveness vary with mastery of specialized techniques and a related body of knowledge, i.e., what is the role of *training?* (4) What is the nature, speed, durability, pervasiveness, safety, and efficiency of the therapeutic amelioration and change that may be effected in the treatment of mental disorders of public health interest, i.e., how *effective* is psychotherapy?

The questions posed to the researcher by the policy-maker and the clinician overlap, particularly in the area of treatment effectiveness; however, the policy-maker has special concerns, among them patient eligibility.

It is recognized that the ultimate decision regarding eligibility for insurance coverage of treatment does not depend on a research-based resolution of the mental health–illness or problems-in-living dichotomy. Eligibility for *reim-*

bursement is a social policy decision. Eligibility for *treatment* is a clinical judgment. Moreover, the weight placed by society on improving the citizen's sense of well-being or increasing the individual's social effectiveness may not be equal.

The health insurance eligibility question is primarily one of value judgment, usually reinforced by political and professional pressures. While I have preferences and convictions, they are not pertinent to my present purpose and will not be further discussed here.

I propose to summarize some answers that research has provided to the aforementioned four questions of the clinician and the policy-maker. Comments on the first three issues—(1) spontaneous remission, (2) placebo effects, and (3) role of training—will be based on our own assessment of the research literature[2] and on the report of the President's Commission on Mental Health.[3] The fourth issue, effectiveness with particular categories of disorders, will be addressed by information derived solely from the commission's report.

Spontaneous Remission

The persistent, recurring question of whether psychotherapy effects are greater than those attributable to spontaneous remission rates continues to be resurrected. This sort of global question presupposes that the improvement rates of all psychotherapy forms, independent of the techniques employed or the particular patient classes treated, are comparable and that all patient classes have comparable rates of so-called spontaneous remission. No such assumptions are warranted. Just as there is no single entity of mental disorders, there is no single spontaneous remission rate (see reference 4, pp. 240–242, and references 5–7). The rate of improvement without formal treatment varies from patient category to category and with the criteria used,[8] source of rating,[9] and measures.[10,11]

A considerable body of research evidence has now been amassed based on studies in which relatively homogeneous groups of patients were randomly assigned to treatment or to no-treatment or wait-list control groups. Such studies attempt to control for the spontaneous remission effect as well as the possible "regression toward the mean" effect. "Regression toward the mean" is a plausible concern since it is recognized that patients tend to enter therapy when they are at a low point with regard to their own chronic, spontaneously fluctuating disorder.

A review of controlled studies permits the conclusion that psychodynamic therapies, client-centered psychotherapy, cognitive therapies, and behavioral therapies have achieved results which are superior to no-treatment procedures. The findings, based on diverse studies using diverse criteria, offer an affirmative global answer to the question of whether psychotherapies are more effective than spontaneous remission rates.[12–16]

A recent review summarized nearly 700 published and unpublished studies, each of which included an untreated group. This design permitted the estimate of relevant rates of spontaneous recovery in each study. It was found that in over 90% of the experiments, the psychotherapy group improved more than the control group. The median person receiving psychotherapy was better off than 80% of the untreated controls.[17] The authors conclude that their survey of research findings overwhelmingly validates the benefit of psychotherapy.[18]

Placebo Effects

The observation that research has demonstrated that a range of psychotherapies are more effective than is the mere passage of time leaves open the question of whether the effects are due primarily to placebo, i.e., suggestion, expectation, hope, cajolery, etc.

This is an area that has not yet been well studied. However, such literature as is available does suggest that treatment effects are usually more powerful than those found in the placebo-control group. [12,13,16,19] The review of psychotherapy research summarized by Glass and Smith[17] concludes that the "placebo effect" was less than half as large as the effects of the other elements in the psychotherapy relationship.

Efforts to control for the placebo effect are, nonetheless, difficult since they presuppose knowledge of the precise mechanisms whereby the so-called specific treatment intervention achieves its potency.[20,21] Such knowledge is not in fact usually available. The placebo in psychotherapy research should ideally be "inert" with regard to such hypothesized specific mechanisms. The usual placebo control study attempts to control for the effects of attention, but this may not be an adequate control either for the other "nonspecific" elements[22-24] that appear to characterize all forms of therapy or for the hypothesized specific elements of the particular therapy under examination.

One of the important dimensions that appears to increase the potency of placebo-controls is its degree of plausibility as a treatment form to the subjects of the study. The more credible the placebo-control intervention, the more closely the placebo effects resemble those of the treatment form with which it is compared.[25] Of increasing interest is the identification of the mechanisms whereby placebos achieve their effects.

It is generally assumed that placebo effects are artifacts and that their positive influences must be substracted from the observed effects of treatment to arrive at the effects attributable to treatment *per se*. This presupposes that placebos operate only in one direction, namely, improvement. Yet it has been observed that some patients in placebo groups tend to become worse (see, e.g., references 20, 22, and 26). Could not some of the reported negative effects of psychotherapy also, then, be due to placebo effects? Similarly, since placebo effects are presumed to be due to suggestion, might not the cognitively oriented therapist now reason that some patients who fail to respond to treatment may simply be giving themselves suggestions that counter the potential effectiveness of psychotherapy? (Shades of psychoanalytic invective regarding the resistant patient!)

My point is simply that the control of placebo effects is a quite complex problem. The definitive answer to the question of the relative role of placebo in various forms of psychotherapy has yet to be achieved.

Perhaps my favorite comment on the difficulty of differentiating the role of placebo—i.e., separating the nonspecific from the so-called specific elements of psychotherapy—is that of Martin Orne,[27] who pointed out that in order for the nonspecific elements to be effective in psychotherapy, the patient must first believe in the potency of its "specific" elements.

Training and Experience

Psychotherapy is not a profession but rather a varied and sometimes ill-defined set of practices engaged in by members of a number of different professions. Each profession requires that its members be trained first and primarily to do something else: medicine, psychology, social work, nursing, or religious ministering. In short, psychotherapy represents ancillary activities engaged in by various professionals whose preparation in the area of psychotherapy may be quite variable.

It is not surprising, therefore, that in the absence of a standardized training program for all psychotherapists across the various professions, the public and the policy-maker should seek assistance from the researcher in distinguishing the possible differences in effectiveness among schools and professions due to differences in training.

Research, unfortunately, provides but little sound evidence on this matter. Comparisons across professions and schools have revealed no characteristic differences (see, e.g., references 12, 28, and 29). While those trained in the application of specific techniques in the treatment of specific problems appear to be more effective in the use of such techniques than those not so trained, there is little evidence that experts of different schools are differentiable in their relative treatment effectiveness.[14,19] Even more troublesome are the findings that some professionally trained therapists, when contrasted with some untrained or minimally trained therapists, appear to achieve comparable results with comparable patients.[30]

Quite apart from the nature of the therapist's training, it is widely believed that length of experience enhances the therapist's "expertness." Careful reviews of the literature suggest only that the therapist's experience level is related to the quality of the therapeutic relationship, but evidence regarding its association with outcome is far less clear.[31,32]

Effectiveness with Specific Categories of Patients

The following is based on the presentation of psychotherapy research evidence as summarized in the report of the President's Commission on Mental Health.[3] In abstracting the salient research findings from the commission's report, I shall purposely abstain from offering any critique in order better to approximate the information as it may appear to the lay reader in its pristine unqualified form.

Schizophrenia

"Treatment [of schizophrenia] by various types of psychotherapy is as yet of unestablished efficacy, although in combination with drug treatment psychotherapy may facilitate recovery and social adaptation" (p. 1694). Examination of "many psychosocial forms of intervention, including milieu therapy, formal individual psychotherapy, formal group therapy, activity groups and 'total push' programs [reveals that] these programs have generally failed to yield results that are equivalent or superior to chemotherapy. In combination with drugs, certain additive or interactive effects appear possible. However, improved personal and social adjustment in the hospital tend to have little or no relationship to subsequent adjustment or length of time in the community. An encouraging exception is a combination of chemotherapy and social learning that has recently been shown to yield improved post-hospital as well as in-hospital functioning with chronic inpatients. For the most part, however, the durability of inpatient treatment effects has been disappointing" (p. 1763).

The foremost contribution of psychosocial treatments has been shown to be improvement in social adjustment, which occurs only when these treatments are combined with maintenance chemotherapy. The benefits of the additional psychosocial treatment, however, seem to take many months to emerge. "There is some evidence that suggests that certain chronic schizophrenics respond adversely to psychological treatments . . ." (p. 1766).

Affective Disorders

"The application and modification of social learning theories to depression have yielded not only etiologic theories, but specific treatment approaches. Although the evidence is in preliminary form, careful experiments have yielded very promising results with depressed patients using such techniques as cognitive/behavioral therapy and social skill therapy" (p. 1702).

"Serious interpersonal conflicts persist long after resolution of symptoms of depression in women, and perhaps in men also. Treatments are currently being designed and tested which address these interpersonal and social problems that are associated with depression" (p. 1703).

Alcoholism

"Follow-up studies generally indicate that failure or success appears independent of the type of treatment received, whether inpatient or outpatient" (p. 1731). It is a general impression that self-help groups such as Alcoholics Anonymous (AA) offer the most successful treatment, but scientific evidence is lacking. What is clear, however, is that many alcoholics are unsuited for AA (p. 1731). There is no ready cure for this severe and pervasive problem.

Drug Abuse

The effectiveness of psychological treatments independent of drug treatment is not established. "The efficacy of innovative treatments such as biofeedback, behavior modification, and behavior therapy has yet to be definitively assessed" (p. 1740).

Neuroses and Personality Disorders

Fears and Phobias. Moderate to severe disabling fears may now be treated by some forms of behavior modification. Systematic desensitization and *in vivo* desensitization or exposure appear to be especially effective. Treatment appears to be more effective when provided in group rather than individual treatment settings. Agoraphobia appears difficult to treat but may be responsive to treatment consisting of 2 or 3 days of prolonged exposure to feared situations. Treatment may be facilitated by the administration of minor tranquilizers, which are then gradually withdrawn (p. 1715).

Obsessive-Compulsive Neuroses. "Although treatment successes are occasionally reported in the literature, there is very little evidence suggesting that drugs or psychotherapy are successful with severe obsessions or compulsions" (p. 1717). ". . . the evidence from initial controlled experiments indicates that preventing the rituals from occurring in a benign atmosphere is an effective treatment for compulsive behavior" (p. 1717). There is less evidence for the effectiveness of this technique in treating obsessions (p. 1717).

Childhood Disorders

Infantile Autism. "Behavioral techniques have been used with dramatic effect for teaching spoken language. However, the procedures are extremely time consuming and costly and, worse yet, may be limited to teaching the child to imitate sounds rather than to develop the complex communicative skills he lacks. Clearly, no great or even modest treatment promise can be held by mental health professionals for children with Infantile Autism" (p. 1708).

Antisocial Disorders. It is estimated that 35–40% of antisocial young-sters will become antisocial adults. The use of the usual psychotherapeutic interventions to prevent this course seems of little use. Effective treatment may require a complete environmental restructuring. ". . . so far, short of removal from an antisocial family, no early psychiatric intervention has been shown to alter the course of this serious disorder" (p. 1709).

Hyperactive Children. While behavioral treatment programs have been of some use, medication has repeatedly been shown to be more effective in dramatically reducing the most disabling symptoms of hyperactive children. "There is no cure nor prevention for the disorder" (p. 1709).

Anxiety Disorders of Childhood. "Though tradition holds that insight psychotherapy is especially well-suited to the treatment of anxiety disorders in children, research data bearing on this important clinical issue are lacking" (p. 1709).
Behavioral techniques have been useful in the treatment of childhood phobic disorders and separation anxiety. In cases of severe separation anx-iety, brief periods of antidepressant medication have been found effective" (p. 1709).

Depression in Childhood. ". . . there is no established therapy for so-called depressed children" (p. 1709).

Learning Disabilities. ". . . in the few studies which have examined the long-term benefits of treatment, gains obtained immediately after the intervention fail to be maintained over time, even for as brief a period as 6–9 months" (p. 1709).

In short, according to the research summaries prepared by the Presi-dent's Commission on Mental Health, evidence regarding the effectiveness of psychotherapy suggests that with patients who present some of the most severe social and public health problems, psychotherapy appears to play but a supportive, habilitative, and rehabilitative role rather than a primary treat-ment role; psychotherapy does not alone appear to be an effective treatment for the symptoms of schizophrenia, manic-depression, autism, alcoholism, or drug abuse. Further, psychotherapy has not yet been shown to be particularly effective in the treatment of severe obsessive-compulsive behaviors in adults nor in the treatment of children with hyperactivity, anxiety, depressive prob-lems, or learning disabilities. The disorders with which psychotherapy may be particularly useful are anxiety states—e.g., fears and phobias—and some nonpsychotic forms of depression. Note, however, that here the reviewers refer primarily to the effectiveness of behavior therapy rather than the usual psychotherapies.

Let us quickly review the answers that researchers have given to these four major questions of the practitioner and the policy-maker: (1) Spontaneous remission effects do not account for the changes observed in treated patients. (2) Studies that controlled for placebo effects suggest that changes associated with treatment are greater than those attributable to placebo. The concept of a placebo control remains ambiguous and, therefore, so does its testing. (3) The role played by specialized training and length of therapist experience in outcome has not been empirically confirmed. (4) While psychotherapy is applied to a wide range of emotional and social disorders, it appears to be most effective as a treatment approach with some forms of anxieties and nonpsychotic depressions. Psychosocial interventions may also be useful in teaching social skills and in habilitating and rehabilitating patients requiring such assistance. Used in combination with drugs, it may also be of help in the treatment of the more severely ill patient.

Discussion

How may these findings impress members of the researchers' new audience? The practitioners will not and should not easily accept the modest assessment of their effectiveness. I anticipate that many practitioners will protest that the listing of problems by discrete diagnostic categories tends to obscure the fact that the preponderance of patients present problems of depression and/or anxiety—problems that the PCMH report acknowledges as appearing to be treated quite effectively. A further problem that inheres in the use of classical diagnostic rubrics is that such classification fails to accommodate the vast numbers of patients/clients treated by most psychotherapists in their day-to-day practice—namely, those who seek and receive assistance for "disabling problems in living," including marital difficulties and vocational uncertainties.

While these anticipated objections have merit, we can hardly blink the fact that many classes of patients (albeit totaling a relatively small number) are not yet satisfactorily treated.

Administrators may not find the available research answers reassuring. Indeed, the evidence may merely create a further dilemma. While research findings may not appear to endorse the efficacy of some service programs, there is mounting social pressure to increase the availability of such services.

In addition, the research evidence regarding the indeterminate role of training will do little to clarify the relative roles of the professional and the paraprofessional. It is not surprising, but it is nonetheless dismaying, that a member of the President's Commission on Mental Health (see reference 33, p. 6) has already announced his decision to "extract mental health and mental health caregiving from the clutches of professionalism."

The policy-maker and the clinician both share the unhappy responsibility of having to make important decisions on the basis of inadequate data. Indeed, they cannot suspend their obligations pending the hoped-for but elusive day when the researchers will provide them with ultimate and definitive answers. In the absence of clear and credible scientific evidence in support of the unique and effective contributions of each of the disciplines offering psychotherapy—psychiatry, psychology, social work, psychiatric nursing, and the clergy—it is inevitable that these disciplines will seek other means of persuading the policy-maker. Each discipline will seek to insure its professional integrity and economic survival by offering its most persuasive arguments, including political pressure. To be sure, pressure will be couched in terms of concern with the welfare of the patient/client. Such ethical motivations have usually led to efforts to guard the public from the presumed deficiencies and inadequacies of members of the helping professions other than one's own. Each discipline—including, of course, our own—may be expected to strive to mobilize the forces of sheer numbers, prestige, and political influence. I regret that the various disciplines, particularly psychology and psychiatry, appear to be headed for a cyclical renewal of their periodic internecine scuffles. We seem destined to pursue, for yet a while longer, our all too familiar "dogma eat dogma" existence.

The tacit assumption that underlies much of the anxiety provoked by the promise and threat of National Health Insurance is that the primary protagonists will be the members of the currently recognized mental health professions. This view overlooks the potential major role of the nonpsychiatrically trained physician. It has been reported that in the United States nonpsychiatrically trained physicians see approximately 60% of all patients who have been identified as suffering from diagnosed mental health problems.[1] Most of the care provided is pharmacological or "supportive" ("therapeutic listening"), and few referrals to mental health practitioners are ever made. The implications of this for the quality of patient care and costs of National Health Insurance to society bear pondering.

How can the researcher more usefully respond to the PCMH autopsy of what most of us believed was still a healthy body of research? Since the field of psychology has contributed disproportionately to the production of the available research corpus, we may understandably take a rather proprietary interest in its proper care and treatment.

What guidance can we offer to the policy-maker and the practitioner to assist them in interpreting the responses that research has given to their questions? Our advice depends, of course, on how seriously we take our own pronouncements and generalizations. The problem of the credibility of generalizations in the field of psychotherapy is shared by all disciplines within the behavioral and social sciences, which must function primarily in the inductive mode. By careful examination of individual instances we attempt to arrive at generalizations that appear best to fit the data. Since we cannot hope to study all instances and cannot be certain that our sampling of the population is adequate, our conclusions must remain tentative.

In my view, the problem is particularly acute in the field of psychotherapy because of the inherent difficulty in deriving supportable conclusions from a literature that is essentially noncumulative. It cannot now be known with any degree of certainty whether the patients, interventions, goals, and measures are comparable from study to study. In view of this fact, I am prepared to place only modest reliance on the present conclusions of the PCMH report regarding psychotherapy. I think that we can assure the non-researchers that psychotherapy has shown some evidence of potency; however, our research has not yet been designed or conducted in a manner that can provide truly responsive answers to their questions. The best that I can say after years of sniffing about in the morass of outcome research literature is that in my optimistic moods I am confident that there's a pony in there somewhere.

The basic question, then, is what must we as researchers do in order to respond more usefully to the pragmatic questions that now face the field. First, I think that it is necessary for us to accept the responsibility to provide more responsive research data to the practitioner and the administrators. We cannot, as a field, remain in the aloof stance caricatured in the familiar picture of the basic scientist who prefers to seek after truth untrammeled by the noisy yammerings of the secular world. The fact is that in the practical world in which we must find support for our research we can only hope to settle for half-aloof.

I wish now to offer some recommendations that I believe may provide the field with a greater likelihood of achieving more useful and interpretable research data regarding psychotherapy outcome.

Emphasis on Clinical Trials Research

I propose that the National Institute of Mental Health be authorized to support and implement new initiatives in the conduct of such clinical trials research as may now be feasible and to support research that will increase the feasibility of subsequently conducting clinical trials studies. Such research should reflect the maximum involvement of the research community in the advisory process. The support of such research should in no way deflect from the continued support of independently initiated, high-quality research on the mechanisms of psychological interventions, nor should it reduce the support for the development and preliminary testing of new and established treatment forms. Such continued independent research is prerequisite to the more definitive clinical trials research program. It is cautioned that the NIMH does not have, nor should it seek, any regulatory functions. It is further urged that policy-makers recognize that clear and compelling research evidence, which constitutes only one of the bases for policy decisions, will not quickly become available. Careful long-term research is required to produce answers to complex research questions. A crash program cannot be expected to yield definitive answers.

I base this lengthy recommendation, in part, on my conviction that small-scale, independently initiated and conducted, uncoordinated research is inherently unable to provide reliable answers to the urgent "applied" questions of the field. Independently initiated research projects have contributed substantially to a body of "basic" knowledge regarding the processes and mechanisms of therapy, provided clinical insights, developed hypotheses, contributed to refinement of research methodologies, and provided preliminary tests of promising treatment techniques and approaches.

Such studies have not, however, provided answers to the questions now being asked with increasing insistence: What kinds of changes are affected by what kinds of techniques applied to what kinds of patients by what kinds of therapists under what kinds of conditions? The problem does not inhere in any limitations of the independent investigator's competence, or even in the complexity and difficulty of the research area. The problem lies instead in the lack of coordinated planning that can permit the gradual acquisition of cumulative knowledge. No single study, no matter how carefully designed and executed, can hope to "control" for or investigate systematically the plethora of variables whose influences on outcome may be confounded with and obscure the effects of treatment.

It is necessary that cooperating investigators each adopt an agreed-upon minimal set of standardized measures for describing and assessing such variables as the nature of the problem being treated, the characteristics of the treatment interventions, and the techniques for assessing the nature, quality, speed, and durability of patient change. The conduct of such large-scale studies requires centralized coordination following the achievement of "technical consensus" based on extensive consultation with the most knowledgeable investigators in the field.

A research program illustrative of this approach may be found in a currently planned, NIMH multiinstitutional "collaborative" study aimed at assessing the effectiveness, efficiency, and safety of two or more pretested psychological approaches to the treatment of carefully defined classes of disabling depressions. The effects of the selected interventions, offered singly or in combination with a designated pharmacologic agent, are to be studied and contrasted with suitable control groups.

Increased Research Attention on the Standard Forms of Psychotherapy

Specifically it is recommended that the researcher attempt to study psychotherapy as it is practiced within community facilities and in private practice. Particular emphasis is to be placed on assessing the effects with specified patient groups of well-described "brief" and "long-term" treatment interventions.

This recommendation grows partly out of the observation that there appears to be a remarkable disparity between the amount of research conducted on behavior therapy and psychotherapy. This may be due to the fact that behavior therapies are more amenable to rigorous study than are the psychotherapies. In any event there appears to be an inverse relationship between the frequency with which a treatment form is actually used by practitioners and the frequency with which that treatment is studied. A related point is that research tends to be conducted primarily in academic institutions, laboratories, or chronic patient wards in large public hospitals; yet most of the psychological treatments are offered in multiservice clinics, military clinics, community mental health centers, general medical care settings, general hospitals, and private practice. The effect of this disparity is that different kinds of patients and perhaps even different qualities of treatment may be characteristic of the research settings. To make our research findings more useful to the practitioners and the policy-makers, this discrepancy should be corrected.

Facilitation of Research on Innovative Therapies

The NIMH should undertake to fund the independent study of those new treatment techniques deemed promising. The mechanisms of grants and contracts are to be used in establishing community psychosocial treatment research organizations competent to provide such services. Such research organizations should have the technical ability to investigate the mechanisms and processes associated with the new treatment procedure as well as its effectiveness. No "standard-setting" or regulatory functions would be implied or authorized.

This recommendation is aimed at dealing with the fact that clinicians who develop new procedures and techniques frequently do not have ready access to researchers who can collaborate with them in scientifically testing the benefits of their innovations.

Unlike the fields of drug and somatic interventions, the psychotherapies (as distinct from behavior therapies) are almost always developed by clinicians rather than researchers. The developers, for the most part, do not usually have the skills, resources, or opportunities to subject their therapy form to objective, independent study. At present, the initiative is left to the clinician, who must voluntarily seek a collaborative relationship with researchers at universities. Cooperation of investigators is often difficult to obtain.

The need for independent assessment of newly developed treatment techniques is frequently overlooked in the field of psychosocial interventions. It is a well-recognized principle that the inventor or developer of a technique cannot be expected to be free of bias; yet in psychological treatment research it is generally the innovator of a technique who is expected to undertake to demonstrate the utility of his/her procedures.

It is appropriate that the clinician who *volunteers* to cooperate in such a study should have the opportunity to do so, provided, of course, that preliminary study suggests that the technique is of potential value.

Acquisition, Evaluation, and Dissemination of Research Information

The ADAMHA and the NIMH should be supported in their initiative to create advisory groups to assess and evaluate on a periodic basis the published research in the field of psychosocial treatment and to prepare appropriate evaluative reports. Such activity should represent the involvement of the research community to a maximum degree in order that such assessments and recommendations represent the best "technical consensus" rather than the views of a particular federal agency, individual scientist, or professional interest group.

Currently, scientific communication is best among researchers and academicians, or those with a direct incentive to keep up with the latest information in their areas. Scientific communication with practitioners, policymakers, and the public is attenuated. While the researcher may be able to interpret published research findings and to recognize the limits of generalizability and interpretability, the clinician and the layman may be less equipped or less inclined to do so. It is necessary, therefore, to establish a mechanism for providing authoritative information to the practitioner, the policy-maker, and the public, regarding the validity and significance of new findings from research and their readiness for wide clinical application.

Specifically, it is necessary to assess the clinical significance of new findings and the adequacy of the research that underpins it. It is necessary to establish a system whereby the informed opinions of most knowledgeable authorities in the field can be brought to bear on the assessment of the current and past research output. On the basis of such a consensus, evaluated information should be disseminated regularly to practitioners and the public regarding such questions as: the generalizability of findings to other samples of patients, therapists, and settings; implications regarding costs; and ethical and social considerations.

Apart from the content, you may have noted two facts about this list of recommendations that may strike the reader as odd: First, the recommendations appear to be primarily addressed to federal administrators, and second, I appear successfully to have resisted the opportunity to exhort my colleagues to go forth and do better. The fact is that our individual research efforts are good and are getting better. I shall, however, reserve the right to offer a suggestion primarily of a strategic sort. Before doing so, I wish to return to the first point—the fact that my recommendations appear to be directed primarily toward officials of the federal government and only secondarily to fellow researchers.

I have done so wittingly, mindful of the fact that the federal government is in a very real sense the source of research support not only for those of us on the payroll but rather for all investigators whose work is supported by grants and contracts. The national government supports approximately 89% of all research in the field of mental health, while state governments contribute but 8% and private sources account for only 3%. As researchers we are all, therefore, immediately and sometimes painfully affected by governmental laws and policy decisions.

And now a word primarily to the researcher rather than to our collective sponsors. While I am reluctant to dwell on technical issues with this audience, which is all too intimately acquainted with the technical problems that beset our field, there is one issue that bears underlining. It appears that some of our studies may be inadvertently designed in a manner that may effectively preclude the investigator's having the opportunity to reject the null hypothesis. I refer to the fact that group comparison studies often include fatuously heterogeneous groups and measures of low reliability and uncertain validity. Measurement error coupled with the variance due to differences among patients within the groups being studied tends to produce estimated population variances of such size as to reduce the likelihood that statistically significant differences between group means can be found. An apparent finding of "no differences" may take on unfortunate significance to the policy-maker who lusts after cost-effectiveness evidence. Thus, comparisons of the relative effectiveness of short-term and long-term therapies, or drugs and psychotherapies, or the advantages of employing professional or nonprofessional therapists may by virtue of inadequate research designs lead to profound overinterpretation or a "no difference" finding.

While I have laid heavy emphasis in one of my earlier recommendations on the conduct of clinical trials research, I do not wish to give the impression that I am unaware of its complexities and dangers. More particularly, I wish to urge that such studies not be designed simply as "horse races" to see which therapy wins. It is past time for us to abandon research aimed solely at identifying "the most effective form of therapy." We must seek instead to determine what kinds of interventions produce what kinds of changes in particular patients. (You are by now all familiar with the rest of that litany.) Clinical trials research will be useful to the degree that it permits the study of interactions among patients, therapists, and therapies and the identification of relevant process variables. Research evidence that promises the greatest generalizability is that which furthers our understanding of the mechanisms whereby particular kinds of changes are effected. Generalizations to discrete mechanisms may be even more useful than efforts to generalize findings to schools of therapy, professions, or diagnostic categories of patients.

In the past, in confronting some of the problems I have posed here, researchers have proposed that it is premature to study outcome until the processes and mechanisms have been better understood. Others have suggested the opposite—that it may be premature to focus on process studies until we have clearer evidence of the nature and quality of outcome. I believe they are both right. In view of this, I believe we have no choice but actively to pursue process studies as part of well-coordinated outcome studies. In this manner a coherent body of knowledge in this field may finally begin to emerge.

References

1. Regier DA, Goldberg ID, Taube CA: The *de facto* U.S. mental health services system: A public health perspective. *Arch Gen Psychiatry* 35:685–693, 1978.
2. Parloff MB, Wolfe BE, Hadley SW, Waskow IE: Assessment of Psychosocial Treatment of Mental Health Disorders: Current Status and Prospects, Report to the National Academy of Sciences, Institute of Medicine, Washington DC, 1978.
3. President's Commission on Mental Health: Report to the President, 1978, vol 4. Washington DC, US Government Printing Office, 1978.
4. Bergin AE: The evaluation of therapeutic outcome, in Bergin AE, Garfield SL (eds): Handbook of Psychotherapy and Behavior Change. New York, John Wiley & Sons Inc, 1971.
5. Subotnik L: Spontaneous remission: Fact or artifact? *Psychol Bull* 77:32–48, 1972.
6. Lambert MJ: Spontaneous remission in adult neurotic disorder: A revision and summary. *Psychol Bull* 83:107–119, 1976.
7. Beiser M: Personal and social factors associated with the remission of psychiatric symptoms. *Arch Gen Psychiatry* 33:941–945, 1976.
8. Malan DH: The outcome problem in psychotherapy research: A historical review. *Arch Gen Psychiatry* 29:719–729, 1973.
9. Strupp HH, Hadley SW: A tripartite model of mental health and therapeutic outcomes: With special reference to negative effects in psychotherapy. *Am Psychol* 32:187–196, 1977.
10. Mintz J: What is "success" in psychotherapy? *J Abnorm Psychol* 80:11–19, 1972.
11. Kiesler DJ: The Process of Psychotherapy. Chicago, Aldine Publishing Co, 1973.
12. Meltzoff J, Kornreich M: Research in Psychotherapy. New York, Atherton Press, 1970.
13. Luborsky L, Singer B, Luborsky L: Comparative studies of psychotherapies. *Arch Gen Psychiatry* 32:995–1008, 1975.
14. Sloane RB, Staples FR, Cristol AH, Yorkston NJ, Whipple K: Short-Term Analytically Oriented Psychotherapy vs. Behavior Therapy. Cambridge Mass, Harvard University Press, 1975.
15. Beutler LE: Psychotherapy: When what works with whom. Unpublished manuscript, Baylor College of Medicine, Houston, 1976.
16. Smith ML, Glass GV: Meta-analysis of psychotherapy outcome studies. *Am Psychol* 32:752–760, 1977.
17. Glass GV, Smith ML: Statement to the Senate Finance Committee Regarding the Benefits of Psychotherapy, August 15, 1978.
18. Smith ML, Glass GV, Miller TI: The Benefits of Psychotherapy. Baltimore, Johns Hopkins University Press, 1981.
19. Bergin AE, Lambert MJ: The evaluation of therapeutic outcomes, in Garfield SL, Bergin AE (eds): Handbook of Psychotherapy and Behavior Change, ed 2. New York, John Wiley & Sons Inc, 1978.
20. Shapiro AK: Placebo effects in medicine, psychotherapy, and psychoanalysis, in Bergin AE, Garfield SL (eds): Handbook of Psychotherapy and Behavior Change. New York, John Wiley & Sons Inc, 1971.
21. Miller NE: Biofeedback and visceral learning. *Ann Rev of Psychol* 29:373–404, 1978.
22. Frank JD: Persuasion and Healing: A Comparative Study of Psychotherapy, Rev ed. Baltimore, Johns Hopkins University Press, 1973.
23. Marmor J: The nature of the psychotherapeutic process revisited. *Can Psychiatr Assoc J* 20:557–565, 1975.
24. Rosenzweig S: A transevaluation of psychotherapy—A reply to Hans Eysenck. *J. Abnorm Soc Psychol* 49:298–304, 1954.
25. Kazdin AE, Wilcoxon LA: Systematic desensitization and nonspecific treatment effects: A methodological evaluation. *Psychol Bull* 83:729–758, 1976.
26. Goldstein AP, Heller K, Sechrest LB: Psychotherapy and the Psychology of Behavior Change. New York, John Wiley & Sons Inc, 1966.

27. Orne M: Psychotherapy in contemporary America: Its development and context, in Freedman DX, Dyrud JE (eds): American Handbook of Psychiatry, ed 2, vol 5. New York, Basic Books, 1975.
28. Henry WE, Sims JH, Spray SL: The Fifth Profession. San Francisco, Jossey-Bass, 1971.
29. Bergin AE, Suinn RM: Individual psychotherapy and behavior therapy. *Ann Rev Psychol* 26:509–556, 1975.
30. Strupp HH, Hadley SW: Specific versus nonspecific factors in psychotherapy: A controlled study of outcome. *Arch Gen Psychiatry* 36:1125–1136, 1979.
31. Auerbach AH, Johnson M: Research on the therapist's level of experience, in Gurman AS, Razin AM (eds): Effective Psychotherapy: A Handbook of Research. New York, Pergamon Press, 1977.
32. Parloff MB, Waskow IE, Wolfe BE: Research on therapist variables in relation to process and outcome, in Garfield SL, Bergin AE (eds): Handbook of Psychotherapy and Behavior Change, ed 2. New York, John Wiley & Sons Inc, 1978.
33. Willie CV: *APA Monitor*, May 1978, p 6.

Jack Weinberg*
and Theodora Fine

This commentary both affirms many of the recommendations contained in Dr. Upton's white paper and additionally attempts to paint a portrait of the prospective problems older population groups may face in the wake of a National Health Insurance program that fails to provide coverage for nervous, mental, or emotional disorders. While we accept as a given the fact that the elderly do not have exactly the same hopes, needs, abilities, or problems as any other generation of Americans, we do believe that some of the problems and, indeed, some of the recommendations contained herein will parallel those faced by all who, suffering from a mental disorder, will seek help under a future federal health insurance program that takes as its minimum benefit package today's Medicare program. As the white paper notes, such is the case in nearly all of the major proposals considered in the 96th and 97th Congress

*Jack Weinberg, M.D., died on March 1, 1982. To the best of my knowledge, this paper, on which he collaborated with Ms. Fine, is his last published work. A former president of the American Psychiatric Association (APA) (1978–1979) and chairman of the APA's Council on Aging (1979–1981), Dr. Weinberg concerned himself, for much of his career, with the mental health care needs of the elderly. He deeply felt that the elderly should be entitled to complete mental health care and he devoted his professional efforts to achieving that end, fighting, among other things, the inequities of Medicare as that program discriminates against the elderly, denying them financial access to treatment for nervous, mental, or emotional disorders. I think this paper elucidates the principles and causes for which Dr. Weinberg stood and the policies and programs toward which he worked. I hope the paper will contribute to a national health policy that takes full cognizance of mental illness as it affects the elderly; I also hope it will lead to legislation that removes current prejudicial barriers to mental health care for the elderly and entitles them to receive a full range of treatment for emotional disorders. I know this would be Dr. Weinberg's wish—ED.

This commentary is based in part on testimony presented before the Senate Special Committee on Aging, "Aging and Mental Health: Overcoming Barriers to Service," May 22, 1980.

Jack Weinberg • Director, Illinois Mental Health Institutes, Chicago, Illinois 60612.   Theodora Fine • Assistant Director of Government Relations, American Psychiatric Association, Washington, D.C. 20002.

and to be considered in the upcoming Congress by the key House and Senate committees with purview over federal health insurance programs.

That we are becoming an increasingly older population is no longer in doubt. Every day, the ranks of the elderly are swelled by 1400 Americans, and that number is escalating.[1] Our nation's population of older persons currently exceeds the total population of the state of California, and in the coming year, we can expect that every one in eight persons in this nation will be over the age of 65. In the past 80 years, the numbers of the aged have nearly tripled: from 4% of our population to over 11%. Current projections point to an aged population of 33.2 million by 2010 and an overwhelming 51.6 million by 2030, as the products of the post-World War II baby boom reach age 65.[2]

That our existing federal health care system was designed over 15 years ago to meet the acute health care needs of the elderly is also not in doubt, nor is the fact that the program has expanded geometrically in both cost and services. Medicare and Medicaid, two of the most costly "uncontrollables" in the federal budget, form the basis for the health care now afforded the vast majority of the aged in our nation. Indeed, such costly programs in the past few years have borne, and in the future will bear, the brunt of fiscal concern and examination as the federal government—both executive and legislative branches—seeks means of controlling federal expenditures. We can expect cutbacks.

However, that the *current* system of care, expansive and broad-ranging though it may be, *fails* to meet the treatment needs of the almost 25% of all elderly who suffer from mental illness is not at all in doubt.[3] Of a total of over $240 million spent in 1975, Medicare expended only 2% of its Part A expenditures (hospitalization) and less than 1% of its Part B expenditures (supplemental benefits) for the treatment of emotional disorders.[4] This was based as much on existing Medicare reimbursement structure as on the failure by primary care physicians to diagnose mental illness, assuming care was sought in the first place.

If, as suggested in the white paper, "National Health Insurance . . . promises to compromise and sacrifice mental health care" for many Americans, we need only look at the historical treatment of the elderly under Medicare to ascertain just how such "compromise" and "sacrifice" are to be carried out and what serious and damaging repercussions such a decision may well entail—not just for the elderly, but for all Americans seeking care for an emotional disorder under any system other than a truly comprehensive health plan, offering full mental health benefits at par with all other medical benefits. The litany of historical failures of policy-makers to consider the mentally ill in their national health care plan legislative initiatives, coupled with both the failure to follow up on almost two decades of recommendations by informed experts as well as by the elderly themselves and the inadequate and incomplete record of action on legislation designed to begin to meet the needs of the mentally ill elderly, gives credence to Dr. Upton's critical accusation that "for many Americans, access to adequate mental health care will be denied rather than promoted by NHI. . . ."

Over 15 years ago, Congress enacted the Older Americans Act, which has as its centerpiece the assurance of dignity and independence for the elderly—for *all* the elderly. Apparently these rights were not considered when Medicare was developed, for it restricted severely the treatment opportunities for those elderly suffering from mental disorders, adversely affecting their ability to be assured of dignity and independence. Medicare failed to recognize, particularly with respect to the mentally ill elderly, the enormous benefits that may be accrued as the result of appropriate, necessary, full-course outpatient treatment in lieu of hospitalization wherever appropriate, whether through the traditional private sector or through public sector-oriented home health care or community mental health center programs. Thus, outpatient care for the mentally ill elderly was restricted to $250 per year from federal coffers (matched by an unprecedented 50% copayment from the patient, in contrast with the more traditional 20% copayment found in Medicare for other medical services). Community mental health centers (CMHCs) established several years previously were given the mandate to provide care to the elderly, but not the Medicare reimbursement necessary to do so, and home health care was severely limited. Day hospitalization services are not covered at all, nor are full-scale physical and psychiatric evaluations.

The lack of relatively inexpensive short-term outpatient mental health services severaly tests the resources of both the elderly person and his or her family.[5] It raises the dual dilemma of Medicare: the absence of adequate outpatient care reimbursement coupled with the emotional stress presented by the inability to meet out-of-pocket medical costs for such care. The result may lead to far more costly, longer-term institutionalization, which is reimbursible at a higher level.

Thus, Medicare has compromised severely the clear federal direction under the Older Americans Act calling for a life of dignity and independence.

While we have seen some improvements in Medicare in general over the past 15 years of experience with the program, not once has Congress effectively moved to broaden the restricted benefits under the program for the mentally ill.* Not once has Congress included equivalent coverage under its

*This is not to suggest that efforts have not been undertaken in both the House and Senate to ameliorate the dislocation caused by inequitable coverage of nervous, mental, or emotional disorders under the Medicare program. In the 95th Congress, Senator Clifford Case introduced American Psychiatric Association-developed legislation, S 3131, which would have lifted the 190-day lifetime inpatient limit for psychiatric disorder treatment, eliminated the $250 annual ceiling on federal reimbursement for outpatient psychiatric care, and brought the unprecedented 50% patient-borne copayment to the 20% out-of-pocket level required for all other treatment costs.

The 96th Congress brought further efforts on both the House and Senate sides. Congressman Tom Downey introduced a House version of the Case legislation, and Senator John Heinz proposed catastrophic health plans, phased-in national plans, or comprehensive national plans. Services provided in a Health Maintenance Organization's basic benefits were thought to include inpatient psychiatric care; now the Department of Health and Human Services has reinterpreted HMO law to the contrary.[6] And now, both the "consumers" and the "providers" of psychiatric care find themselves confronted with yet another damaging and dangerous hurdle: the proof that the treatment rendered is "safe and efficacious" before even the current limited benefits may be utilized. (See S 3029, Senators Matsunaga and Inouye, 96th Congress, and the Upton discussion of safety and efficacy.) Patients and providers of treatment for mental illness find themselves again segregated from access to benefits and reimbursement-afforded illnesses and treatments of physical disorders. This can do little for dignity and independence of those elderly who may be caught in yet another trap of seeking help for an unfortunately stigmatizing medical condition and finding it nonreimbursable.*

---

offered substantially similar legislation in the Senate. (Only the Downey bill was reintroduced in the 97th Congress.) At the same time, the administration proposed incremental improvements in the Medicare mental illness benefit, raising the outpatient ceiling to $750 and ending the discriminatory copayment features. The measure was adopted by the House of Representatives and sent to the Senate, where it ultimately "died" in the wake of "safety and efficacy" of mental health treatments legislation.

Prospects under the new administration, coupled with the economic picture as viewed from Capitol Hill, make adoption of these improvements unlikely in the 97th or 98th Congress.

*The Board of Trustees of the American Psychiatric Association adopted the following resolution in the wake of the debate on "safety and efficacy of mental health treatments" legislation:

WHEREAS, the Congress in response to APA legislative activities which have urged non-discriminatory reimbursement for the treatment of mental illness, has considered such legislation; and

WHEREAS, one body of the Congreee, the House of Representatives has, in great measure responded positively to such APA legislative activities through the adoption of not only non-discriminatory coverage under Medicaid through the Child Health Assurance Program (H.R. 4962), but also improved incrementally Medicare coverage for the treatment of mental illness by increasing the annual outpatient Federal reimbursement ceiling from $250 to $750 with an 80-20 copayment (increased from 50-50); providing reimbursement to Community Mental Health Centers but only where patients are under the case management of a physician; and providing reimbursement to clinical psychologists but only where patients have been referred by a physician (H.R. 3990); and

WHEREAS, the Senate Finance Committee has been identified by the JCGR as considering the development of legislation, commonly referred to as an efficacy of mental health services amendment, which will effectively impede the APA's efforts by requiring treatment to be safe, efficacious and appropriate in order to be eligible for reimbursement under Medicare and Medicaid; and

WHEREAS, there has now been introduced in the senate legislation which would establish a Presidential Commission to evaluate the safety, efficacy and appropriateness of mental health services to determine their eligibility for reimbursement under Medicare and Medicaid (S. 3029) and for which hearings have

Ironically, over the same 15 years, increasing public attention has been paid to the needs of the mentally ill elderly. The 1971 White House Conference on Aging urged legislative changes to meet the needs of the mentally ill elderly, both in service system modifications and in reimbursement.[7] The Social Security Administration, during the first term of President Nixon, recommended removing the restrictions under both Parts A and B of Medicare, which discriminate against the treatment of the mentally ill elderly. Similar sentiments were registered by the President's Task Force on the Aging as well as the President's Task Force on the Mentally Handicapped.[8] No changes were made in the law.

The Senate Special Committee on Aging has held hearings during the 1970s and into 1980 on problems of the mentally ill elderly. In its November 1971 report[9] the committee stated: "Public policy in mental health care of the elderly is confused, riddled with contradictions and shortsighted limitations, and in need of intensive scrutiny geared to immediate and long-term action." Regrettably, that committee has no legislative authority nor does the House Select Committee on Aging, which held a conference on the same issue, reaching many of the same conclusions. Both the Senate Finance Committee and the House Ways and Means Committee, which have legislative jurisdic-

---

been scheduled for September 29, 1980 by the Senate Health Subcommittee of the Finance Committee and at which hearings the APA has been invited to testify; and

WHEREAS, the APA believes that in the best interest of patient treatment practices, such treatment to the maximum extent possible should have as its basis scientific validation of treatment safety and efficacy but does not support legislation which would establish a new, duplicative Federal bureaucracy to evaluate the safety, efficacy and appropriateness of medical treatment to determine whether there should be reimbursement for medical treatment otherwise determined by the medical profession as reasonable and necessary in the best interest of the patient.

NOW THEREFORE BE IT RESOLVED, that the APA continue to express to the Congress its opposition to S 3029 or any legislative initiative which would provide a discriminatory response to the need for treatment of mental illness as contrasted to treatment for physical health problems through inappropriate linkages of reimbursement with the conduct of findings of research into the safety, efficacy and appropriateness of mental illness treatment.

AND, NOW BE IT FURTHER RESOLVED, that the APA believes the most appropriate way to achieve such a determination is through the APA Commission on Psychiatric Therapies which will review the somatic, dyadic, group, familial and social therapies in current use by a thorough and critical examination of the literature (including reports of other APA components), as to techniques, duration, results, costs, and other characteristics; to correlate and analyze the findings for the purpose of eliciting the common vectors that are therapeutically effective as distinguished from procedures that are extraneous or counterproductive. Moreover, the Commission will be naming therapies, describing therapies, evaluating outcome data, collecting data, interviewing patients and therapists, observing therapists, etc., and when the largest common denominator is found, all material will be integrated for use in recommending standards and evaluating approaches to psychiatrists and other mental health professionals.

tion over the Medicare program, have considered the matter. Organizations dealing with aging, recognizing the plight of the mentally ill elderly as an area of importance, have begun to take an active role in the fight for equitable and appropriate mental health care. Still, no changes have been made, although Medicare may well form the base benefit package for National Health Insurance, thereby affecting us all—not just the elderly.

Naturally, many of us in the field of geriatric psychiatry were gratified to learn that the Carter administration, when first in office, expressed interest— indeed, concern—about the problems facing the mentally ill in general. We were equally gratified to note that the President's Commission on Mental Health, the group given the spearheading responsibility for this interest, stated in its preliminary report,[10] "In our society, individuals must have the opportunity to have their suffering alleviated insofar as possible and . . . no individual who needs assistance should feel ashamed or embarrassed to seek or receive help." We believed this statement marked a commitment to the mentally ill elderly that paralleled the historic commitment made under the Older Americans Act.

Our positive beliefs were reinforced further as we read the final report and recommendations of the President's Commission[11] a year later regarding the appropriate means of meeting the mental health needs of the elderly, one of the four groups determined by the commission to be underserved, unserved, or inappropriately served by our existing system of mental health care. Our gratification came as a result of our belief that, at long last, the recommendations and promises of the past to help meet the treatment needs of the mentally ill elderly would be implemented, and would bring such individuals into the mainstream of our health care system over a decade and a half after Congress had adopted the Older Americans Act, with its commitment to assuring the elderly a life of independence and dignity. At last, we believed, this forgotten segment of our population would not be relegated to either the back wards or the back alleys, but could step forward for treatment and then return to being or become productive, producing, contributing members of society.

However, since the publication of that report, we have seen few changes in the law, with the notable exception of the congressionally amended provisions for the elderly contained in the Mental Health Systems Act (PL96-398), and services are still almost entirely a promise, not a reality. As current law is drafted, discrimination exists. As new catastrophic health insurance legislation is proposed, discrimination continues. Federal regulations continue the discrimination, as does the failure of appropriate House and Senate committees to consider legislation aimed at eliminating the discrimination.

Assurances that "suffering is alleviated insofar as possible"[10] will be no more than lip service until a wholesale series of alterations is made to restructure the current Medicare program into an integrated system that delivers *all* medical care on an equal basis. Such changes will be clearly articulated hereinafter, and this commentary will touch upon many of the considerations in the white paper, including the concept of triage, the "who provides care" issue, the appropriateness and extent of coverage, and, most important, the end to discriminatory public and private reimbursement practices regarding treatment of emotional disorders.

To provide perspective on the issue, we shall first paint a portrait of the mentally ill elderly: who they are, how many they are, what their general problems are. Next, we will explain in greater detail the barriers that exist between these individuals and appropriate treatment opportunities, and we will provide recommendations that may begin to help assure that the elderly are afforded a full range of appropriate treatment services and access to such services, should they require treatment of a nervous, mental, or emotional disorder. These recommendations can, and indeed should, form a sound basis with respect to this one population group for the comparable recommendations in the white paper.

The Need for Service

With 95% of them residing in the community, most older Americans have little or no evidence of mental disorders, and though 86% have chronic health problems of all sorts, fewer than one-fifth of the group have serious problems.[12] However, the elderly, in comparison with other age groups, in general have an increased incidence of serious physical disease, a greater likelihood of becoming physically isolated, and a higher probability of lost status through loss of income, jobs, etc. Significant numbers, therefore, are at risk of developing psychiatric symptoms or illnesses. Older persons are more apt to develop depressions, organic brain syndromes, mental reactions as side effects to medication, and certain paranoid reactions.[13] The predominant number of elderly suffer not from a single acute-term illness but from a constellation of problems, both physical and emotional, which, while treatable, do not have the same characteristics as short-term acute illnesses.

Though constituting only 11% of the population, the elderly contribute over 25% of the nation's suicides.[12] The elderly lead the World Health Organization's list of incidences of new cases of psychopathology at 236.1 cases per 100,000 population (compared to 93.0 in the next lower age category). Psychoses increases after 65, and even more so after 75.[12] Organic brain disorders in severe form affect over 1 million elderly, and appear in less severe forms in an additional 2 million persons.[13] Senile dementia is seen today as the fourth leading cause of death in the nation.[14] All in all, 15 to 25% of older persons demonstrate significant symptoms of mental illness.[11] Because the fastest-growing segment of the American population is the group over 75 years of age, we can expect that the number of elderly with significant nervous, mental, or emotional disorders will increase significantly over the next decade.

Notwithstanding this clear statistical base, which demonstrates the increased risk for mental disorder, the elderly have been chronically underserved by both the private and public health care sectors: Only 4% of Community Mental Health Center patients are elderly; the elderly represent but 2% of the population receiving care from private practitioners and clinics[15]; in fact, less than 1.5% of the direct cost expenditures for mental illness is provided for older persons residing in the community.

The data are particularly disconcerting because the considerable majority of these disorders is treatable and reversible. Indeed, the President's Commission on Mental Health noted that as many as 25% of those individuals determined to be "senile" actually have treatable reversible conditions.[11] Specific examples of treatable "senility" include reversible confusional states due to physical disorders (myxedema, occult pneumonia, medication side effects), all of which are correctable and treatable depressions, masquerading as organic brain syndrome. Early diagnosis and treatment of emotional disorders can minimize their impact, delaying or preventing a worsening of the conditon.

These facts have been thoroughly studied, have been stated and restated, and are well established. The Age Discrimination Study of the United States Commission on Civil Rights reports that the elderly are grossly underserved in comparison to other age groups within federally supported Community Mental Health Centers. The President's Commission on Mental Health Task Panel on the Elderly[11] states that the elderly are "unserved, underserved, or inappropriately served." The Secretary's Committee on the Mental Health and Illness of the Elderly[16] and the United States House of Representatives Select Committee on Aging's National Conference on Mental Health and the Elderly[17] confirmed these findings and conclusions.

Yet the situation persists, and persists as the result of a combination of factors: reimbursement structures under federal health programs; the fragmented, disorganized system of health care and social service delivery system available to the elderly; widespread misunderstanding of the cost of treating the mentally ill in general and the elderly in particular; an inadequate number of psychiatrists, other physicians, and nonphysician mental health professionals interested and trained to provide care to the elderly (coupled with problems in the area of just *who* would provide what services to this group); and the continuing fear and stigma that still haunt the public's conception of mental illness. All of these areas are addressed in Dr. Upton's white paper and we herein concur.

Barriers and Access to Care

We know today the prevalence of mental illness among the elderly. We now know that, with adequate treatment opportunities, the vast majority of these elderly suffering from some form of mental disorder will improve. We also know that with timely, early intervention through routine screening (or through preventive care before such screening), some difficulties may be avoided altogether.

At this juncture, it is important to review why there are barriers to the delivery of care, why the mentally ill elderly are not adequately served by our existing, predominantly federal system of health care delivery. The reasons are multiple and complex: They include the relative lack of value placed on the elderly in our society; the stigma of mental illness in general; the lack of accessibility to and availability of needed services; insufficient means of financing such services; poor coordination of such services; and a lack of understanding of the nature and treatability of late-life mental disorders on the part of physicians and nonphysician health professionals, the elderly themselves, and their families. Each of these barriers to the provision of appropriate and necessary care to the elderly is detailed below and must be grappled with if it is to be eliminated as new health policy and law regarding care for the mentally ill under national or catastrophic health insurance is developed.

The "ageism" that continues to exist within our society is best characterized by the perception that the elderly have served their purpose in life and may therefore be consigned to the shelf. As Robert Butler, M.D., director of the National Institute on Aging, has pointed out, this belief, this "ageism" which pervades the mental health community as well, acts as a major deterrent to caregiving. He further notes:

> Many psychiatrists and other mental health specialists share our culture's negative attitudes toward older people, the pervasive prejudice I have called ageism which is the process of systematically stereotyping and discriminating against people because they are old. Old people are categorized as senile, rigid, and old-fashioned in morality and skills. Ageism allows those of us who are younger to see old people as "different." We subtly cease to identify with them as human beings, which enables us to feel more comfortable about our neglect and dislike of them.[18]

Coupled with the myriad other factors cited above, this "ageism" forms the basis for our failure to provide needed care to the mentally ill elderly.

But if ageism controls many of our attitudes toward the elderly in general, it is abundantly clear that an elderly person afflicted by emotional disorder is in double jeopardy. As detailed in the President's Commission on Mental Health Report, articulated in newspaper and journal articles, and included in television documentaries over the past few years, the stigma of mental illness in general is still with us. The movement from the institution to the community continues without adequate attention to the constellation of services required by such individuals (although the Mental Health Systems Act, PL 96-398, proposes to make some start at providing the necessary continuity of care).* In part, this may be explained by the trend to deinstitutionalize too

---

*House Health Subcommittee Chairman Henry Waxman, in speaking in support of the adoption of the Mental Health Systems Act on the floor of the House of Representatives, stated: "The special provisions for the elderly [contained in the act] are made in hopes of returning this group

quickly without adequate preparation at the community level, but a major portion of the problem is the result of our feeling that somehow the mentally ill are not human, do not need care, are outside society. The elderly person is thus stigmatized twice: once by the fact of being old in an ageist society, and once again by the fact of mental illness.

Due to the stigma popularly attached to mental illness and due also to their private fears relating to it, most people are reluctant to seek mental health care. Indeed, the mentally ill person is more likely to delay or reject early treatment for his complaint than he would be in seeking help for a physical illness. Add to this the fact that today's elderly belong to a generation that has traditionally viewed psychiatry and mental illness with an almost superstitious dread. To many of them, senility is a normal aspect of aging; to be gloomy and without hope for the future is a natural state, not a manifestation of depression. Moreover, it is often assumed that the mentally healthy older person grows more pessimistic, rigid, and irascible with age. In the case of the mentally ill elderly, the problem is not predominantly one of whether there is or is not mental dysfunction, but rather the belief that the problem cannot be treated or the quality of life be improved (or worse, that it is not worth treating or improving).

Such erroneous belief structures must be erased. Without ending the stigma of mental illness, placing it in its proper perspective, namely, that it is often a treatable disease that may be ameliorated in the same way as many physiological difficulties may be resolved, we will continue to be frustrated, not only in meeting the treatment needs of those already diagnosed as mentally ill but also by the vast numbers of individuals who are too proud, or too frightened, to accept the fact of mental illness and to receive treatment for that illness.

The stigma of mental illness is heightened further because the discrimination has become institutionalized—written in the Medicare law, written in the restrictive language for treatment of mental illness contained in the health

---

to full and functional daily lives." Those provisions specifically include (a) a set-aside of 40% of the funds allocated under Section 204 of the bill specifically for the elderly, (b) the mandate for a differential diagnosis, (c) required outreach, and (d) appropriate numbers of trained personnel in nursing homes to meet the needs of the mentally ill elderly in such facilities. Congressman John Paul Hammerschmitt, speaking specifically about the mandated differential diagnosis, noted that it is an "effective screen to prevent mistreatment of an underlying physical problem and to identify physical disorders which could prove fatal. On the advice of experts in the field of geriatric psychiatry, we expect that at a minimum a medical differential diagnosis shall consist of a general physical and neurological examination, an adequate blood chemistry workup, and an inventory of both prescribed and over-the-counter medications."

Other provisions that will have a positive effect upon the mentally ill elderly are contained in Section 202, pertaining to the chronic patient, wherein a predischarge treatment plan and a community-based case manager are mandated before a patient may be discharged into the community, and in Section 206, which requires that appropriate training be made available to nursing home personnel to manage the special problems of the mentally ill housed in such facilities.

insurance legislation that has been before Congress during the past few years, and written in the restrictive measures contained in most private health insurance plans. All suggest that mental illness is grossly different from physical illness—not treatable, not reversible, and not equally reimbursable when treatment is provided.* Such stigmatizing, compounded by the pervasive ageism of our society, renders care to the mentally ill elderly virtually impossible.

Because we have ignored the situation confronting the mentally ill elderly for so long, the treatment system today is badly fragmented. It is based on the Medicare assumption, a badly flawed assumption, that most illnesses are ones that require *acute inpatient treatment* for *short periods of time*, and that if longer-stay care is necessary, the most appropriate location for such care is a nursing home. As articulated in the literature time and time again, the aged do better when able to remain in their homes in their communities, with adequate outpatient, day hospitalization, or home health care, than when hospitalized or institutionalized.

Greater flexibility, other than that provided under existing Medicare law, is necessary if we are to meet the various needs of our older population in a manner that is both appropriate and cost-effective.† We cannot rely upon the current system, which, unfortunately, stresses the wrong types of care and encourages abuse of the very population it is designed to serve.

Of particular concern is the situation regarding the deinstitutionalization of the elderly into nursing homes or foster care facilities. While such action removes the financial burden from the state by relocating the population from the state hospital, it does not *per se* constitute appropriate and adequate care. Very often, no discharge plan is developed that will follow the patient and chart the care he requires once he is deinstitutionalized. Moreover, more often than not, foster care facilities, nursing homes, and welfare hotels do not

---

*A *New York Times* article of January 27, 1980, cites a memorandum sent by the Department of Health, Education and Welfare (now, Department of Health and Human Services) on the subject of Medicare reimbursement for an elderly person's psychiatric care, which reads: "It is understood, that those symptoms attributable to the chronic brain symdrome condition [the scientific name for senility] are not expected to remit and that treatment directed to this end will be ruled non-covered." In response to such directive, Dr. Monica Blumenthal, its recipient, noted, "Physicians generally agree that these problems are hallmarks of illnesses, most of which are amenable to treatment and to cure." Thus, the Medicare interpretation has simply reinforced the erroneous belief that treatment of mental illness in the elderly is not a worthwhile or productive undertaking.

†Dr. Robert Butler, director of the National Institute on Aging, pointed out in *Aging and Mental Health*,[12] "There is also no proof that the deductible features of Medicare deter unnecessary use of health services. Instead, the exclusions may actually increase the government's bill by discouraging preventive and early rehabilitative care. . . . Some old people get themselves checked into a hospital just to get a physical examination (basing it on some physical complaint) because this will not be paid for on an outpatient basis." The same situation is true for mental health coverage: other physical complaints often form the basis for hospitalization or outpatient visits, thereby raising the cost of Medicare coverage and possibly masking the psychiatric illness with physical symptoms—all in an effort to secure Medicare coverage.

provide the continuity of psychiatric services required by the deinstitutionalized. Indeed, fewer than 1% of all patients residing in nursing homes
have access to psychologic or psychiatric assessment and treatment.[19] Nursing homes are discouraged from specifying in a patient's record that the
patient is in care for a primary diagnosis of mental illness, for if more than
50% of the patients have such diagnoses, the nursing home may lose its
certification. Indeed, fewer than 10% of patients in a sample of 60 nursing
homes in nine states were identified as having mental or emotional disturbances. However, when a team of mental health professionals investigated
their clinical status, more than 70% of these patients did evidence some degree of diagnosable dementia.[19]

Though multiple layers of federal, state, and local regulations have accu-
mulated, nowhere does accreditation of a nursing home depend on its guar-
anteeing staff training in interpersonal relations, psychosocial assessment
and management, or uses and adverse effects of psychotropic medications;
nowhere is a nursing home required to provide psychiatric consultation. (Recent proposed federal regulations, which continue to ask the very questions
they have asked previously and for which they have repeatedly received
answers, still provide few if any changes in the nursing home situation.) The
results of this are unnecessary suffering for patients, and rejection, abuse,
and avoidable transfer of patients whose disorders could be treated.

An exchange of several years ago before the Senate Special Committee on
Aging[20] plainly demonstrates the actual and potential dangers of the deinstitutionalization movement when the major (if not only) placement alternative is the nursing home:

> DR. WEINBERG: I criticized . . . the idea of transferring inordinately large numbers
> of people into nursing homes from mental hospitals. I was amazed when . . . the
> new Governor of the State of Illinois . . . announced he was going to release 7000
> elderly patients into the community. I didn't know who made the important clinical
> decision that those 7000 people were not mentally ill.
> SENATOR PERCY: Don't you imagine that there is the possibility that the operators of
> these nursing homes organized into an association and an officer . . . put pressure
> on the State and other government officials to release patients so they want to fill
> beds? They have got stockholders' reports to show. They have got empty beds and
> they are going to fill them with bodies and maybe those bodies are going to have to
> come out of the mental hospitals. Don't you think that sets the pressure up then to
> fill those beds?
> DR. WEINBERG: It certainly does. May I reveal something personally, that when I
> was asked to supervise this program and it was announced, someone in my family
> was approached by a nursing home operator, asking my brother, to be exact, to
> approach me to direct patients into his home and that he would offer me a stipend
> of $100 per head. This actually happened and appalled both my family and me.

There must be alternatives, and among the best is avoiding institutionalization in the first place through early and appropriate intervention.

But even if our elderly mentally ill are allowed to remain in their homes in
their communities and are provided the kind of physical and emotional en-

vironment that is conducive to successful treatment, poor coordination of services, inappropriate care rendered by those not specifically trained to meet the particular needs of the mentally ill elderly, and inaccessibility to services still combine to thwart the delivery of care. For example, statewide responsibility for planning mental health services for the elderly is often not clearly defined. Departments on Aging may expect Departments of Mental Health to take the leadership role, and vice versa. While provisions in the Mental Health Systems Act may somewhat ameliorate this problem as it applies to the planning of treatment for the chronically mentally ill who have been deinstitutionalized, nothing assures that the mentally ill elderly will not "fall through the cracks" of this system.

Because of inordinate delays and poor coordination, the private sector often is unable to provide the comprehensive multidisciplinary evaluations requisite to an accurate differential diagnosis. For example, the disturbed elderly patient who attempts to see a primary care physician and a psychiatrist may not have a complete evaluation for several weeks—during which time his mental/physical condition may deteriorate. Even where comprehensive evaluation programs do exist, many agencies and the elderly themselves are unaware of them. What is more, Medicare will not reimburse for evaluation.

Compounding the problem is the fact that, regrettably, the general practitioner to whom the elderly patient turns for treatment often does not have the requisite training to appropriately segregate the physical from the emotional disorder. All too often, medications proffered for physical symptomology actually exacerbate the emotional disorder. (Examples include the inappropriately aggressive treatment of mild hypertnesion with drugs that may exacerbate depression and the injudicious use of antiparkinsonian agents that can produce a severe confusional state. The issue of differentiating physical from mental disorders is critical since treatable geriatric depression may present as multiple somatic complaints, and conversely, acute confusion may be due to a considerable medical problem.)

Further, the nonphysician mental health professional, in contrast to the psychiatrist, is not able to ascertain the critical distinction between a physical and an emotional etiology, and consequently may fail to provide an appropriate diagnosis. The critical interplay of physical and mental illnesses among the elderly makes the role of the psychiatrist as the "point man" for diagnosis and treatment all the more compelling. However, he is seldom consulted directly by an elderly patient, and not substantially more frequently by other physicians or mental health professionals.

We believe that, if nonphysician mental health professionals are to deliver care to the mentally ill elderly and if Medicare reimbursement to such nonphysicians is to be made available, certain limitations must first be defined relative to the types of care they are qualified to deliver. In this connection, it is critical to emphasize the unique role and function of the psychiatrist, who is not only trained to do psychotherapy but is also trained to make differential diagnoses, to prescribe medication, and, if need be, to hospitalize a patient for treatment. The kind of help that each professional offers is dependent upon his own background, training, professional attitudes, knowledge, and skills. They are not interchangeable.

NIMH director Herbert Pardes, has noted[21] that "the mental health care system is based on a team concept with services delivered by many types of mental health specialists, but where psychiatric supervision and overall medical responsibility is often essential." We concur in that assessment in general, and with respect to the elderly, we concur unequivocally. A similar perspective has been articulated in the Mental Health Systems Act, wherein a differential diagnosis for the elderly is mandated—a diagnosis that can only be performed by a psychiatrist—assuring that psychotherapeutic treatment of an emotional illness in the elderly is not only medically necessary but also consistent with the medical diagnosis. It places the psychiatrist at the "point" position in the triage, a position from which the key medical staff has been too long absent in rendering care for mental illness.

The Community Mental Health Center remains the primary treatment program outside the private sector to which an elderly mentally ill person can turn for community-based care. However, as mentioned previously, fewer than 4% of the patients seen as CMHCs are elderly.[15] Clearly, the absence of Medicare reimbursement is part of the problem. Yet another problem is the failure to diagnose mental illness in the elderly—again based on the stereotyped picture of the elderly as "senile," rigid, and confused, but not mentally ill—resultant in part from the inadequate understanding of and training in the problems of the elderly by nonphysicians who staff such programs.

There is generally no central clearinghouse (formal or informal) where information concerning community-based treatment programs for the mentally ill elderly can be obtained. Further, a lack of supportive services and information for families of the patients, to assist them in helping an elderly relative, highlights yet another glaring deficiency. Dr. Carl Eisdorfer points out in one recent study that 70% of intact families were willing without help to provide intensive personal care and services to severely disabled elderly persons returning home from the hospital for the first time. However, only 38% of these same relatives were willing to provide care without social supports after the second hospitalization.[22] Mechanisms such as respite care and day hospitalization, which would overcome such difficulties, exist; they are simply not utilized in an appropriate fashion. The network and information are there but are being severely underutilized, again perhaps because the stigma of mental illness overrides concern and the willingness to help.

In the final analysis, however, the subject of barriers to care ultimately devolves to issues of flawed Medicare reimbursement mechanisms, which serve as the critical, essential, and basic problem facing the mentally ill elderly today as well as that facing policy-makers now seeking to develop any workable National Health Insurance program aimed at meeting the needs of the mentally ill in the future. Reimbursement problems prohibit CMHCs from providing care required by the mentally ill elderly. Reimbursement problems restrict the willingness of private psychiatrists to accept elderly patients. Reimbursement problems have encouraged the use of state hospitals and nursing homes in lieu of either outpatient home-based care or hospitalization in a private psychiatric hospital or the psychiatric unit of a general hospital. Reimbursement problems have restricted the growth in the number of geriatric psychiatrists and general physicians who have greater in-depth knowledge of the mental health problems of the elderly.

It is critical to note that, in speaking of the treatment of mental illness and reimbursement, we are not speaking of the health/happiness/achievement of potential/social welfare continuum. We are speaking of treatments of illness as aggressive as many life-saving physical health care techniques, not programs that seek to expand consciousness or raise the awareness of the general well public. We are defining mental illness in much the same way as it is articulated in the white paper in that we do not view generic "helping" as identical to treating mental illness *per se*. Such delineation forms the basis for what we believe are appropriate reimbursement changes, the same changes set forth in the white paper—the elimination of the restrictions now placed on psychiatric treatment under Medicare.

In one of its recommendations, the President's Commission on Mental Health[10] articulated the basic underpinnings necessary in providing insurance benefits for those suffering from mental illness, whether under Medicare or any other federally developed catastrophic or comprehensive national health insurance program. It stated that "There should be minimal patient-borne cost sharing for emergency care. In all other instances, patient-borne cost sharing, through copayments and deductibles for evaluation, diagnosis and short-term therapy, should be no greater than for a comparable course of physical illness."

Moreover, the Task Panel on Cost and Finance of Mental Health of the President's Commission[10] specifically noted that "the financing of mental health services is far from parity with the financing of other medical services and this discrimination against mental health services is serving as a barrier to access to care." The panel concurred in the appropriateness and importance of parity of funding and agreed that the funding of services should be independent of whether the diagnosis had been for a mental or a physical disorder.

National Institute on Aging director Robert Butler[23] pointed out that "Medicare coverage for psychiatric disorders is unrealistically limited and was inserted as a kind of afterthought. . . . The system obviously affords inadequate coverage."

That Medicare's current approach is penny-wise and pound-foolish is clear, particularly in light of the data that have been and are continuing to be amassed indicating that the provision of treatment for mental disorders can have a cost-saving effect upon overall health care costs. The provision of treatment to the mentally ill elderly has a similar positive cost benefit. One longitudinal Texas study (1973–1977) demonstrated that access to needed treatment for mental illness resulted in a reduction in mean length of stay of over-65 patients in inpatient facilities from 111 days to 53 days, a halving of hospital stays that resulted in a cost-reduction of more than $1.1 million.[10]

Elimination of the currently restrictive practices under Medicare not only will enable the elderly to receive the care they need but will enable most of those diagnosed as mentally ill to return to active participation in the social and economic activities of our society—ultimately at a saving to the federal government, rather than as an added burden.

As the 97th Congress convenes, we find ourselves at a historic crossroad. We find the willingness to provide some type of new direction to federal health care policy. We find the psychiatric profession ready and able to work to assure that safe, effective, and appropriate care is rendered to those Americans suffering from mental illness. We find members of the House and Senate interested in, and committed to changing, the historic discrimination against the treatment of the mentally ill elderly under Medicare. We have the option today to work toward change within this structure, or alternatively, to seek the simple solution, which is to "sit it out" for the time being, to take no active role in trying to change current Medicare discrimination that deprives one in every nine Americans of the access to psychiatric care should it be needed and, in doing so, sows the seeds of continued discrimination, not just against today's Medicare population but against any American who may find himself suffering from mental illness in the future.

We concur in the activist spirit of the white paper, which seeks to define what we should do now, what is needed now, and how best to go about doing it.

References

1. Butler RN: Address before the National Conference on County Resources Development for Aging Citizens. Washington DC, January 10, 1977.
2. U.S. Department of Commerce, Bureau of the Census: Status. Washington DC, US Government Printing Office, 1976, pp 23–38.
3. Cohen GD: Prospects for mental health and aging, in Birren JE, Sloane RB (eds): Handbook of Mental Health and Aging. Englewood Cliffs NJ, Prentice-Hall, 1980, p 972.
4. United States Department of Health and Human Services, Health Care Financing Administration: Orally transmitted data, 1978.
5. American Psychiatric Association, American Psychological Association, et al: Draft Report of the Mini-Conference on Mental Health of Older Americans. California, 1980, p 26.
6. United States Department of Health and Human Services, Public Health Service: Health maintenance organizations; requirements for a health maintenance organization. Fed Reg 45–213:72524, October 31, 1980.
7. 1971 White House Conference on Aging: Toward a National Policy on Aging, Final Report. Washington DC, US Government Printing Office, 1971.
8. Social Security Administration, Office of Research and Statistics: Financing Mental Health

Care Under Medicare and Medicaid, Research Report 37. Washington DC, US Government Printing Office, 1971.

9. United States Senate, Special Committee on Aging: Mental Health Care and the Elderly: Shortcomings in Public Policy. Washington DC, US Government Printing Office, 1971, p 3.

10. President's Commission on Mental Health: Preliminary Report to the President. Washington DC, US Government Printing Office, 1977.

11. President's Commission on Mental Health: Report to the President. Washington DC, US Government Printing Office, 1978.

12. Butler RN, Lewis MI: Aging and Mental Health: Positive Psychosocial Approaches, ed 2. St. Louis, CV Mosby Co, 1977.

13. Task Force on the 1981 White House Conference on Aging: Providing and Coordinating Mental Health Services for the Elderly. Prepublication manuscript of official position paper of the American Psychiatric Association, Washington DC, 1981.

14. Katzman R: The prevalence and malignancy of Alzheimer's disease. *Arch Neurol* 33:217–218, 1976.

15. Cohen GD: Mental health services and the elderly: Needs and options. *Am J Psychiatry* 133: 65–68, 1976.

16. United States Department of Health and Human Services: Report of the Secretary's Committee on the Mental Health and Illness of the Elderly. Washington DC, US Government Printing Office, 1977.

17. United States House of Representatives, Select Committee on Aging: Report of the National Conference on Mental Health and the Elderly. Washington DC, US Government Printing Office, 1979.

18. Butler RN: Psychiatry and the elderly: An overview. *Am J Psychiatry* 132:893–900, 1975.

19. Glasscote RN, et al: Old Folks at Homes: A Field Study of Nursing and Board and Care Homes. Washington DC, Joint Information Service of the American Psychiatric Association and National Mental Health Association, 1976.

20. United States Senate, Special Committee on Aging: Hearing on Trends in Long-Term Care, Field Hearing, Illinois. Washington DC, US Government Printing Office, 1971.

21. Pardes H: Future needs for psychiatrists and other mental health personnel. *Arch Gen Psychiatry* 36:1401–1408, 1979.

22. United States Senate, Labor and Human Resources Subcommittee on Aging: Hearing on Alzheimer's Disease and Related Disorders. Washington DC, US Government Printing Office, 1980.

23. Butler RN: Why Survive: Being Old in America. New York, Harper & Row, 1975.

Index